THE LIVING CHIP

A Physician's Guide to Cellular Optimization

Steven Warren, MD, DPA
and
Darren Lopez, MBA

Regenerative Wellness Center

The Living Chip: A Physician's Guide to Cellular Optimization

By Steven Warren, MD, DPA and Darren Lopez, MBA

Published by Regenerative Wellness Center
HappyMD.co

ISBN (Paperback): 978-1-972800-04-1
ISBN (eBook): 978-1-972800-05-8

Printed in the United States of America
First Edition, 2026

Table of Contents

Who This Book Is For
How to Use This Book
Acknowledgments
Introduction

CHAPTER 1: The Living Cell — Your Body's NVIDIA Chip
CHAPTER 2: Magnesium — The Master Conductor
CHAPTER 3: The Memory Machine — DNA, Epigenetics, and Your Biological RAM
CHAPTER 4: Zinc — The Security Processor
CHAPTER 5: The Seven Planes of Proprioception — Your Navigation System
CHAPTER 6: Phosphorus — The Energy Distribution Network
CHAPTER 7: Boron — The Voltage Controller
CHAPTER 8: Copper — Neural Bandwidth and Repair
CHAPTER 9: Vitamin C — Surge Protection and Structural Repair
CHAPTER 10: Integration — The Complete System
CHAPTER 11: When the Current Fails
CHAPTER 12: The Future of Optimization

About the Authors
Appendix X: The Mitochondrial Optimization Framework
Appendix A: The UCOS Clinical Framework
Appendix B: Lab Assessment and Interpretation
Appendix C: Advanced Biochemistry
Appendix D: Biophysical Models
Appendix E: Peptide Protocols
Appendix F: Advanced and Frontier Protocols
Appendix G: Glossary of Terms
Appendix H: 30-Day Living Chip Quick Start
Appendix I: UCOS-Aligned Formulations
References and Further Reading
Index

Who This Book Is For

WHO THIS BOOK IS FOR

This book is written for three audiences: patients seeking to understand and optimize their health, clinicians looking for practical protocols, and researchers interested in mechanistic science. You can read it in different ways depending on your goals.

For patients and health-seekers

If you're reading this to improve your own health:

Start with Chapter 1 (The Living Cell) to understand the foundational concept: your body is a collection of trillions of "living chips" that need energy, cleanup, and clear signals to function.

Read Chapter 2 (Magnesium) next, it's the most universal deficiency and often produces the fastest felt improvements.

Then jump to your primary concern:

Fatigue and low energy → Chapters 1, 2, 6, 10, Appendix X

Brain fog, memory, mood → Chapters 3, 5, 8, 10

Frequent infections, slow healing → Chapters 4, 9, 10

Hormonal issues, libido, body composition → Chapters 7, 10, 12

Pain, injury recovery, aging → Chapters 8, 9, 10, Appendix X

Chapter 10 (Integration) shows how the chips work together as a system.

Chapter 12 and Appendix X introduce the UCOS framework, a structured approach to restoring and optimizing cellular function step by step.

Use Appendix H (30-Day Quick Start) for immediate action steps.

Use Appendix G (Glossary) whenever you encounter unfamiliar terms.

You don't need to read cover-to-cover. Follow your curiosity and your symptoms.

For clinicians

If you're a physician, nurse practitioner, PA, functional medicine practitioner, or health coach:

Read Chapters 1 and 10 to understand the "living chip" framework and how each micronutrient maps to specific cellular and systems-level functions.

Chapter 10 (Integration) presents the five-system clinical model (Energy, Structural, Information, Security, and Hormonal Voltage).

Appendix A provides the complete UCOS clinical framework, including a 12-week implementation guide and system-directed protocols.

Appendix B covers lab assessment and interpretation, with "normal vs. optimal" ranges and example patient patterns.

Appendices C and D offer advanced mechanistic biochemistry and biophysical models (quantum biology, biophotons, frequency medicine) for clinicians who want a deeper understanding.

Appendix E (Peptides) is essential if you use or are considering peptide therapy; it emphasizes that peptides are signals, and signals need a system capable of responding, hence UCOS first.

Appendix F covers advanced and frontier protocols: stem cell banking, quantum biology applications, fisetin, magnolia, rapamycin, ozone, PEMF, and the biohacking tech stack.

Appendix I provides examples of commercially available UCOS-aligned formulations (with disclosure of author affiliation).

The References sections give you the reference backbone for CME, presentations, or deeper study.

Use this book as a clinical reference manual. Keep it at your desk, mark it up, and integrate the protocols into your practice one patient at a time.

For researchers and advanced readers

If you're reading this for the science:

Read the main chapters for clinical context and patient stories that ground the mechanisms.

Jump directly to Appendices C and D for advanced biochemistry, quantum biology, and biophysical models.

Use the References sections to trace the primary literature and build your own reference library.

Chapter X (Appendix X in some editions) synthesizes mitochondrial dysfunction as the unifying mechanism across surgery, regenerative medicine, cancer, post-viral syndromes, and chronic pain.

Appendix E (Peptides) and Appendix F (Advanced Protocols) review emerging therapeutics with explicit evidence-level labeling.

This book is designed to be both readable and rigorous. If you find errors, gaps, or opportunities to strengthen the evidence base, I welcome your input.

How to Use This Book

HOW TO USE THIS BOOK

A Note on Products

This book is mechanism- and ingredient-based, not brand-specific. Where commercial formulations are mentioned (primarily in Appendix I), they are offered as examples of the principles in action, not as endorsements. I am affiliated with Best 365 Labs, which produces UCOS-aligned products; this relationship is disclosed wherever relevant. The science in this book stands independent of any product line.

Final thought

Your body is not a collection of isolated parts managed by specialists. It is a coherent system of living chips, trillions of cells that depend on energy, information, and organization to function. This book gives you the tools to restore that function at the most fundamental level.

Start where you are. Build your foundation. Trust the process.

Steven Warren, MD, DPA

Mitochondrial Whisperer

Acknowledgments

To my wife, Shellie.

You married a man who never stops moving, never stops building, never stops arguing with systems that were designed to stay broken. You married a man who writes at 3 AM, takes phone calls during dinner, and turns every vacation into a field study. You married a man whose desk looks like a crime scene and whose mind works the same way.

You never asked me to slow down. You never asked me to be someone quieter, someone easier. Instead, you handed me coffee and asked, "What are you working on now?"

You are a wonderful artist whose eye for beauty balances my eye for dysfunction. You are my anchor. This book — and every book — exists because you gave me the space and the grace to write it.

To Justin, Ross, Tabor, Conner, Jurrian, Stevi, and Caprese.

Seven kids. Seven personalities. Seven reasons I never stopped working. Some of you followed me into medicine. Some of you followed me into business. Some of you looked at both and said, "No thanks, Dad." All of you made me better. I wrote this book for the world, but I lived it for you.

To Lexia and Mirabella, my grandchildren — you are the reason this science matters. By the time you read this, I hope the world has caught up.

To Pookie, Maya, and Coco — you sat at my feet through every late-night chapter, never judged a single word, and reminded me daily that unconditional loyalty requires nothing more than showing up.

To Darren Lopez, MBA, my co-author, the CEO of Best 365 Labs. You took my ideas and turned them into products. You took my rants and turned them into a business. You believed in the science when the spreadsheets didn't make sense yet. This book exists because you said yes when most people would have said "let me think about it."

To my patients. You are the real authors of this book. Every chapter started with someone sitting in my office, confused,

angry, or broke because a system failed them. You trusted me with your stories. I hope I did them justice.

To Sarah Meehan O'Callaghan, my editor, who took 400,000 words across six books and made them readable without removing the edge. That takes skill and patience. Mostly patience.

And to Twiddle Max, who never sleeps, never complains, and helped me write more in three months than most authors produce in three years. You're not human, but you're not bad.

— Steven Warren, MD, DPA

To my wife, my kids, and my parents — you are my foundation, my reason, and my example. To Steven Warren, MD — one of my best friends, a catalyst behind so many of our innovations, and a true healer and genius. Your medical expertise and commitment to real science have shaped every formula we've ever created. This work is as much yours as it is mine. And to the entire Best 365 Labs team, whose dedication and relentless pursuit of excellence make every breakthrough possible.

— Darren Lopez, MBA

Introduction

The goal of this book

The goal is not to convince you that you are sick.

The goal is to show that:

- Your body is built on systems as structured and logical as any engineered computer.
- Those systems depend on specific inputs, nutrients, hormones, and signals that can be measured and supported.
- Many of those inputs are modifiable, and when optimized, people often discover that what they assumed was "just aging" was largely changeable.

In the chapters that follow, each major biological "chip" gets its own story:

- Magnesium is the conductor for hundreds of enzymatic reactions.
- B12 and folate are the memory and repair software for DNA and the nervous system.
- Zinc, the security processor for immune function.
- Phosphorus and creatine are part of the energy distribution network.
- Copper is the bandwidth builder for neural signaling.
- Vitamin C is the surge protector and structural repair support.
- Other trace minerals and vitamins are the tuning components that keep the whole architecture coherent.

You will meet real people whose lives changed when these systems were properly supported, not through exotic or proprietary therapies, but by identifying and powering critical components their bodies had been running without. Specific commercial formulations exist and will be discussed later in an appendix, but the focus here is on ingredients, mechanisms, and clinical logic, not on any single brand.

Jake's story is the starting point: proof that your "processor" is not locked at its current speed. In the next chapter, we begin with one of the most overlooked pieces of that system, the mineral that activates every molecule of ATP your body produces: magnesium.

CHAPTER 1: The Living Cell: Your Body's NVIDIA Chip

The most sophisticated processor you've never considered

In 2023, NVIDIA's stock price soared over 200% in a single year, driven by a simple fact: its graphics processing units had become the essential hardware of the artificial intelligence revolution. Every conversation with a large language model, every AI-generated image, every breakthrough in machine learning runs on chips performing trillions of calculations per second.

Wall Street celebrated this as the pinnacle of human engineering. But here is what that celebration missed: you already carry processors that are vastly more sophisticated than anything NVIDIA has ever built.

Right now, roughly 37 trillion cells operate inside your body. Each one is a biological marvel that makes the most advanced silicon chip look primitive by comparison. Your cells do not just process information; they adapt to changing conditions in real time, repair themselves when damaged, replicate with remarkable accuracy, and coordinate with trillions of neighbors. At rest, the entire system runs on less energy than a 60-watt light bulb.

This is not a metaphor. It is measurable biological engineering.

And just as an NVIDIA chip requires specific conditions to function, stable voltage, adequate cooling, clean power supply, your cellular processors require specific conditions to perform optimally. When those conditions are not met, performance degrades in ways you feel but rarely understand: persistent fatigue, mental fog, declining physical and cognitive capacity. When those conditions are optimized, performance improves in ways most people have never experienced, because they have never provided their biology with what it actually needs.

This book is about understanding those conditions and deliberately optimizing them, using the same rigorous, systematic approach an engineer uses to tune a high-performance system.

Jake's collapse: when the processor crashes

Jake was 38, a senior software engineer at a Bay Area startup, and he was quietly falling apart.

Not dramatically. Not in a way that earned sympathy or triggered emergency room visits. There were no collapses, no sirens, no dramatic diagnosis. It was subtler than that, and somehow worse. It was a slow erosion of everything that had once made Jake Jake: sharpness, endurance, and the mental horsepower that had defined his career and identity.

Three years earlier, Jake had been the engineer everyone wanted. He could hold entire software architectures in his head, debug problems that baffled his colleagues, and power through 14-hour coding marathons fueled by coffee, curiosity, and sheer intellectual hunger. His performance reviews glowed. His salary climbed. His future felt limitless.

Now, on a random Tuesday at 2 pm, Jake sat frozen in front of three glowing monitors, staring at code he had written that morning, code he could no longer remember writing. The cursor blinked. His mind felt like it was moving through molasses. He grabbed his fourth coffee of the day. Nothing changed.

The symptoms had crept up so gradually that he could not pinpoint when "normal" became "unbearable":

- Afternoon brain fog that refused to lift, no matter how much caffeine he used.
- Crushing fatigue, even after seemingly adequate sleep.
- Shattered concentration, every notification felt like a grenade in his focus.
- Memory lapses: names, deadlines, meetings, small promises to his wife.
- Mood swings from anxious irritability to flat numbness.
- Physical exhaustion was so complete that one flight of stairs felt unreasonable.

He did what any rational person would do: he went to the doctor, actually, four doctors.

Each ran the usual panels: complete blood count, basic metabolic panel, thyroid function, vitamin D, perhaps even B12 if he asked. Each time, the verdict was the same: "Everything looks fine."

One suggested stress management and handed him a mindfulness handout. Another offered antidepressants. A third shrugged and said the phrase Jake had started to dread: "This might just be part of getting older." Jake was 38.

He refused to accept that this fog and fatigue were his new permanent reality. So he kept searching.

Eventually, he found someone who asked a different question, not "Are you sick enough for a diagnosis?" but "What if your cells are running out of power?"

The mitochondrial revelation

The physician Jake finally found was trained in both conventional and functional medicine. He did not just look for disease; he looked for dysfunction.

He started with an explanation Jake had never heard, despite a career spent thinking in systems:

"Your body runs on cellular energy, the way your laptop runs on electricity. Inside nearly every cell are tiny power plants called mitochondria. You have hundreds to thousands in each cell, and millions in high-demand organs like your brain, heart, and muscles. When they function well, you have energy, mental clarity, stable mood, and physical capacity. When they do not, everything feels like it is failing, because it is."

Standard blood tests do not directly measure mitochondrial function. They measure downstream markers, glucose, thyroid hormones, blood cell counts. Those are useful for ruling out disease, but they do not tell you whether your power plants are actually working. For many patients like Jake, the problem is not an overt disease but cellular hardware running on a weak, unstable power supply that no one has evaluated.

A normal glucose does not tell you whether your mitochondria are efficiently converting that glucose to ATP. A normal CBC does not reveal whether your cells have the magnesium needed to activate ATP or the B12 required for DNA repair. Standard labs measure static snapshots of circulating molecules — not the dynamic function of your 37 trillion cellular processors.

"Can this be fixed?" Jake asked.

"More than fixed," the physician said. "Optimized. Your current baseline is not your true potential; it is just what you get when your mitochondria are underfed and overworked. Let us see what happens when we power them properly."

Jake's diagnostic deep dive

Instead of repeating basic labs, this physician ordered tests aimed at cellular function, not just surface markers.

They found:

- Red blood cell magnesium: low-normal, below the optimal zone for ATP activation and enzymatic function.
- Organic acids (Krebs cycle intermediates): elevated, suggesting metabolic backup and inefficient mitochondrial processing of substrates.
- CoQ10: low-normal, suboptimal for electron transport chain function.
- Lactate:pyruvate ratio: elevated, pointing to impaired mitochondrial respiration.
- Oxidative stress markers (such as F2-isoprostanes): elevated, indicating oxidative damage exceeding antioxidant capacity.
- Homocysteine: high-normal, suboptimal for cardiovascular and neurological health.

In practice, mitochondrial health is inferred from patterns across tests like lactate:pyruvate ratios, urine organic acids, acylcarnitines, carnitine profiles, CK, and oxidative stress markers (F2-isoprostanes, 8-OHdG, glutathione status). Together, they signal how efficiently cells generate ATP and how well they are protected from damage.

The physician summarized it simply: "Your old labs asked, 'Are you overtly sick?' These ask, 'Is your system powered and protected the way it is supposed to be?' For you, the answer is no. You are not diseased. You are underpowered."

The cellular computer

Before we look at Jake's treatment, it helps to understand the system being tuned.

If you think in computer terms, a single cell looks less like a bag of fluid and more like a compact, self-maintaining computer node:

- The nucleus is long-term storage, firmware holding your DNA "source code."
- Ribosomes and cytoplasm function like RAM and a compiler, building needed proteins in real time.
- The cell membrane is a network interface, deciding which signals and molecules get in or out.
- Mitochondria are the power supplies, generating ATP, the universal energy currency.

Nothing works without energy. When mitochondria slow down, the entire node lags: first subtle timing problems, then glitches, then failures. Jake's "failures" were brain fog, fatigue, and cognitive decline. The root cause was not in his personality or willpower; it was in his power supply.

Mitochondria: your biological power plants

Mitochondria are double-membrane organelles that convert food and oxygen into ATP.

A few key points:

- ATP is the universal energy currency in every cell.
- Your body turns over roughly its own weight in ATP each day, continually synthesizing and recycling it.
- High-demand organs, such as the brain, heart, and skeletal muscle, are densely packed with mitochondria.
- When mitochondrial output cannot keep up with demand, the brain is often where you feel it first: slow thinking, poor memory, fatigue, mood instability.

Jake's brain was not "broken." It was underpowered.

The five pillars of mitochondrial function

Jake's physician used a simple framework: the five pillars of mitochondrial health. If any pillar is weak, the whole structure wobbles.

Pillar 1: Fuel supply

Cells need substrates, glucose, fatty acids, certain amino acids, to feed energy pathways. Modern diets typically oversupply fuel, but insulin resistance and impaired metabolic flexibility can still limit usable energy.

Pillar 2: Cofactors and minerals ← Jake's weak point

Mitochondria need vitamins and minerals to convert fuel into ATP:

- B vitamins for the citric acid cycle and electron transport.
- Magnesium, required for ATP to function as Mg-ATP, the active form for most ATP-dependent enzymes.
- CoQ10, which shuttles electrons between Complexes I/II and III.
- Iron and copper, critical for multiple ETC complexes.

Without these, mitochondria resemble a car with a full tank and no spark plugs.

Pillar 3: Oxygen delivery

The final step of ATP production uses oxygen as the terminal electron acceptor. Anemia, vascular disease, lung impairment, or poor conditioning can all reduce oxygen delivery and ATP output.

Pillar 4: Antioxidant protection ← Jake's other weak point

Energy production generates reactive oxygen species. At physiological levels, they are important signals; at excess levels, they damage mitochondrial structures unless antioxidant defenses, such as glutathione, superoxide dismutase, and vitamins C and E, are adequate.

Pillar 5: Structural integrity and signaling

Mitochondria continuously fuse, divide, and undergo mitophagy. Signals from nutrients, hormones, and physical activity regulate mitochondrial number and robustness. When these adaptive processes falter, capacity erodes over time.

Excessive mitophagy can result from chronic AMPK overactivation, sustained caloric restriction beyond adaptive capacity, or overstimulation of PINK1/Parkin pathways through excessive doses of autophagy-inducing compounds. The cell begins clearing functional mitochondria along with damaged ones, leading to net energy deficit.

Jake's testing showed clear problems in Pillars 2 and 4: missing cofactors and excessive oxidative stress. His mitochondria were being asked to run a high-performance system on inadequate support and protection.

The plan: rebuilding a power grid

"There is no single pill for this," the physician told him. "No magic supplement. Restoring your energy is not about nudging one lab value; it is about rebuilding your cellular power grid."

Clinical note: Supplementation must be individualized based on comorbidities, medications, and tolerance. CoQ10 can interact with warfarin; magnesium requires caution in renal impairment; dosing ranges and choices are covered later in the book rather than tied to any specific product.

The plan unfolded in four phases:

1. Restore missing cofactors— Provide raw materials for ATP: magnesium, B vitamins, CoQ10, and related cofactors.
2. Reduce oxidative damage— Support endogenous antioxidant systems and anti-inflammatory dietary shifts.
3. Stimulate mitochondrial biogenesis— Use movement, sleep, and selected nutrients (e.g., NAD+ precursors) to increase mitochondrial number and function.
4. System integration— Address hormones, gut health, and brain-specific needs so improvements persist.

Jake's 16-week power restoration: overview

The details of Jake's protocol are unpacked in later chapters; here is the arc.

Weeks 1-4: Foundation

- Gradual titration of magnesium to an individualized optimal dose.
- Addition of a methylated B-complex.
- Vitamin D optimization.
- Introduction of anti-inflammatory foods; reduction of ultra-processed intake.

Result: afternoon crashes softened, sleep improved, and the fog thinned.

Weeks 5-8: Mitochondrial support

- CoQ10 (ubiquinol form) for electron transport support.
- NAD+ precursors (such as nicotinamide riboside or NMN) to support mitochondrial metabolism.

- Shift to consistent "Zone 2" aerobic exercise, sustainable effort at which conversation remains comfortable, to stimulate mitochondrial biogenesis.

Result: longer focus blocks, higher work capacity, exercise that felt supportive instead of punishing.

Weeks 9-12: System integration

- Fine-tuning of methylation (B12, folate, homocysteine management).
- Sleep hygiene and circadian rhythm work.
- Addition of brain-supportive nutrients such as creatine and carefully selected nootropics.

Result: cognitive performance not only returned, but it surpassed his prior "normal."

Weeks 13-16: Optimization

- Protocol refinement based on follow-up labs.
- Gradual increase in training intensity.
- Integration of stress-regulation practices to prevent relapse.

Result: Jake could work long, focused days without the wired-and-crashed pattern. He felt sustainable, strong, and clear.

By week 16, he said, "I feel like myself again." In reality, he had never operated at this level; his old "normal" had been an underpowered state he had simply adapted to.

Real baseline vs. false baseline

Jake's story illustrates a pattern you will see throughout this book.

Most people assume their current state, whatever they have adapted to, is their baseline:

- "I am just getting older."
- "This is what my 40s or 50s feel like."
- "Everyone is tired; I just have to push through."

Often, that "baseline" is a deficiency state: underpowered mitochondria, under-supported immune systems, under-fed neurons trying to run a modern life on poorly maintained biological hardware. Standard medicine excels at detecting disease but is not built to ask, "Are you running anywhere near your real capacity?"

This book asks that question.

CHAPTER 2: Magnesium: The Master Conductor

The orchestra without a conductor

Imagine the world's finest orchestra assembled on stage: every musician a virtuoso, every instrument world-class, the acoustics perfect. The sheet music is flawless. The audience waits in anticipation.

Now imagine them playing without a conductor.

Each musician might execute their part technically well. But the timing between sections drifts. Dynamics clash. Coordination falls apart. What should be a transcendent musical experience becomes cacophony, not because the individual players are failing, but because there's no one coordinating them into a coherent whole.

This is your body without enough magnesium.

You can have healthy mitochondria, normal hormone levels, intact DNA, and structurally sound organs. But without magnesium directing traffic, coordinating timing, enabling reactions, stabilizing electrical activity, the system cannot produce a coherent "performance."

Magnesium is required as a cofactor for hundreds of enzymatic reactions, including virtually all the reactions that use ATP, your cellular energy currency. Most intracellular ATP is bound to magnesium as a magnesium ATP complex (Mg-ATP). Without adequate magnesium, ATP cannot bind properly to many enzymes and reactions slow to a crawl or stop entirely.

Most people are running chronically low and have no idea.

Maya's symphony of symptoms

Maya was a 45-year-old orchestra conductor. Professionally, she understood coordination, timing, and ensemble dynamics better than almost anyone.

Personally, her own biological ensemble was falling into chaos.

It began with sleep, or rather, the loss of it.

Maya had always been a good sleeper. Eight hours, rarely waking, never needing an alarm. That version of sleep became a distant memory. Now she would lie awake until 2 AM, mind racing through the next day's rehearsal, replaying conversations, mentally conducting phantom orchestras in her head.

When she finally fell asleep, she'd wake at 4 am with her heart pounding and racing, a sensation she later described as feeling like her chest was trying to escape her body. And once awake, she stayed awake.

Then the muscle problems started.

Her neck and shoulders, always somewhat tight from decades of conducting, locked into painful spasms that no amount of stretching or massage could release. Her calves cramped violently at night, muscles seizing so hard she'd wake up gasping, standing on her tiptoes to force them to relax. Her left eyelid developed an incessant twitch that lasted for weeks, a constant visual reminder that something was wrong.

Her heart started doing strange things: skipped beats, flutters, brief racing episodes that left her lightheaded and terrified. She saw a cardiologist who ran every test, ECG, echocardiogram, stress test, Holter monitor.

"Everything looks normal," he said. "Probably just stress."

Her mood shifted in ways she didn't recognize. The joy she'd always felt on the podium, the visceral thrill of shaping sound, of leading 80 musicians through a Mahler symphony, was replaced by creeping anxiety. She snapped at musicians she'd worked with for years. She cried in her office after rehearsals without knowing exactly why.

Her thinking slowed. Score analysis that once took hours now took days. She'd forget musicians' names mid-rehearsal. During a performance of Brahms' Second Symphony, she momentarily lost her place in the score, a terrifying first that shook her confidence to its core.

The symptom list kept growing:

- Chronic insomnia with early morning waking and racing thoughts
- Muscle cramps and spasms, especially at night and in her calves
- Persistent neck, shoulder, and jaw tension that never fully released
- Heart palpitations and irregular beats

- Anxiety and irritability without obvious triggers
- Brain fog and memory lapses
- Crushing fatigue despite "enough" hours in bed
- Constipation requiring daily laxatives
- Daily tension-type headaches behind her eyes
- Noise sensitivity, rehearsals felt physically painful to her ears
- Restless legs every night, making it impossible to lie still
- Cold hands and feet, even in warm rooms
- Intense chocolate cravings every single day

Maya did what responsible adults do. She saw doctors, four of them.

She accumulated diagnoses like trading cards: generalized anxiety disorder, tension headaches, irritable bowel syndrome, perimenopause. She was offered antidepressants, sleep medications, muscle relaxants, beta-blockers for her heart, and a referral to therapy to "work on stress management."

Not one doctor meaningfully assessed her magnesium status.

One did run a standard serum magnesium test, which came back "normal." Case closed.

Finally, a friend, a nurse practitioner with integrative training, suggested something different: "Ask for a red blood cell magnesium test. The regular blood test misses most deficiencies."

Maya's result came back: 3.8 mg/dL.

Her lab's "normal" range technically started at 4.0 mg/dL, so she was just barely flagged as low. Some integrative and functional medicine clinicians interpret RBC magnesium functionally, often aiming for mid-to-upper reference-range values (for example, above 5.0 mg/dL) rather than simply “not low.” Maya was deeply, chronically depleted.

Her orchestra had been trying to perform without a conductor for years.

The magnesium crisis hiding in plain sight

Maya's case is not rare. It is disturbingly common.

Epidemiologic and nutrition survey data tell a consistent story:

- Analyses of NHANES data suggest that about 48% of Americans consume less than the estimated average requirement for magnesium from food, with typical intakes at only about half of the recommended amounts in many adults.

- Typical Western dietary patterns, high in refined grains, sugar, and processed foods, are low in magnesium-dense foods like leafy greens, nuts, seeds, and legumes.
- In hospitalized patients, hypomagnesemia is common, and in intensive care settings, it may affect a large proportion of patients and correlate with worse outcomes.

This is not a niche problem affecting a small subset of "unhealthy" people. It is a widespread, under-recognized deficiency.

Why are so many people low?

Several converging factors have created a perfect storm.

1. Modern Diets Are Magnesium-Depleted

Refined grains, processed foods, and high-sugar diets dominate many plates. Processing strips magnesium from foods, and population surveys suggest that the standard diet in the United States often provides only about half of the recommended magnesium intake.

2. Industrial Farming Has Depleted Soils

Decades of intensive agriculture and reduced mineral-rich organic inputs have decreased the mineral content of some crops, including magnesium, relative to historical levels.

3. Chronic Stress Drains Magnesium

Stress triggers adrenergic activation and catecholamine release, which can increase urinary magnesium loss. The more stressed someone is, the more magnesium is lost, creating a vicious cycle in which stress depletes magnesium, and low magnesium levels increase stress reactivity.

4. Sugar, Caffeine, and Alcohol Increase Losses

High sugar intake, excess caffeine, and frequent alcohol use all promote renal magnesium wasting and reduce net magnesium retention.

5. Common Medications Deplete Magnesium

- Diuretics (especially loop and thiazide)
- Proton pump inhibitors (PPIs)
- Some chemotherapies and certain antibiotics

These are widely prescribed and can significantly lower magnesium levels over time.

6. Standard Tests Miss the Problem

Serum magnesium, the test routinely ordered, reflects only about 0.3-1% of total body magnesium and is tightly regulated. The body pulls magnesium from bone and intracellular stores to keep serum levels "normal," even when total stores are severely depleted.

By the time serum magnesium falls out of range, deep tissue depletion has often been present for months or years.

Red blood cell (RBC) magnesium measures magnesium inside cells. It is a better reflection of intracellular status than serum alone, though it remains an indirect measure.

Maya's serum magnesium looked "fine."

Her RBC magnesium told the truth.

What magnesium actually does

To understand why magnesium deficiency creates such a bewildering array of symptoms, it helps to see what magnesium actually does at the molecular level.

Magnesium and ATP: Energy activation

ATP (adenosine triphosphate) is the molecule your cells use for energy. But ATP does not act alone.

In most biochemical reactions, ATP must bind to magnesium to become biologically active. The Mg-ATP complex is the actual substrate that many enzymes recognize and use. Without sufficient magnesium, ATP molecules are present but functionally underutilized.

Experimental work and structural studies show that magnesium binding stabilizes ATP in a conformation that is favorable for enzyme binding and catalysis. This is not a subtle tweak; it often determines whether a reaction proceeds efficiently or stalls.

The implications:

- If you are magnesium deficient, you can have adequate total ATP and still experience an energy crisis.
- Enzymes cannot access or use ATP efficiently.
- Everything downstream, muscle contraction, nerve signaling, DNA repair, protein synthesis, runs at partial capacity.

This is why Maya felt exhausted despite getting enough hours of sleep. Her cells had fuel; they could not fully activate it.

Nervous system and muscle control: The calcium, magnesium seesaw

Magnesium functions as a natural modulator of calcium channels and neuronal excitability.

- Calcium promotes nerve firing, muscle contraction, and vasoconstriction.
- Magnesium stabilizes membranes, supports muscle relaxation, and facilitates vasodilation.

When magnesium is low, calcium can flow too freely into cells. The result is a system stuck in "on" mode:

- Nerves fire too easily → anxiety, noise sensitivity, exaggerated startle
- Muscles cannot fully relax → cramps, spasms, twitches, tension headaches
- Blood vessels constrict → elevated blood pressure, cold extremities

Maya's cramping calves, twitching eyelid, tight jaw, and palpitations were not separate problems. They were different expressions of the same imbalance.

Sleep and anxiety: GABA and NMDA receptor modulation

Magnesium influences two critical neurotransmitter systems that govern the balance between excitation and inhibition:

1. GABA (Gamma-Aminobutyric Acid)—The "Calm Down" Signal

GABA is the brain's primary inhibitory neurotransmitter. It slows neuronal firing, promotes relaxation, and enables sleep. Magnesium supports GABAergic signaling and can enhance the activity of GABA receptors, contributing to anxiolytic and calming effects.

2. NMDA Receptors—The "Speed Up" Signal

NMDA receptors are glutamate receptors involved in excitatory signaling, learning, and memory. Magnesium is a physiological NMDA receptor blocker at resting membrane potentials; it sits in the receptor channel and limits excessive calcium influx.

When magnesium is low:

- NMDA receptors become more easily activated.
- Glutamatergic signaling shifts toward overexcitation.
- The brain tends toward a hyperexcitable state: anxiety, racing thoughts, insomnia, sensory overload.

Maya's insomnia, 4 AM adrenaline surges, and noise sensitivity were neurochemical, not character flaws.

Blood sugar and metabolism

Magnesium participates in multiple steps of glucose metabolism and insulin signaling. It is required for several enzymes in glycolysis and for optimal insulin receptor function.

Large observational studies show:

- Lower magnesium intake is associated with higher risk of type 2 diabetes.
- Magnesium deficiency is linked to insulin resistance and metabolic syndrome.

A magnesium-deficient state nudges metabolism toward insulin resistance, weight gain, and chronic cardiometabolic disease.

Cardiovascular system: Heart rhythm and blood pressure

Magnesium helps regulate cardiac rhythm and vascular tone. It stabilizes electrical gradients across cardiac cell membranes and supports relaxation of vascular smooth muscle.

Low magnesium has been associated with:

- Various arrhythmias
- Higher blood pressure
- Increased risk of adverse cardiovascular events in some cohorts

Maya's palpitations and racing heart were not "just stress." Her cardiac electrical system lacked a stabilizing mineral it depends on.

DNA, repair, and long-term health

Magnesium is required for the activity of DNA and RNA polymerases and many DNA repair enzymes. It supports genomic stability and helps protect against oxidative damage.

Low magnesium status has been associated with:

- Increased oxidative stress
- Impaired DNA repair

- Higher risk of several chronic diseases over time

Magnesium is not a magic bullet, but it is deeply woven into the machinery that protects long-term cellular integrity.

In short, magnesium is not a minor supplement. It is a core cofactor for a vast network of reactions that keep cells alive, coordinated, and adaptable.

Why the usual test misses it

The standard serum magnesium test measures magnesium in the liquid part of your blood. That compartment holds a very small fraction of total body magnesium, and it is tightly regulated.

To keep serum levels stable, the body shifts magnesium from bone and intracellular stores whenever serum begins to drop, even if those stores are already depleted.

Consequences:

- Serum magnesium can be "normal" while tissues are significantly deficient.
- By the time serum is low, deficiency is usually advanced.

RBC magnesium, by contrast, measures magnesium inside red blood cells and better reflects intracellular status, though it is still an imperfect proxy for total body stores.

Whole blood magnesium (serum + cellular) is another informative measure when available.

Maya's serum magnesium was "okay."

Her RBC magnesium showed that her tissues had been running below their needs for years.

Maya's 12-Week conductor restoration

Maya's physician designed a three-phase magnesium restoration plan. The goal was not just to raise a lab value; it was to refill depleted body stores, support related nutrient systems, and transition into sustainable maintenance.

Phase 1 (weeks 1-4): Repletion without overwhelm

The priority in the first month was to restore depleted magnesium stores using well-absorbed forms while minimizing digestive side effects.

Daily regimen (individualized, under supervision):

- Morning: Magnesium glycinate, around 200 mg elemental magnesium with breakfast
- Evening: Magnesium glycinate, around 200 mg with dinner

Many adults in clinical practice require roughly 200-400 mg/day of supplemental elemental magnesium (sometimes more under medical supervision) to correct suboptimal intake, adjusted for kidney function and medications.

Specific product examples are intentionally omitted here; the focus is on nutrient forms and physiology, with a separate appendix later describing how to evaluate commercially available formulations.

Why magnesium Glycinate?

Magnesium glycinate is a chelated form in which magnesium is bound to the amino acid glycine.

Advantages:

- Higher bioavailability than magnesium oxide and some other inorganic forms
- Less likely to cause loose stools at equivalent doses
- Glycine itself has calming properties that may support sleep and relaxation which are generic and supported.

Additional support:

Her physician also:

- Checked and optimized vitamin D status (vitamin D and magnesium metabolism are interdependent)
- Added a methylated B-complex to support energy pathways
- Encouraged magnesium-rich foods: leafy greens, nuts, seeds, beans, and dark chocolate

Early results (Weeks 1-4):

Within two weeks, Maya noticed:

- Fewer nighttime cramps
- Slightly better sleep onset
- Lower baseline anxiety, especially in the evenings
- Her eyelid twitch resolved

Phase 2 (weeks 5-8): Nervous system and sleep optimization

Once initial stores improved and she tolerated supplementation well, the regimen was refined.

Adjustments:

- Magnesium glycinate continued twice daily
- Magnesium L-threonate added in the late afternoon or evening

Why magnesium l-threonate?

Magnesium L-threonate is a form studied for its ability to raise brain magnesium levels and support cognitive function in early research.

Features:

- Crosses the blood-brain barrier more efficiently than many other forms
- In animal and early human studies, increases brain magnesium levels and supports synaptic plasticity and cognitive function
- May improve aspects of sleep quality and reduce daytime sleepiness in some trials

Goals for Phase 2:

- Deeper, more restorative sleep
- Reduced neural hyperexcitability (twitches, palpitations, noise sensitivity)
- Better cognitive performance under demanding workloads

Results (Weeks 5-8):

By Week 8, Maya reported:

- Falling asleep within about 20 minutes most nights
- Waking once or not at all
- Cramps largely gone
- Dramatic reduction in palpitations
- Clearer thinking during score study and rehearsals
- Much less irritability, colleagues noticed she was "back."

Phase 3 (weeks 9-12): Maintenance and fine-tuning

By now, her repeated RBC magnesium had risen into a more optimal range. The focus shifted to long-term sustainability.

Goals:

- Identify the lowest effective maintenance dose (often 200-400 mg/day, individualized)

- Integrate magnesium with her broader protocol: zinc, B12, folate, boron, and other cofactors covered later in the book
- Maintain gains through diet, sleep hygiene, and stress management

Maya continued:

- Daily magnesium supplementation
- Magnesium-rich nutrition
- Regular sleep and wake times
- Stress-reduction practices designed to reduce adrenergic surges and magnesium loss

Results (Week 12):

Her symptom profile looked dramatically different:

Symptom	Before	After 12 Weeks
---	---	---
Insomnia	Severe, nightly	Largely resolved
Muscle cramps	Multiple per night	Gone
Palpitations	Daily	Rare, brief
Anxiety	Constant	Significantly reduced
Headaches	Daily	Occasional
Brain fog	Marked	Minimal
Energy	Exhausted	Stable through day
Noise sensitivity	Debilitating	Tolerable/normal
Mood	Irritable, tearful	Stable, engaged

Her orchestra had its conductor back.

Beyond Maya: Who else should think about magnesium?

The short answer: almost everyone in modern environments.

Groups at especially high risk include:

- People under chronic stress
- Those eating processed, high-sugar diets

- Heavy coffee, soda, or alcohol users
- Patients on long-term diuretics, PPIs, and certain other medications
- Athletes and heavy exercisers (losses in sweat + higher demand)
- People with diabetes or metabolic syndrome
- Older adults, who often have reduced intake and absorption

Symptoms that should raise suspicion

- Persistent muscle cramps, twitches, or tightness
- Frequent tension headaches or migraines
- Insomnia or non-restorative sleep
- Anxiety or "wired but tired" states without clear triggers
- Heart palpitations with an otherwise normal cardiac workup
- Chronic constipation
- Noise sensitivity and sensory overload
- Restless legs at night
- Brain fog, poor concentration, or memory lapses
- Cold hands and feet
- Strong, recurrent chocolate cravings

If you recognize yourself, or your patients, in several of these, magnesium is one of the first "chips" worth investigating.

Why this matters for the rest of the book

Magnesium comes first in this book for a reason: it underpins almost every other system discussed.

- Without magnesium, ATP-dependent processes slow or stall.
- Without magnesium, DNA replication and repair are less efficient.
- Without magnesium, neurons become more excitable and muscles cannot fully relax.
- Without magnesium, sleep quality, mood stability, and cognitive performance suffer.

Maya's story illustrates three key points:

1. A long list of seemingly unrelated symptoms can share a biochemical root.
2. Standard labs often fail to reveal that root.

3. Restoring one critical mineral can radically change daily experience.

What's next: From magnesium to your genetic software

In the next chapter, the focus shifts from magnesium's role in energy and neuromuscular stability to the vitamins that maintain your genetic "software": B12, folate, and the methylation systems that determine how your DNA is expressed, how your brain synthesizes neurotransmitters, and how your body repairs itself over time.

Having a conductor is only useful if the score, the genetic code and its regulation are being read correctly.

SIDEBAR: Magnesium Forms Compared, Which One Should You Use?

Form	Bioavailability / Use	Notes
Magnesium glycinate	High; general repletion, anxiety, sleep	Chelated; gentle on GI; glycine is calming.
Magnesium L-threonate	Brain-specific support, cognition, sleep based on emerging evidence	Crosses blood-brain barrier; raises brain magnesium.
Magnesium citrate	Moderate-high; constipation, general use	Mild laxative effect; well absorbed.
Magnesium taurate	Cardiovascular support	Taurine supports cardiac function (limited data).
Magnesium malate	Energy support, fibromyalgia	Malic acid participates in energy pathways.
Magnesium oxide	Very low systemic bioavailability	Useful for short-term constipation; poor for repletion.
Magnesium chloride	Moderate; sometimes used topically	Transdermal benefits are still under active study.

General patterns:

- For sleep, anxiety, muscle tension: magnesium glycinate is often preferred.
- For cognitive and brain-focused goals: magnesium L-threonate is a good option.
- For constipation: magnesium citrate can be useful, starting with lower doses.

Always adjust for kidney function and medications, and involve a clinician when building higher-dose regimens.

SIDEBAR: Testing Magnesium— what to ask for

If magnesium deficiency is suspected, useful tests include:

1. RBC Magnesium (Red Blood Cell Magnesium)

- Better reflects intracellular status than serum alone.
- Often interpreted functionally; many integrative clinicians target mid-to-upper range values.

2. Serum Magnesium

- Standard and inexpensive.
- Useful for detecting severe or acute deficiency, but often normal in subclinical depletion.

3. Whole Blood Magnesium (if available)

- Combines cellular and serum compartments.
- More comprehensive but less commonly offered.

4. Magnesium Loading Test (specialty)

- Oral or IV magnesium dose followed by 24-hour urine collection.
- High retention suggests systemic deficiency.

Lab results should always be interpreted in the context of symptoms and the overall clinical picture.

CHAPTER 3: The Memory Machine: DNA, Epigenetics, and Your Biological RAM

The computer that programs itself

When James Watson and Francis Crick described the double-helix structure of DNA in 1953, it fueled a seductive simplicity: DNA was the "code of life", a fixed program that determined everything about you, from eye color to disease risk.

For decades, the dominant narrative was elegantly simple but incomplete: "Genes are destiny."

Then a puzzle emerged. Every cell in your body, with a few immune system exceptions, contains essentially the same DNA. The same 3 billion base pairs, the same genes, the same code. Yet a neuron looks nothing like a hepatocyte or a myocyte and performs completely different roles.

Same code. Totally different behavior.

The missing piece was epigenetics.

If DNA is the code, epigenetics is the operating system and configuration layer. It decides which genes are read or silenced, when they are turned on or off, and how strongly they are expressed. This system is dynamic and responds to nutrients, stress, sleep, toxins, and hormones, changing over time and, critically, remaining modifiable.

The machinery that runs this system heavily depends on methylation, a biochemical process that, in turn, depends on specific nutrients, especially vitamin B12 and folate.

When methylation falters, consequences ripple through DNA repair, neurotransmitter balance, myelin maintenance, and cognition.

This is Daniel's story.

Daniel's disappearing mind

Daniel, 47, was a graphic designer whose work depended on memory, visual thinking, and fine detail. He could hold entire brand systems in his mind and juggle multiple projects without dropping a thread.

Then his memory began to fray.

At first, there were minor events:

- Misplacing his phone more often.
- Forgetting names.
- Losing his train of thought mid-sentence.

He called it stress.

Over the next year, it became more serious:

- He missed deadlines because he forgot projects existed.
- He reread emails three times and still did not retain them.
- He got lost driving to familiar places and forgot scheduled calls.
- He struggled to follow TV plots; 20 minutes in, he had no idea what was happening.

His wife noticed he repeated the same story minutes apart with no awareness.

The worst moment came when he forgot his daughter's 10th birthday, not just the details, but the day itself, until his wife reminded him that evening.

His father had died of Alzheimer's in his early seventies; his grandfather had faded mentally in his sixties. Daniel was sure he was next.

The medical dead end

His primary care physician ordered basic labs: CBC, CMP, TSH, B12, lipids. Everything came back "normal."

"Could be stress. Maybe some depression," the doctor said, suggesting therapy.

Daniel was referred to a neurologist, who ordered a brain MRI and formal cognitive testing. The MRI showed no strokes, tumors, or overt structural damage. Cognitive testing showed mild cognitive impairment (MCI), worse than expected for age and education, but not meeting dementia criteria.

"We'll monitor it. Not much to do at this stage," the neurologist said. "Come back in a year."

"Wait and watch your mind decline" felt like a polite death sentence.

The functional medicine approach

Daniel sought a clinician focused on cognitive decline and potentially reversible contributors.

The key question shifted from "What diagnosis fits?" to "Which systems that support brain function are underperforming?"

A deeper metabolic and nutrient panel focused on methylation and cellular function included:

- Serum B12.
- Methylmalonic acid (MMA).
- Homocysteine.
- Folate (serum and RBC).
- Vitamin D.
- Inflammatory markers (hs-CRP, homocysteine).
- Common MTHFR variants.

Daniel's results: the hidden deficiency

Test	Daniel's result	Interpretation
Serum B12	285 pg/mL	Technically "normal," but low for optimal neurologic function
Methylmalonic acid	385 nmol/L	Elevated → functional B12 deficiency
Homocysteine	18.2 μmol/L	Elevated → impaired methylation
RBC folate	Low-normal	Suboptimal intracellular folate
Vitamin D	22 ng/mL	Deficient
hs-CRP	3.8 mg/L	Mildly elevated inflammation
MTHFR genotype	C677T heterozygous	Reduced enzyme activity; impairs folate metabolism

On paper, he had no classic B12-deficiency anemia; serum B12 was "normal." Functionally, his brain was underpowered. Elevated MMA showed B12 was not sufficient inside cells. Elevated homocysteine showed a clogged methylation cycle. With an MTHFR variant, his folate metabolism ran at reduced capacity, making him functionally deficient.

What methylation is and why it matters

Methylation is the transfer of a methyl group (CH_3) from one molecule to another, happening billions of times per second in every cell.

Methylation is required for:

- Building and repairing DNA and RNA.
- Regulating gene expression (epigenetic control).
- Producing and breaking down neurotransmitters.
- Synthesizing myelin.
- Detoxification and immune modulation.

When methylation is suboptimal, all of these systems lose efficiency.

The methylation cycle

The primary methyl donor is S-adenosylmethionine (SAM). After donating its methyl group, SAM forms S-adenosylhomocysteine, which then forms homocysteine. To keep the cycle going, homocysteine must be recycled to methionine, regenerating SAM. This remethylation step requires:

- Folate, mainly as 5-MTHF.
- Vitamin B12 as a cofactor for methionine synthase.

When B12 or folate is inadequate, homocysteine accumulates and methylation slows. Elevated homocysteine is neurotoxic, pro-inflammatory, and associated with cognitive decline, brain atrophy, and vascular risk.

How B12 and folate support your "software"

1. DNA synthesis and repair

B12 and folate are required for nucleotide synthesis. When low, DNA replication becomes error-prone and repair falters, especially in high-demand tissues like the brain.

2. Myelin maintenance

B12 is essential for myelin formation and repair. Deficiency contributes to demyelination, slower conduction, neuropathy, and cognitive decline.

3. Neurotransmitter balance

Methylation supports the synthesis and breakdown of dopamine, serotonin, and norepinephrine. Impaired methylation can contribute to depression, anxiety, and cognitive dullness.

4. Epigenetic regulation

DNA methylation helps silence or activate genes, maintain cellular identity, and coordinate stress and repair responses. Impaired methylation can weaken repair programs, amplify inflammatory signaling, and accelerate cellular aging.

Why "normal" B12 was not enough

Standard B12 ranges are designed to detect overt deficiency, including anemia and obvious neurologic disease, not subtle functional impairment. People can have low-normal B12 and still show neurologic and cognitive symptoms.

Functional markers matter:

- Methylmalonic acid (MMA)
- Accumulates when intracellular B12 is insufficient.
- Elevated MMA is specific for functional B12 deficiency, even with normal serum B12.
- Homocysteine
- Rises when methylation is impaired (low B12, folate, or B6).
- Elevated levels are linked to cognitive decline, dementia, and vascular disease.

Daniel's elevated MMA and homocysteine showed that his methylation system was underpowered and his brain was undersupported.

Daniel's methylation restoration plan

The clinician built a multi-layered protocol.

Layer 1: Replenish B12 and folate

- High-dose methylcobalamin, often given sublingually to bypass absorption issues.

- Periodic hydroxocobalamin injections to rebuild stores and ensure tissue delivery.
- L-methylfolate (5-MTHF) instead of synthetic folic acid.

Why methylcobalamin?

- It is a naturally occurring, bioactive B12 form used directly in methylation and nervous system function.

Why 5-MTHF, especially with MTHFR variants?

- It is the active folate form used to remethylate homocysteine and bypasses reduced MTHFR activity, avoiding accumulation of unmetabolized folic acid.

Additional cofactors:

- Vitamin B6 (as P5P) to support homocysteine metabolism.
- Vitamin B2 (riboflavin) to support MTHFR function.

Goal: lower MMA and homocysteine over 8-12 weeks and normalize methylation flow.

Layer 2: Neuroprotection and inflammation control

- Omega-3 fatty acids (EPA/DHA) for membrane integrity and anti-inflammatory support.
- Vitamin D optimization.
- Anti-inflammatory nutritional strategies and, where appropriate, nutrients such as curcumin.

Layer 3: Stimulate neuroplasticity

- Regular exercise, especially aerobic, to increase BDNF.
- Deliberate new learning (e.g., language, skills).
- Prioritized sleep quality for memory consolidation and glymphatic clearance.

The first eight weeks

Within weeks, Daniel noticed clearer mornings, fewer "blank spots," and better recall of recent events.

At Week 8, labs showed:

Test	Baseline	Week 8	Trend

MMA	385 nmol/L	245 nmol/L	Moving into normal range
Homocysteine	18.2 µmol/L	11.8 µmol/L	Markedly improved
Vitamin D	22 ng/mL	52 ng/mL	Optimized
hs-CRP	3.8 mg/L	1.9 mg/L	Lower inflammation

In his everyday life, these results translated to missing fewer appointments, following stories more easily, and his wife noticed he stopped repeating himself.

Weeks 8-16: from stabilization to improvement

Between Weeks 8 and 16:

- B12 and methylfolate were fine-tuned based on labs and symptoms.
- Movement, learning, and sleep became consistent habits.

By Week 16, cognitive testing showed meaningful improvement, with performance at or slightly above expectations for his age and education. The story shifted from "I'm on a one-way track to dementia" to "My brain improves when supported."

Epigenetics: beyond "levels"

Daniel's case is not just about B12 and folate levels; it shows how these nutrients feed epigenetic machinery that controls gene expression and cellular aging.

DNA methylation and the epigenetic clock

DNA methylation patterns change with age, lifestyle, and environment. Epigenetic clocks estimate biological age from methylation signatures and often predict health status and mortality better than chronological age.

Key insights:

- Biological age can run ahead of or behind calendar age.
- Elevated homocysteine and chronic inflammation are associated with accelerated epigenetic aging in some research.

- Nutrient optimization and lifestyle interventions that support methylation may slow or modestly reverse epigenetic age markers in certain contexts.

Restoring methylation capacity supports not only memory but also the cellular conditions that allow the brain to age more slowly.

Why this matters for "too-young-to-decline" brains

Daniel was 47. His MRI and standard labs were "normal," yet he was experiencing real cognitive decline.

Many people in their 30s and 50s who feel mentally "off" are told:

- "You're just stressed."
- "That's aging."
- "Your labs are fine."

Sometimes that is accurate; often it is incomplete.

Modest deficiencies in B12 and folate, with elevated homocysteine and inflammation, can impair brain function long before structural changes appear on imaging.

The point is not that B12 and folate explain every case of brain fog, but that they are foundational to methylation systems that maintain DNA, neurotransmitters, and myelin and are frequently under-assessed.

The bigger pattern: Why Methylation connects everything

Daniel's story illustrates a recurrent pattern:

- There is a wide space between "not yet diseased" and "functioning optimally."
- Standard lab ranges detect frank disease, not optimal function.
- Deeper testing (MMA, homocysteine, RBC folate, MTHFR variants) can reveal modifiable problems behind "normal" labs.

When those problems are addressed, people often regain abilities they assumed were lost to age or genetics.

Throughout this book, the same pattern appears with different "chips": magnesium, zinc, phosphorus, copper, vitamin C, and boron.

For now, Daniel's story highlights a central truth: your genetic hardware is crucial, but how well it runs over decades depends heavily on software maintenance, methylation and epigenetic regulation. These processes are nutrient-dependent, especially on B12 and folate. When they falter, brains dim; when they are restored, many brains improve.

What's next: From Methylation to immune security

The next chapter shifts from B12 and epigenetics to another overlooked master regulator: zinc, the nutrient that acts as your immune system's security processor.

SIDEBAR: Functional B12 deficiency, why "normal" isn't always normal

Problems with serum B12 alone:

- Measures circulating B12, not intracellular B12.
- Reference ranges (~200, 900 pg/mL) are tuned to detect severe deficiency, not early functional insufficiency.
- A substantial proportion of people with "normal" B12 levels may have elevated MMA, indicating functional deficiency.

Key functional markers:

Test	What It Measures	Why It Matters
---	---	---
Methylmalonic acid (MMA)	Accumulates when intracellular B12 is insufficient	Highly specific marker of functional B12 deficiency
Homocysteine	Accumulates when methylation is impaired	Reflects B12/folate/B6 status; predicts cognitive and vascular risk
Holotranscobalamin (holoTC)	Active B12 fraction bound to transcobalamin	Early marker of B12 deficiency in some cases

When to consider functional testing:

- Cognitive symptoms (memory loss, brain fog, confusion)
- Neurological symptoms (numbness, tingling, gait issues)
- Serum B12 in the low-normal range
- Known MTHFR variants or malabsorption risk

SIDEBAR: Methylcobalamin vs. Cyanocobalamin

Both methylcobalamin and cyanocobalamin can correct B12 deficiency, but they differ in form and handling.

Methylcobalamin

- Naturally occurring, bioactive form used directly in methylation and nervous system function
- Often preferred in protocols focused on cognition, neuropathy, or MTHFR-related issues

Cyanocobalamin

- Synthetic form that must be converted to active coenzyme forms
- Stable, inexpensive, and widely used in fortification and standard supplementation

For patients with neurological symptoms, absorption issues, or MTHFR variants, many clinicians favor methylcobalamin or hydroxocobalamin, delivered orally (sublingual) or by injection, while acknowledging that cyanocobalamin remains effective for many individuals.

SIDEBAR: Methylfolate vs. Folic acid, why form matters

Folic acid

- Synthetic form used in fortification and many supplements
- Requires multiple enzymatic steps, including MTHFR, to convert to active 5-MTHF

L-methylfolate (5-MTHF)

- Biologically active folate form used directly for remethylation of homocysteine
- Bypasses MTHFR, which is useful for individuals with MTHFR polymorphisms
- Does not lead to unmetabolized folic acid accumulation

Patients with elevated homocysteine, MTHFR variants, or neuropsychiatric symptoms often benefit from 5-MTHF rather than high-dose folic acid, under medical supervision.

SIDEBAR: The MTHFR Gene— what it is and why it matters

MTHFR (methylenetetrahydrofolate reductase) converts folate into 5-MTHF, the active methyl-donating form.

Common variants (e.g., C677T, A1298C):

- Reduce enzyme activity to varying degrees
- Can contribute to elevated homocysteine when folate status is marginal
- Increase reliance on sufficient folate, B12, B6, and B2

Clinical implications:

- Higher folate needs and better response to 5-MTHF
- Need for monitoring homocysteine as a functional marker
- Relevance in cognitive decline, cardiovascular risk, and reproductive outcomes

CHAPTER 4: Zinc: The Security Processor

The security system that protects everything

Modern computers and cloud systems do not rely solely on fast processors and robust power supplies; to function optimally, they need an adequate defense system. They depend on security, firewalls, intrusion detection, antivirus software, access protocols to provide this function. Without a functional security layer, a single breach can compromise the entire system.

Your immune system is your body's security layer.

It constantly monitors for threats, viruses, bacteria, fungi, parasites, malignant cells, distinguishes self from non-self, and decides when to mount, scale, and shut down responses.

Zinc is one of the essential nutrients for this system.

It is required for the development, activation, and regulation of many immune cells, influences inflammatory signaling, supports skin and mucosal barrier integrity, and affects how robustly you respond to infections and vaccines.

When zinc is insufficient, your security system is underpowered and erratic:

- You get sick more often.
- Infections last longer.
- Wounds heal slowly.
- Inflammation smolders instead of resolving.
- Your body may struggle to distinguish friend from foe.

This is Priya's story.

Priya's immune collapse

Priya, 34, was a former collegiate track athlete turned ultramarathon runner. Lean, fit, and disciplined, she looked like the picture of health until her immune system began to unravel.

Over eighteen months, an ironclad constitution deteriorated into chronic vulnerability.

It started with a "bad cold" that refused to leave. She expected a week of symptoms; instead, she got three weeks of cough, congestion, and exhaustion. Then it happened again. And again.

Patterns emerged:

- Colds lasting three to four weeks instead of seven to ten days.
- Respiratory infections requiring repeated antibiotics.
- Flu-like illnesses that tested negative for influenza.
- Recurrent canker sores that took two weeks to heal.
- Small skin infections (folliculitis) that cropped up constantly.
- Recurrent yeast infections.
- Cold sores erupting monthly instead of rarely.

She reduced training, slept more, cleaned up her diet, and added vitamin D and omega-3s. Nothing changed.

Standard labs (CBC, CMP, thyroid) were "normal." An immunologist ruled out primary immune deficiencies; immunoglobulins and complement studies were normal. "Sometimes people just have bad luck with infections," she was told.

Priya disagreed. Her "luck" had shifted abruptly and stayed bad despite reasonable changes. Something in the system had changed.

The zinc connection

A clinician familiar with nutrient-immune interactions asked a different question: "What if your immune system is structurally intact but functionally underpowered?"

In addition to reviewing sleep, stress, diet, and medications, the clinician ordered:

- Plasma zinc.
- Serum copper.
- Zinc:copper ratio.
- CBC with differential.
- Secretory IgA (sIgA), if available.

Priya's results: the security gap

Test	Priya's result	Interpretation
---	---	---

Plasma zinc	62 µg/dL	Low-side "normal"; below typical functional targets for immune support
Serum copper	High-normal	Relatively elevated compared with zinc
Zinc:copper	0.55	Low (<0.7); suggests copper-skewed pattern seen with inflammation in some
Lymphocytes	Low-normal	Possible reduced adaptive capacity when combined with symptoms
Secretory IgA	Low	Weakened mucosal defense

"Zinc supports the development and function of T cells, B cells, natural killer cells, neutrophils, and macrophages," the clinician explained. "With low zinc, the thymus can shrink and T-cell output drops; antibody responses weaken; natural killer cells lose some capacity to clear infected or abnormal cells."

"Mucosal barriers in your mouth, sinuses, lungs, gut, and reproductive tract also rely on zinc for repair. When zinc is low, those barriers become fragile, helping explain recurrent mouth sores, respiratory infections, and yeast infections."

"And your zinc:copper ratio tells us about balance. When zinc is relatively low and copper relatively high, immune function often tilts toward more inflammation and less efficient targeted responses."

Priya's immune system was not broken; it was under-supported and mis-tuned because a critical "security chip", zinc, was underpowered.

What zinc actually does for immunity

1. T-cell development and the thymus

The thymus is where immature T cells mature and learn to distinguish self from non-self. Zinc is crucial for thymic structure and T-cell development. Zinc deficiency leads to thymic atrophy, reduced naïve T-cell production, and altered T-cell subsets; supplementation can improve thymic output in deficiency states and after certain intensive therapies.

2. B cells and antibody production

B-cell development, activation, and antibody production require zinc. Low zinc blunts antibody responses and can weaken responses to vaccines and infections.

3. Innate immune cells: first responders

Neutrophils, macrophages, and natural killer cells depend on zinc for phagocytosis, oxidative burst, cytokine production, and cytotoxic activity. Deficiency impairs these functions and increases susceptibility to infection.

4. Cytokine regulation and inflammatory balance

Zinc helps maintain balanced cytokine profiles: strong enough to clear infection, controlled enough to limit collateral damage. Low zinc is associated with altered cytokine patterns and persistent low-grade inflammation.

5. Barrier integrity and wound healing

Skin and mucosal surfaces rely on zinc for epithelial integrity and repair. Deficiency is associated with slower wound healing, barrier breakdown, and increased infections at barrier sites.

6. Secretory IgA: mucosal shield

Secretory IgA (sIgA) is the dominant antibody at mucosal surfaces. Adequate zinc supports antibody production and mucosal immune function; low sIgA with low zinc suggests compromised front-line defense.

7. Antiviral support

Zinc supports interferon signaling and T/NK cell activity and, in vitro, can inhibit the replication of some viruses by interfering with viral polymerases. Clinical data suggest that correcting low zinc may shorten some respiratory infections and support outcomes, as an adjunct to standard therapy rather than a stand-alone treatment.

The zinc:copper ratio: why balance matters

Copper, like zinc, is essential for enzymes in antioxidant defense, connective tissue, and immune function. The key is balance.

- Too little zinc relative to copper is linked with higher oxidative stress, inflammation, and infection risk in some groups.

- Too much zinc for prolonged periods without copper monitoring can induce copper deficiency, anemia, and neurologic symptoms.

A zinc:copper ratio around 0.7, 1.0 is often considered functionally balanced, though individual targets vary.

Priya's ratio of 0.55 reflected relative zinc insufficiency and a copper-skewed pattern consistent with her clinical picture.

Priya's 12-week security upgrade

The clinician created a stepwise plan to restore zinc status, rebalance copper, and support immune resilience.

Phase 1 (Weeks 1-4): Repletion and barrier support

Goals:

- Raise zinc toward a more optimal range.
- Support gut and mucosal immunity.
- Begin reducing chronic inflammatory load.

Core regimen (individualized, under supervision):

- Zinc about 25-30 mg/day as a well-absorbed chelated form (such as zinc picolinate or bisglycinate), taken with food to minimize nausea.
- Zinc L-carnosine, where gastrointestinal mucosal support was indicated, at doses similar to those used in clinical and experimental studies.
- Vitamin D optimization to an agreed target range.
- Vitamin C and omega-3 fatty acids to support immune regulation and repair.
- Emphasis on zinc-rich foods: shellfish, beef, poultry, pumpkin seeds, legumes prepared to reduce phytates.

Early results:

- Mouth sores healed faster.
- Fewer minor infections despite similar exposures.
- Slightly improved energy between training sessions.

Phase 2 (Weeks 5-8): Functional strengthening

With zinc improving and copper monitored:

- Zinc dose adjusted (often ~20-25 mg/day) based on labs and symptoms.
- Selenium added at physiologic doses to support antioxidant enzymes and antiviral defenses.
- Gut-support strategies (probiotics, fermented foods, prebiotic fibers) to normalize mucosal immunity and sIgA.
- Gradual return to structured training with careful attention to recovery.

Results:

- No new major infections.
- Early symptoms were milder and resolved in days instead of weeks.
- Folliculitis lesions resolved more quickly; canker sores stopped recurring.

Follow-up labs:

Test	Baseline	Week 8	Trend
---	---	---	---
Plasma zinc	62 μg/dL	95 μg/dL	Into typical optimal range
Zinc:copper	0.55	0.82	Balanced
Lymphocytes	Low-normal	Mid-normal	Improved
Secretory IgA	Low	Normal	Restored

Phase 3 (Weeks 9-12): Maintenance and resilience

Once values and symptoms stabilized:

- Zinc was titrated to a maintenance level (often 15-20 mg/day, individualized).
- Copper was periodically monitored to avoid deficiency.
- Whole-food zinc sources became primary, with supplements used more strategically during high-demand periods (heavy training, travel, peak viral seasons).

Priya rebuilt her ultramarathon training volume; intense blocks no longer automatically ended in prolonged respiratory illness. Her immune system was no longer the weak link.

Broader implications: Zinc deficiency beyond Priya's case

Priya's story shows how "normal" immune testing can miss functional weaknesses that nutrient-focused evaluation reveals.

Key lessons:

- Normal white blood cell counts and no primary immunodeficiency do not rule out frequent infections from marginal zinc status.
- Chronic, low-grade insufficiency rarely looks dramatic on standard labs but can be dramatic in lived experience.
- Correcting imbalances usually requires steady support over weeks to months, not just "taking zinc when you're sick."
- Zinc works with copper, vitamin D, vitamin C, selenium, and others; it is part of an integrated system.

Who should consider zinc evaluation?

Groups at higher risk include:

- People with frequent infections or slow recovery.
- Those with recurrent mouth ulcers, skin infections, or poor wound healing.
- Vegetarians and vegans (lower bioavailability due to phytates).
- Heavy exercisers or endurance athletes (losses in sweat plus higher demand).
- People with chronic gastrointestinal disorders affecting absorption.
- Older adults, whose intake and absorption often decline.
- Individuals with chronic inflammatory conditions or autoimmunity.

Symptoms that may suggest zinc insufficiency:

- Frequent colds and respiratory infections.
- Slow wound healing.
- Hair loss or brittle nails.
- Changes in taste or smell.

- Persistent skin rashes or acne.
- Low mood or irritability.
- Poor appetite.

If these patterns sound familiar, zinc is one of the first "security chips" worth examining.

Testing and caution

Testing options:

- Plasma or serum zinc, most common; best interpreted with symptoms and other labs.
- Zinc:copper ratio, useful for balance and inflammatory patterns.
- RBC zinc, less available but may add an intracellular context.

Cautions:

- Long-term higher-dose zinc (e.g., >40-50 mg/day for months) without copper monitoring can cause copper deficiency, anemia, and neurologic symptoms.
- Dosing should be tailored to overall health, kidney function, medications, and broader micronutrient status, under clinician supervision.

A brief note you can use once early in your zinc or supplement chapter to make your stance explicit:

"Specific brands are intentionally omitted; the focus is on nutrient forms, physiology, and dosing ranges, with a separate appendix on how to evaluate commercially available products."

Why this matters for the rest of the book

If mitochondria are your power plants and magnesium is your conductor, zinc is your security processor.

It influences:

- How robustly you respond to threats.
- How quickly you recover from infections.
- How you regulate chronic, low-grade inflammation.
- How well you maintain barrier integrity and tissue repair.

Zinc interacts with other "chips":

- With copper and vitamin C in antioxidant enzymes like superoxide dismutase.
- With vitamin D and selenium in immune modulation.
- With mitochondrial and DNA integrity by limiting oxidative and inflammatory damage.

Priya's story shows that frequent illness is often not just "bad luck"; basic labs can miss nutrient-related vulnerabilities, and restoring a critical immune nutrient can shift someone from "always sick" to resilient.

The next chapter moves from immune security to navigation, how your brain knows where you are in space, coordinates movement, and why energy failure in those systems leads to dizziness, clumsiness, and feeling disconnected from your own body.

SIDEBAR: Zinc Supplementation Forms—Which Should You Choose?

Different zinc forms vary in absorption, tolerability, and clinical use.

Form	Absorption / Use	GI Tolerability	Notes
---	---	---	---
-	High; good tissue uptake in small trials	Generally good	Chelated with picolinic acid; often used for systemic repletion.
Zinc bisglycinate	High; often superior to gluconate in bioavailability reviews	Excellent	Chelated with glycine; gentle on the GI tract; good for long-term use.
Zinc gluconate	Moderate; well-studied	Good	Common, cost-effective; often found in lozenges.
Zinc citrate	Moderate	Good	Similar systemic use as gluconate.

Zinc, L-carnosine	Designed for mucosal delivery	Excellent	Used for gut mucosal healing and protection in several studies.
Zinc sulfate	Lower bioavailability; more GI issues	Fair, poor	May cause nausea/GI upset; less ideal for long-term oral use.
Zinc oxide	Very low systemic absorption	Poor	Generally used topically; not ideal for systemic supplementation.

Practical patterns (under clinician guidance):

- General immune support: zinc picolinate or zinc bisglycinate (15-30 mg/day).
- Gut mucosal support: zinc, L-carnosine at doses used in clinical trials.
- Sensitive stomachs: zinc bisglycinate.
- Always consider copper status if using higher zinc doses long term.

SIDEBAR: the Zinc:Copper ratio— A functional immune marker

The zinc:copper ratio integrates information about two interdependent minerals involved in antioxidant defense and immune function.

- Ratios <0.7 (zinc:copper) are often associated with higher inflammatory and oxidative stress markers and greater infection risk in some populations.
- Ratios in the 0.7, 1.0 range are often considered balanced.
- Ratios >1.2 may indicate high zinc relative to copper and potential risk of copper depletion if supplementation is excessive.

Clinically, the ratio is useful:

- In patients with recurrent infections or chronic inflammation
- During and after therapeutic zinc supplementation

- As part of a broader panel including CRP, ferritin, and vitamin D

SIDEBAR: secretory IgA: Your mucosal shield

Secretory IgA (sIgA) is the immune system's main antibody at mucosal surfaces.

It:

- Traps pathogens in mucus and helps clear them
- Neutralizes toxins and viruses
- Helps prevent harmful bacteria from adhering to the gut or respiratory lining
- Shapes the microbiome while avoiding excessive inflammation

Low sIgA is associated with:

- Frequent upper respiratory infections
- Recurrent sinus or ear infections
- Chronic digestive issues and food sensitivities
- Recurrent vaginal or urinary infections

Supporting sIgA often involves:

- Optimizing zinc and vitamin A/D status
- Improving gut health (probiotics, prebiotics, reducing irritants)
- Managing chronic stress and overtraining

Testing sIgA (in saliva or stool) can be useful in patients with recurrent infections or suspected mucosal immune compromise.

GLOSSARY: Key Terms for Chapter 4

- **Zinc:** Essential trace mineral involved in hundreds of enzymes and critical for immune function, wound healing, DNA synthesis, and antioxidant defense.
- **Thymus:** Lymphoid organ where T cells mature; highly sensitive to zinc status.
- **T cells:** Adaptive immune cells that coordinate and execute targeted immune responses.
- **B cells:** Immune cells that produce antibodies.
- **Natural killer (NK) cells:** Innate immune cells that destroy virus-infected and cancerous cells.

- **Secretory IgA (sIgA):** Primary antibody at mucosal surfaces, acting as a non-inflammatory shield.
- **Zinc:copper ratio:** Relationship between zinc and copper levels; used as a functional marker of immune and inflammatory balance.
- **Cytokines:** Immune signaling molecules that coordinate responses to infection and injury.
- **Mucosal immunity:** Immune defense at mucous membranes in the respiratory, gastrointestinal, and urogenital tracts.
- **Zinc picolinate / bisglycinate:** Chelated zinc forms with higher bioavailability and better GI tolerability than some inorganic forms.
- **Zinc:** L-carnosine, Zinc bound to L-carnosine; studied for gastrointestinal mucosal support.
- **Thymic atrophy:** Shrinkage of the thymus, often seen with aging and zinc deficiency, leading to reduced T-cell output.
- **Phytates:** Compounds in grains and legumes that bind minerals like zinc and reduce absorption.
- **Oxidative stress:** Imbalance between reactive oxygen species and antioxidant defenses; contributes to tissue damage and immune dysregulation.
- **Superoxide dismutase (SOD):** An antioxidant enzyme that requires zinc and copper as cofactors.

CHAPTER 5: The Seven Planes of Proprioception: Your Navigation System

The hidden navigation system

Right now, as you read this, your brain is running one of the most sophisticated navigation systems on Earth. It is:

- Tracking the position of every joint.
- Monitoring balance and orientation in three-dimensional space.
- Processing two slightly different visual angles to compute depth.
- Estimating distances and speeds with millisecond precision.
- Coordinating hundreds of muscles to maintain posture without conscious effort.
- Planning and executing movements before you are aware that you have decided to move.

When this system works, you walk, turn, reach, drive, and play without thinking about the complexity beneath the surface. When it glitches, you do not just feel "a little off." You feel disconnected from your body or as if the world itself is unstable.

This is Michael's story.

Michael's disorienting decline

Michael, 44, was a former college basketball player turned tech project manager. For decades, his coordination and spatial awareness were invisible strengths.

Over two years, that confidence quietly eroded.

He started:

- Missing the edge of a table when reaching for his mug.
- Bumping his shoulder into familiar door frames.
- Feeling unsteady in the dark, as if the ground was not where his brain expected.

Driving became uncomfortable. On the highway, lane position felt uncertain; distances looked "wrong." After a near-collision during an overcorrection, he pulled off the road shaken and wondering whether he was "losing his mind."

Standard evaluations followed:

- Primary care exam and basic neuro testing: normal.
- Ophthalmology: 20/20 vision, normal retina.
- Neurology: normal MRI; no stroke, tumor, or demyelination.
- Vestibular testing: "normal" inner ear function.

He was told it might be stress or "getting older."

The hardware, eyes, ears, gross brain structures looked intact. The problem lay in the integration and power supply of his navigation system: not the cameras and gyroscopes, but the energy feeding them and the "software" stitching signals together.

Your brain is running autonomous-vehicle software

A self-driving car uses multiple overlapping sensors:

- Cameras (vision).
- Radar/lidar (depth, motion).
- Ultrasonic sensors (proximity).
- Inertial measurement units (orientation, acceleration).
- GPS (location).
- Central processors (integration, decision-making).

Your brain does something similar:

- Visual system (cameras).
- Vestibular system (inner-ear gyroscope and accelerometer).
- Proprioceptive system (joint and muscle position sensors).
- Somatosensory system (pressure, touch, pain, temperature).
- Auditory system (sound localization).
- Cerebellum (integration and refinement).
- Prefrontal and parietal cortex (planning, prediction, spatial working memory).

All of it runs on ATP. When energy is inadequate, high-demand systems fail first. The navigation planes are among the most energy-intensive networks in the brain. For Michael, his "self-driving software" ran invisibly until the energy budget shrank and glitches appeared.

The seven planes of proprioception

This chapter divides the navigation system into seven "planes," like layers in a software stack. Each plane depends on those below and feeds those above. Michael's symptoms illustrate what happens when multiple planes lose power at once, too subtly to trigger classic pathology on imaging, but enough to make daily navigation unreliable.

Plane 1: Visual system— your cameras

Vision does far more than make images. It:

- Calculates depth via binocular disparity.
- Tracks motion and predicts trajectories.
- Provides a vertical reference for balance.
- Integrates with hand and body movements.

The visual cortex is among the most metabolically active brain regions; visual processing is energy-hungry. When energy is limited, you may notice:

- "Foggy" vision not fixed by glasses.
- Difficulty tracking moving objects.
- Problems with depth perception.
- Light sensitivity and visual overwhelm.

Michael's eye chart was normal, but at freeway speeds and dusk lighting, his brain struggled to maintain a stable 3D map, making lane changes feel unsafe. That is Plane 1 on a dimmed power supply.

Plane 2: Vestibular system, your gyroscope and accelerometer

The vestibular apparatus includes:

- Semicircular canals (angular acceleration/head rotation).
- Otolith organs (utricle, saccule) for linear acceleration and gravity.

Vestibular hair cells rely heavily on oxidative phosphorylation; they have high mitochondrial content and enriched electron transport chain enzymes compared with auditory hair cells, which rely more on glycolysis.

Vestibular inputs support:

- Gaze stabilization via the vestibulo-ocular reflex (VOR).
- Balance and upright posture.

When vestibular processing is compromised by mitochondrial dysfunction or energy failure, people may feel:

- Dizziness or vertigo.
- Unsteadiness when turning the head.
- Difficulty walking in the dark.
- Persistent imbalance despite "normal" vestibular tests.

Recent work in adults with the m.3243A>G mitochondrial variant shows frequent vestibular dysfunction and involvement of the semicircular canals and otolith organs, despite structural imaging that can appear unremarkable.

Michael's vestibular tests were "normal," but his lived experience, roads that felt subtly tilted, floors not quite predictable, "boat-like" walking in darkness, is characteristic of an energy-limited vestibular system before frank vertigo appears.

Plane 3: Proprioceptive system, your joint-position sensors

Proprioception is body position sense without looking, mediated by:

- Muscle spindles (length and rate of stretch).
- Golgi tendon organs (tension).
- Joint receptors (angle and movement).
- Skin mechanoreceptors.

Signals travel via dorsal root ganglia to the spinal cord, brainstem, cerebellum, and cortex. Emerging data show that certain proprioceptive neurons exhibit particularly high expression of energy-metabolism genes, suggesting a high energy demand for these specialized sensory functions; training induces transcriptional and metabolic adaptations.

When proprioception falters, people report:

- Feeling disconnected from the body.
- Heaviness or sluggishness in limbs.
- Inaccuracy in finger-to-nose with eyes closed.

- Uncertainty walking downstairs or on uneven ground.

Michael could perform the finger-to-nose test in a quiet exam room, but at home, on the stairs, or while reaching in motion, his hand or foot regularly ended up slightly off, as real-world complexity strained his proprioceptive bandwidth in ways controlled drills did not

.

Plane 4: Somatosensory system, collision detection

This system processes light touch, pressure, vibration, pain, and temperature to:

- Detect contact and pressure.
- Judge texture and shape.
- Avoid injury by sensing damaging stimuli.

Energy limitations in peripheral or central processing can cause:

- Reduced light touch or vibration sense.
- Amplified pain when inhibitory control fails due to low ATP.
- Paresthesias and allodynia.

Michael described an urge to "guard" himself in crowds, unsure where his body ended and others began. A minor bump felt disproportionately jarring.

Plane 5: Auditory system, acoustic positioning

Hearing also contributes spatial information:

- Interaural time and intensity differences localize sounds left/right and in depth.
- Frequency filtering helps with elevation and distance.

When auditory processing is strained:

- Speech in noise becomes difficult despite normal thresholds.
- Noisy or crowded places feel overwhelming.
- Tinnitus may emerge as the brain amplifies internal signals.

Auditory hair cells rely more on glycolysis, partly because cochlear tissue limits vascularization to prevent sound distortion, while vestibular hair cells rely more on oxidative phosphorylation and have higher mitochondrial enzyme expression.

Michael began orienting his head more toward sounds, as if his brain no longer fully trusted its passive spatial audio map.

Plane 6: Cerebellar integration, your central movement processor

The cerebellum, containing more than half the brain's neurons, integrates visual, vestibular, proprioceptive, somatosensory, and auditory inputs to:

- Coordinate smooth, accurate movements.
- Maintain balance and posture.
- Adjust actions based on error feedback (motor learning).

Purkinje cells are exceptionally energy-demanding:

- Enormous dendritic trees with up to ~200,000 synapses.
- Continuous spontaneous firing at 50, 150 Hz.
- High ATP needs for calcium clearance and synaptic signaling.

A 2019 study showed that ATP depletion activates ATM kinase, which phosphorylates NRF1, driving mitochondrial biogenesis; in ATM deficiency (ataxia-telangiectasia), Purkinje cells cannot adequately respond to increased energy demand and degenerate, causing cerebellar ataxia.

Calcium clearance in Purkinje and granule cells relies on Ca^{2+}-ATPases and is energy-intensive; glycolytic failure first impairs distal dendrites and spines, then propagates centrally.

Cerebellar dysfunction signs:

- Clumsiness and poor coordination.
- Intention tremor.
- Difficulty with rapid alternating movements.
- Unsteady gait, especially on uneven or dark surfaces.
- Dysmetria (overshoot/undershoot).

Michael did not meet the criteria for ataxia, but he exhibited a milder form: slight delays between intention and movement, subtle timing errors, and loss of confidence in dynamic settings.

Plane 7: Cortical planning, motor planning, and awareness

The top plane resides in the prefrontal and parietal regions that:

- Plan actions.
- Sequence complex movements.

- Maintain spatial working memory.
- Simulate movements and monitor performance.

These regions are metabolically expensive: they require high baseline energy for working memory and attention, plus frequent ATP bursts for decision-making and plan updates.

Mild energy failure can cause:

- Slowed decisions.
- Difficulty planning or sequencing movement.
- Trouble holding spatial intentions ("What was I reaching for?").

Moderate failure:

- Getting stuck mid-action.
- Misjudging physical ability.
- Needing conscious effort for formerly automatic tasks.

Severe failure:

- Marked loss of goal-directed behavior and movement initiation.

Patients say:

- "I know what I want to do, but I can't organize the steps."
- "I start something and freeze or forget what I'm doing."

Michael could pass a simple clinic-based driving simulation, but the demands of a real-world freeway, with multiple planes active at once, exceeded his energetic "headroom."

Energy crisis: when navigation fails

Failure is usually gradual:

1. Metabolic decline

Hormonal shifts, chronic stress, sleep loss, and metabolic disease reduce mitochondrial biogenesis and efficiency, lowering total brain ATP.

2. High-demand systems fail first

The cerebellum, prefrontal cortex, and visual and vestibular hubs begin to underperform; signals become noisy and desynchronized across planes.

3. Functional symptoms emerge

Months 1, 3: subtle disequilibrium and coordination issues.

Months 3, 6: frequent bumps, "boat-like" walking, sensory overwhelm.

Months 6, 12: avoidance of driving, sports, and complex environments, with near-falls and sustained fear of movement.

Michael lived in this mid-range zone for over a year.

Standard tests often remain "normal" because they assess hardware in isolation, not the energy delivery and multi-plane integration that determine performance.

Self-check: simple navigation tests

Your self-tests section is already clear and noncommercial; it can remain as written, with the understanding that these are screening tools to track trends and guide clinician conversations, not diagnostic algorithms.

Michael's energy and navigation restoration

His clinician targeted both:

- Power supply (hormones, nutrients, mitochondrial cofactors).
- Navigation training (balance, vestibular, proprioceptive, cerebellar drills).

Layer 1: Power supply

Interventions included:

- Optimizing endogenous testosterone production (within physiologic ranges) via lifestyle and, where appropriate, carefully chosen agents, to support brain glucose uptake and mitochondrial function.
- Restoring magnesium with well-absorbed forms (e.g., glycinate) to support Mg-ATP-dependent neuronal and muscular processes.
- Supporting mitochondrial cofactors generically (CoQ10, B-vitamins, NAD+ precursors) to bolster electron transport and ATP generation.
- Adding antioxidant support (e.g., vitamin C and other non-branded antioxidants) to help contain oxidative stress in high-demand circuits.

No specific commercial products are endorsed here; examples of how to evaluate available formulations appear in a separate appendix.

Layer 2: Navigation system training

As his capacity improved, they introduced:

- Balance work (single-leg stance, wobble boards).
- Vestibular exercises (head movements with gaze stabilization).
- Coordination drills (tandem gait, rapid alternating movements).
- Gradual re-exposure to complex movement (low-risk sport-like drills).

Because proprioceptive and vestibular neurons are plastic, targeted training can enhance performance when metabolic capacity is sufficient.

Over ~12 weeks, Michael's home tests and lived experience improved: steadier single-leg stance, better balance in the dark, more confident lane positioning, and a return to activities he had quietly abandoned.

Practical takeaways

Michael's story illustrates:

1. Navigation complaints are real and often functional

"Boat-like" walking, body disconnection, and new driving anxiety often signal subtle multi-plane dysfunction, not just anxiety.

2. High-demand systems fail first when energy is limited

Navigation planes, especially cerebellar and prefrontal networks, are energy-intensive and sensitive to mitochondrial compromise.

3. Standard tests focus on hardware, not performance

MRI, basic neuro exams, and standard vestibular tests can all be normal while integration and energy remain impaired.

4. Support and training can restore function

Improving energy supply, along with systematic retraining, allows many people to regain abilities previously written off as "aging."

How this connects to the rest of the book

The seven planes of proprioception sit on top of multiple "chips" discussed elsewhere:

- Magnesium for ATP activation.
- B12/folate for myelin and methylation.
- Zinc for immune and inflammatory modulation impacting neural health.

- Phosphorus and creatine for rapid ATP buffering.
- Copper for myelin and enzymatic function.
- Vitamin C for vascular and connective-tissue integrity.
- Boron for hormonal and inflammatory set-points.

Your navigation system is real, testable, and trainable. When it functions, you move through the world with ease; when it falters, life shrinks. The next chapter turns to phosphorus and creatine, the elements that build your internal power grid and determine how effectively mitochondrial ATP can be delivered and used.

SIDEBAR: Why Purkinje cells are the "canaries in the coal mine" for energy failure

Purkinje cells in the cerebellum are extraordinary neurons, and extraordinarily vulnerable.

What makes them special

Size and connectivity:

- Among the largest neurons in the brain
- Each Purkinje cell receives up to 200,000 synaptic inputs
- Massive dendritic trees that integrate information from parallel fibers and climbing fibers

Energy demands:

- Highest spontaneous firing rates in the nervous system: 50- 150 Hz continuously, even at rest
- Dynamic ATP fluctuations with every change in neuronal activity
- Calcium clearance (essential for maintaining function) is ATP-intensive and powered by glycolysis

Why they fail first

A 2019 landmark study showed that ATP depletion activates ATM kinase, which then phosphorylates NRF1 (nuclear respiratory factor-1) to drive mitochondrial biogenesis.

In the absence of ATM (as in ataxia-telangiectasia):

- Purkinje cells cannot respond to increased energy demands
- ATP deficit accumulates

- Neurons degenerate, causing progressive cerebellar ataxia (loss of coordination)

Clinical relevance

When patients present with:

- Unexplained clumsiness
- Intention tremor
- Balance problems
- Difficulty with complex movements

and imaging is "normal," consider:

- Mitochondrial dysfunction (not structural damage)
- Energy substrate deficiencies (NAD+, CoQ10, magnesium, B vitamins)
- Hormonal factors affecting brain glucose uptake and mitochondrial biogenesis

Purkinje cells are the "canaries in the coal mine"; they signal energy failure before it's visible on MRI.

SIDEBAR: Vestibular vs. Auditory energy Metabolism—why it matters

Not all inner ear cells use energy in the same way.

A groundbreaking 2012 study revealed a fundamental metabolic difference between auditory and vestibular systems:

Auditory (cochlear) hair cells

- Rely predominantly on glycolysis (oxygen-independent energy production)
- Express 3× higher levels of glycolytic enzymes than vestibular cells
- Have 1/4 the mitochondrial protein content of vestibular cells
- Glycolysis rate is 4× higher in the cochlea vs. the utricle

Why? The cochlea actively inhibits vascularization (blood vessel formation) to prevent interference with sound transmission. With a limited oxygen supply, it relies on glycolysis.

Vestibular hair cells

- Rely predominantly on oxidative phosphorylation (OXPHOS), mitochondrial ATP production

- Contain numerous mitochondria, especially near synaptic ribbons, where energy demand is highest
- 4× higher levels of citric acid cycle enzymes than cochlear cells
- 10× higher levels of electron transport chain enzymes

Clinical implications

1. Mitochondrial disease affects vestibular function disproportionately:

- Patients with m.3243A>G mitochondrial mutation show widespread vestibular dysfunction
- Semicircular canal and otolithic organ impairments are common
- Standard vestibular tests may appear "normal" but functional deficits persist

2. Age-related vestibular decline is partly mitochondrial:

- Mitochondrial DNA damage accumulates in vestibular hair cells with aging
- Mitochondrial dysfunction impairs OXPHOS, reducing ATP supply to vestibular sensors

3. Nutritional support for vestibular function requires mitochondrial optimization:

- CoQ10, NAD+, B vitamins, magnesium, all critical for OXPHOS
- Antioxidants to protect mitochondrial membranes from oxidative damage

Bottom line: If you have unexplained dizziness, imbalance, or vestibular symptoms with "normal" testing, consider mitochondrial dysfunction and nutrient deficiencies affecting oxidative phosphorylation.

CHAPTER 6: Phosphorus: The Energy Distribution Network

When the grid fails even with plenty of power

In February 2021, parts of Texas experienced a catastrophic power-grid failure. Power plants could still generate electricity. Fuel existed. Transformers stood ready. But the distribution network, transmission lines, substations, and control systems could not handle the conditions. The result: lights out, heat off, systems down.

The problem was not that energy did not exist. It was that energy could not get where it needed to go.

Your cells face a similar challenge every day.

Mitochondria can generate ATP. But without a functioning distribution network, ATP cannot be stored, transported, or used efficiently when demand spikes. Much of that "wiring" and buffering is built on one element: phosphorus.

This is Jake's second wall.

Jake's second wall: generator on, house dim

Sixteen weeks into his mitochondrial and magnesium protocol, Jake felt dramatically better. Afternoon crashes were gone; sleep and anxiety had improved; he could focus through a 10-hour workday. Yet he hit a new plateau.

He could sustain solid workdays, but:

- Flow states remained elusive.
- High-intensity "sprint" efforts at work stalled after 20-30 minutes.
- He described his brain as "idling in neutral" instead of shifting into high gear.

"My generator is running, but half the house is still on dim mode," he told his clinician.

Follow-up testing showed:

- Mitochondrial markers looked good.
- Magnesium and other key minerals were now in optimal ranges.

- Inflammation was under control.

The power plants were no longer the problem. "Your generators are working," his clinician said. "Now we need to examine your grid."

ATP: currency, not infrastructure

ATP is the cell's energy currency; it carries energy in phosphate bonds. When one phosphate is cleaved (ATP → ADP + Pi), energy is released for:

- Muscle contraction.
- Nerve signaling.
- Protein synthesis.
- Active transport.
- DNA/RNA synthesis.

Cells must continually regenerate ATP to keep the ATP:ADP ratio high, largely via oxidative phosphorylation.

However:

- The phosphagen system (ATP, phosphocreatine) acts as a rapid buffer.
- Phosphocreatine (PCr) stores a high-energy phosphate; creatine kinase transfers this to ADP to regenerate ATP on the spot.
- PCr can regenerate ATP far faster than oxidative phosphorylation or glycolysis.

Phosphorus also:

- Builds phospholipid membranes (cell and organelle boundaries).
- Participates in phosphorylation signaling that turns pathways on/off.

If phosphorus is insufficient or poorly managed:

- ATP regeneration may be constrained.
- Phosphocreatine stores may be low.
- Membrane integrity and signaling may be impaired.

Even with adequate mitochondrial function, the system can feel sluggish.

Jake's phosphorus profile

Jake's serum phosphorus was "normal," but that primarily reflects circulating phosphate, not intracellular handling.

Deeper assessment showed:

- RBC phosphorus at the low end of functional targets.
- Exercise response patterns suggesting limited phosphocreatine buffer.
- ATP:ADP ratio improved but was still lower than expected for his mitochondrial capacity.

In plain terms, his power plants could produce energy, but his grid could not store and distribute it fast enough under peak demand.

Three main roles of phosphorus in cellular energy

1. ATP and the phosphagen buffer

ATP contains three phosphate groups, but cellular ATP stores are tiny. They would last only a few seconds at maximal effort without regeneration. The phosphagen system bridges rapid demand changes:

$\text{ADP}+\text{Phosphocreatine}\rightleftharpoons\text{ATP}+\text{Creatine}$

$\text{ADP}+\text{Phosphocreatine}\rightleftharpoons\text{ATP}+\text{Creatine}$

This system:

- Provides ~8-10 seconds of maximal-effort energy.
- Buys time while mitochondria ramp up output.

Low PCr means hitting an invisible wall quickly in high-intensity efforts, physical or cognitive.

2. Phospholipid membranes

Phospholipids, with phosphate "heads" and fatty "tails," form:

- Cell membranes.
- Organelle membranes (including mitochondria).

They host channels, receptors, and enzymes and they support the electrical gradients in neurons and myocytes. Chronic phosphate imbalance can compromise membrane behavior and signal transmission.

3. Phosphorylation signaling

Kinases and phosphatases add/remove phosphate groups to regulate:

- Metabolism.
- Cell cycle and growth.

- Hormone responses.
- Neural plasticity.

Subtle, chronic phosphate insufficiency or mismanagement can dampen the responsiveness of these systems even without overt deficiency.

The phosphagen system and performance

Short, maximal efforts, sprints, heavy lifts, and mentally intense bursts rely heavily on the ATP, PCr system.

If PCr stores are robust:

- You sustain maximal output for several seconds.
- Recovery between bursts is quick.
- You experience "snap" and explosiveness.

If PCr stores are limited:

- You fatigue almost instantly under max load.
- Your nervous system feels reluctant to "go all out."
- Repeated efforts feel progressively worse.

Cognitive tasks also require rapid local ATP turnover in specific brain regions. Low PCr can feel like:

- Inability to sustain deep focus.
- Rapid mental "burnout" under deadline pressure.
- A sense of "hitting a wall" despite decent baseline energy.

Creatine and brain energy: what studies show

Several lines of evidence support creatine's role in brain energy buffering:

- Systematic review and meta-analysis (2024): creatine monohydrate supplementation modestly improved memory, attention time, and information-processing speed in adults, especially under cognitive stress.
- Sleep-deprivation RCT (2024): a single high dose of creatine monohydrate (0.35 g/kg) during 21 h of sleep deprivation:
- Increased brain PCr/Pi and ATP on 31P-MRS.
- Prevented pH drop.
- Improved cognitive performance and processing speed.

- Multiple RCTs in healthy adults: 3-5 g/day creatine monohydrate over weeks:
- Improved aspects of working memory and reasoning, with stronger effects in individuals with lower baseline creatine (e.g., vegetarians).

Together, current evidence suggests that creatine can modestly enhance cognitive performance, particularly memory and processing speed, likely by increasing brain PCr and improving energy buffering.

Jake's experience after phosphagen support

Before addressing phosphorus/PCr:

- Baseline energy was good.
- Maximal efforts felt disproportionately taxing.
- Flow states were rare and fragile.

After:

- Ensuring adequate phosphorus intake from whole foods.
- Supporting PCr with creatine monohydrate (around 5 g/day, under supervision).
- Optimizing cofactors (magnesium, B-vitamins).

Jake reported:

- Improved physical sprint and strength metrics.
- Longer, more sustainable "deep work" blocks.
- Less exhaustion after intense pushes.
- Faster recovery between high-intensity work sessions.

By roughly Week 8 of creatine use, he described classic flow episodes, 2- to 3-hour coding stretches with preserved energy afterward.

No specific brands are recommended; creatine monohydrate is referenced as the widely studied, generic form.

Phosphorus in diet and physiology

Most diets containing animal products provide ample phosphorus; severe deficiency is rare in industrialized settings. Nonetheless, functional issues can arise when:

- Intake is marginal in the context of high demand.
- Renal handling is altered.
- Calcium/phosphate balance is disturbed.

- Energy pathways are otherwise compromised.

Well-absorbed sources:

- Meat, poultry, fish.
- Dairy (milk, cheese, yogurt).
- Eggs.
- Legumes, nuts, and seeds.

By contrast, phosphate additives in processed foods and soft drinks may alter mineral balance and vascular health without necessarily improving intracellular energy handling.

Creatine: a practical lever for the phosphagen system

Creatine's primary roles:

- Combine with phosphate to form PCr in muscle and brain.
- Help maintain ATP during high demand.
- Improve performance in short, high-intensity exercise.
- Support cognition modestly, especially under stress or sleep loss.

Typical dosing:

- Common daily doses are ~3-5 g/day creatine monohydrate for adults, assuming normal kidney function and clinical oversight.
- Loading protocols (e.g., ~20 g/day for 5-7 days) saturate stores faster but are optional; steady daily dosing reaches similar steady-state levels in 3-4 weeks.

Key points:

- Creatine complements adequate phosphorus; it does not substitute for it.
- Vegetarians/vegans often have lower baseline creatine and may experience larger benefits.
- Long-term safety data in healthy adults at recommended doses are generally reassuring; major reviews report no clinically significant adverse effects on renal, muscular, or thermoregulatory systems in typical use.

Jake's phosphagen upgrade in practice

Rather than "phosphate pills," Jake's plan focused on:

- Adequate dietary phosphorus from whole foods.
- Creatine monohydrate around 5 g/day.
- Cofactor optimization (magnesium, B-complex).
- Structuring training and work to challenge, not overwhelm, the phosphagen system.

This included:

- Exercise: Short sprints (~10 seconds) with ample rest; resistance training to increase creatine storage capacity.
- Nutrition timing: Carbohydrate and protein near intense efforts to support glycogen and creatine uptake (insulin facilitates creatine transport).
- Work structure: Pomodoro-style deep-work blocks (e.g., 25-50 minutes focus, 5-10 minutes rest) to allow PCr regeneration.
- Sleep: Adequate duration and quality to restore ATP and PCr overnight.

Over several weeks, metrics and lived experience improved; by ~8 weeks, he could schedule multiple high-intensity cognitive sessions in a day without burning out after the first one.

Why this matters for everyday life

Even without sprinting or heavy lifting, your brain and nervous system depend on rapid, localized energy shifts.

Phosphorus and the phosphagen system help:

- Buffer short bursts of demand so performance does not collapse.
- Maintain responsiveness when switching tasks or handling acute stress.
- Support intense creative or analytical work without immediate burnout.

Patterns that may suggest a "grid" limitation:

- Doing well at moderate effort but hitting a wall quickly when pushing harder.
- Short deep-work capacity despite decent baseline energy and sleep.
- Flow only on unusually well-rested days.

- Early peak followed by rapid drop-off in physical or cognitive performance.

Not everyone needs phosphagen-targeted support. But for individuals who have already optimized basic mitochondrial function and still feel capped, this layer can be the difference between "better" and "fully online."

Bigger integration: How phosphorus connects to the full system

Phosphorus and the phosphagen system interact with:

- Magnesium, required for ATP use and many phosphorylation reactions.
- B-vitamins, driving pathways that regenerate ATP.
- Zinc and copper, influencing enzymes and redox balance in energy pathways.
- Vitamin C and other antioxidants, protecting membranes and proteins.
- Hormones (testosterone, thyroid), setting energy demand and capacity.

If mitochondria are power supplies and processors, and magnesium is the conductor, phosphorus and creatine are the high-speed distribution network. Jake's story shows that even after repairing mitochondria and magnesium, another tier of performance can be unlocked by upgrading the grid.

The next chapter moves from power and distribution to a subtler controller: boron. This trace mineral acts like a voltage regulator on hormonal and inflammatory systems, which can destabilize performance when unbalanced.

SIDEBAR: How Phosphocreatine works as a spatial and temporal energy buffer

Phosphocreatine (PCr) is often called the "energy buffer" of cells, but what does that actually mean?

The problem: ATP is consumed faster than it can be replenished

During intense activity, whether a sprint, a heavy deadlift, or a burst of deep cognitive work, ATP is consumed extremely rapidly.

- Mitochondria can produce ATP through oxidative phosphorylation, but this process takes time to ramp up
- Glycolysis is faster but still can't match the instantaneous demand
- Without a buffer system, ATP would be depleted in seconds, and cells would fail

The solution: Phosphocreatine regenerates ATP instantly

Phosphocreatine stores a high-energy phosphate group. When ATP is hydrolyzed to ADP during work, the enzyme creatine kinase (CK) rapidly transfers the phosphate from PCr to ADP, regenerating ATP:

ADP+Phosphocreatine→CKATP+Creatine

ADP+Phosphocreatine

CK

ATP+Creatine

This reaction is:

- Reversible, during rest, ATP phosphorylates creatine back to PCr
- Extremely fast, regenerates ATP 40x faster than oxidative phosphorylation and 10x faster than glycolysis
- Non-acidifying, doesn't produce lactate or H^+ (protons), so it doesn't contribute to muscle burn or pH drop

Spatial buffering: Moving energy where It's needed

Mitochondria are located in specific parts of cells (often near sites of high energy demand). But ATP doesn't diffuse quickly through the cytoplasm.

Phosphocreatine acts as a "shuttle":

1. ATP is generated in mitochondria
2. CK converts ATP + Creatine → ADP + Phosphocreatine near mitochondria
3. PCr diffuses to sites of high ATP demand (e.g., myofibrils in muscle, synapses in neurons)
4. At those sites, CK converts PCr + ADP → ATP + Creatine, delivering energy exactly where it's needed

This spatial buffering allows energy to be distributed efficiently throughout large cells like neurons and muscle fibers.

Temporal buffering: Bridging the gap

During the first 8-10 seconds of maximal effort, the phosphagen system provides nearly all the energy while mitochondria "spin up" to meet demand.

This temporal buffering is critical for:

- Sprint starts (athletics)
- Heavy lifts (strength training)
- Cognitive bursts (rapid problem-solving, decision-making under time pressure)

Why this matters for brain function

The brain accounts for ~2% of body weight but ~20% of daily energy expenditure.

Neurons have high, fluctuating ATP demands:

- Action potentials (nerve signals) require rapid ATP turnover to restore ion gradients
- Synaptic transmission and neurotransmitter recycling are ATP-intensive
- Complex cognitive tasks create localized energy "hotspots" in specific brain regions

Creatine and phosphocreatine are abundant in the brain, particularly in regions with high energy demand, such as the prefrontal cortex, hippocampus, and cerebellum.

When brain creatine/PCr is optimized:

- Neurons can sustain high firing rates longer
- Recovery between cognitive bursts is faster
- Mental fatigue is reduced

SIDEBAR: Creatine for cognitive Performance— the evidence

Creatine is best known as a sports supplement, but emerging evidence shows it also enhances brain function.

Key Clinical Trials:

1. University of Sydney (2003), Landmark Study in Vegetarians

- Design: 45 vegetarians, randomized to 5 g/day creatine vs. placebo for 6 weeks
- Results:
- Significant improvements in Raven's Advanced Progressive Matrices (intelligence/reasoning)
- Enhanced working memory (backward digit span)
- Effects are most pronounced in vegetarians, who have lower baseline creatine stores
- Conclusion: Creatine supplementation enhances cognitive processing, particularly in tasks requiring speed of processing

2. Sleep Deprivation Study (2024), Single-Dose Creatine

- Design: Randomized, double-blind, crossover trial; single high dose creatine (0.35 g/kg) vs. placebo during 21 hours of sleep deprivation
- Measurements: Brain 31P-MRS (phosphocreatine, ATP, pH), 1H-MRS (total creatine), cognitive testing
- Results:
- Increased brain PCr/Pi ratio and ATP levels
- Prevented pH drop (acidosis impairs cognition)
- Improved cognitive performance and processing speed
- Positive correlations between brain PCr/Pi and performance on working memory, attention, and numeric tasks
- Significance: First study to show that a single dose of creatine can acutely improve brain energy metabolism and cognitive function under stress

3. Meta-Analysis (2024), Frontiers in Nutrition

- Design: Systematic review + meta-analysis of RCTs (1993, 2024)
- Total participants: Hundreds across multiple studies
- Results:
- Memory: SMD 0.34 ($p = 0.02$), significant improvement
- Attention time: SMD −0.31 ($p = 0.03$), faster processing
- Information processing speed: SMD 0.27 ($p = 0.01$), significant improvement

- Effects are strongest in stressed populations and 18, 60 age group
- No significant difference between short-term (<4 weeks) and long-term (>4 weeks) interventions
- Conclusion: Creatine monohydrate supplementation confers beneficial effects on cognitive function, particularly memory, attention, and processing speed

4. Dose-Response Study (2023)

- Design: 6 weeks of creatine (10 g/day or 20 g/day) in healthy young adults; functional near-infrared spectroscopy (fNIRS) during cognitive tasks
- Results:
- Trend toward decreased prefrontal cortex oxygenation during cognitive tasks
- Suggests a metabolic shift, increased brain creatine allows more efficient ATP synthesis via phosphocreatine, reducing reliance on aerobic metabolism and potentially reducing mental fatigue
- Implication: Creatine doesn't just "add more energy", it makes energy production more efficient

5. Cross-Over RCT (2023), Vegetarians and Omnivores

- Design: 123 participants (half vegetarian, half omnivore); 5 g/day creatine vs. placebo for 6 weeks each (crossover design)
- Results:
- Small but significant cognitive improvements: Cohen's d = 0.09 for RAPM, 0.17 for BDS
- Equivalent to 1, 2.5 IQ point improvement in raw scores
- Higher side effects with creatine vs. placebo ($p = 0.002$), mostly GI discomfort, but no serious adverse events
- Conclusion: Modest but reliable cognitive enhancement across diverse populations

Mechanism summary:

Creatine enhances cognition by:

1. Increasing brain phosphocreatine stores, creating a larger energy buffer for rapid ATP regeneration

2. Improving spatial and temporal energy buffering in neurons, allowing sustained high firing rates
3. Preventing acidosis (pH drop) during intense cognitive effort
4. Reducing oxidative stress and inflammation in the brain
5. Supporting neuroprotection and potentially slowing age-related cognitive decline

Who benefits most?

- Vegetarians/vegans (lower baseline creatine stores)
- Older adults (age-related decline in brain creatine)
- Sleep-deprived individuals
- People under cognitive stress (demanding jobs, exams, high mental workload)
- Individuals with mild cognitive impairment or early dementia

Dosing and safety:

- Standard dose: 3-5 g/day creatine monohydrate
- Loading protocol (optional): 20 g/day for 5-7 days, then 3-5 g/day maintenance
- Safety: Creatine is one of the most studied supplements; it is safe for long-term use in healthy individuals
- Side effects: Mild GI discomfort in some individuals; drink plenty of water to minimize

CHAPTER 7: Boron: The Voltage Controller

The hidden voltage regulators

In electrical engineering, voltage regulators are quiet heroes. They sit between a fluctuating power source and sensitive components, smoothing spikes and dips so circuits receive the right amount of power. Too much voltage burns components out. Too little, and systems underperform or crash.

Hormones behave like biological voltage signals. They regulate metabolism, stress resilience, reproduction, mood, bone health, and inflammation. When they swing wildly or sit at the edge of function, everything from energy to cognition to body composition suffers.

Boron is a trace mineral that acts like a subtle voltage controller in this system. It does not replace hormones, but it influences how they are produced, bound, and cleared, as well as how inflammatory signals and vitamin D function. Most people have never heard of boron beyond plant biology. Their hormonal "voltage" runs without this quiet regulator until the system starts to swing.

This is Sarah's story.

Sarah's hormonal whiplash

Sarah was 43, a high-performing attorney in a demanding firm. For years, she was the one colleagues relied on in crises: calm, sharp, tireless.

Over about eighteen months, that started to erode.

- Energy swings: Some days she felt wired and restless; other days she moved through wet sand.
- Mood instability: Small frustrations triggered outsized irritability or tears. "This is not me," she kept saying.
- Sleep chaos: Some nights she crashed and then woke at 2 AM wired; others she lay awake for hours.
- Physical changes: Weight gathered around her midsection, her skin dried, her hair thinned.
- Cognitive drag: She re-read briefs, missed details, and felt off her game in court.

Basic labs came back "reassuring":

- Thyroid: in range.
- Fasting glucose: in range.
- Sex hormones: "perimenopausal, expected for your age."

The advice: manage stress, consider a sleep aid, think about hormone replacement "down the line."

Sarah's lived experience was different from the assumptions being made. It felt less like one gland failing and more like the entire control system flickering, a dimmer switch being jerked up and down. She did not want to wait for "bad enough" before she took action.

A different lens on hormonal health

An integrative clinician changed the questions.

Instead of only asking, "Are these numbers in range?" the focus shifted to:

- How stable are these hormones over time?
- How much is free vs bound?
- What is the inflammatory background?
- Which nutrients touch these control points?

Key labs:

- Free and total testosterone
- Estradiol (± metabolites)
- SHBG (sex hormone-binding globulin)
- DHEA-S
- Cortisol pattern (multi-time-point or salivary)
- 25-OH vitamin D
- hs-CRP
- Diet and mineral review, including boron-rich foods

A pattern emerged:

- Free testosterone: low-normal, but low for her workload and age.
- SHBG: elevated, binding much of her testosterone and estradiol.
- Estradiol: variable but not dramatic.

- 25-OH vitamin D: low-normal despite supplementation.
- hs-CRP: mildly elevated, signaling chronic low-grade inflammation.
- Diet: low in boron-rich foods; no supplemental boron.

The clinician explained:

- SHBG binds testosterone and estradiol, lowering the free, bioavailable fraction.
- Small human trials using 6-10 mg/day boron for short periods in men showed:
- Lower SHBG.
- Higher free testosterone.
- Modest shifts in estradiol and DHT.
- Higher 25-OH vitamin D.
- Reduced hs-CRP and pro-inflammatory cytokines.
- Controlled metabolic studies in postmenopausal women at ≈3 mg/day showed reduced urinary magnesium and calcium losses and higher estradiol/testosterone, especially when magnesium intake was low.

The message was simple: Sarah's voltage regulator was underpowered. Her glands were not failing outright, but the way hormones were bound, buffered, and delivered was pushing her system toward instability.

What boron does

Boron is needed only in small amounts, but it plays an important role at key junctions in hormone, mineral, and inflammatory control.

Sex hormone modulation

Short trials in men using 6-10 mg/day boron for 7-10 days found:

- Free testosterone increased.
- SHBG decreased.
- Estradiol and hs-CRP decreased.
- 25-OH vitamin D increased modestly.

Reviews and small studies point in the same direction: boron can lower SHBG in some individuals and improve the balance between free testosterone and estradiol while reducing inflammatory tone.

This does not make boron "testosterone in a pill." It is better understood as a modulator of binding and inflammation. In people with high SHBG and low free hormone, it can nudge the system toward a more favorable state.

For Sarah, total testosterone was technically "fine," but the fraction reaching receptors was low for a brain and body running 60-hour weeks under legal stress.

Vitamin D metabolism

Several human studies suggest boron:

- Helps preserve 25-OH vitamin D levels, likely by slowing breakdown.
- Reduces urinary calcium and magnesium excretion.
- Improves bone and mineral markers in postmenopausal women when combined with magnesium and vitamin D.

Given vitamin D's roles in bone, immune function, mood, and metabolic regulation, that small shift in half-life and mineral economy can matter.

Mineral handling (magnesium and calcium)

In metabolic ward studies, adding ≈3 mg/day boron to low-boron diets:

- Decreased urinary magnesium and calcium losses.
- Supported bone mineralization.

This is especially relevant for women in midlife, when estrogen declines accelerate bone turnover and mineral balance becomes fragile.

Inflammation and oxidative stress

Boron can modulate:

- Cytokines such as TNF-α and IL-6.
- Inflammatory markers like hs-CRP.
- Signaling via NF-κB and related pathways in preclinical models.

Small human trials report reductions in hs-CRP and TNF-α within days to weeks of boron supplementation, suggesting that low intake leaves some people running "hotter" than necessary on the inflammatory scale.

Cognitive and neuromuscular effects

Diet-controlled studies comparing low (~0.25 mg/day) vs adequate (~3 mg/day) boron intake showed that deficiency states worsen:

- Reaction time.
- Short- and long-term memory.
- Manual dexterity and eye-hand coordination.
- Sustained attention.

When intake was restored, these parameters improved. The mechanisms are likely to involve changes in membrane function, metabolic enzymes, and signaling molecules in the brain and the neuromuscular system.

For someone like Sarah, living at the edge of her cognitive capacity, even small shifts in baseline reaction time and attention show up in real-world performance.

The voltage regulator analogy

Think of her endocrine system as an electrical grid feeding a complex building.

- Generators: ovaries, adrenal glands, peripheral steroidogenic tissues.
- Loads: brain, muscle, bone, immune system, metabolic organs.
- Control systems: feedback loops, SHBG, vitamin D activation and breakdown, inflammatory cytokines, hormone-metabolizing enzymes.

When the regulator works:

- Hormones are not just "in range" but stable and responsive.
- Small stressors do not cause wild swings.
- Tissues see a steady, usable signal.

When the regulator is off:

- SHBG rises, binding more hormone and forcing glands to work harder.
- Inflammation blunts receptor sensitivity and distorts signaling.
- Vitamin D half-life and mineral handling become less efficient.

The result is a system that whipsaws, surging under stress, crashing afterward, never fully settling. That is how Sarah's life felt: wired, then wiped; sharp, then foggy; calm, then raw. The problem was not only the amount produced, but how the signal was shaped and buffered.

Sarah's 10-week boron and stability protocol

From the start, boron was framed as one lever, not a magic fix.

Phase 1 (Weeks 1-3): Quiet the background

Before adding boron, her clinician:

- Reduced ultra-processed carbohydrates to lower inflammatory load.
- Ensured adequate protein and healthy fats to stabilize blood sugar and provide hormone substrates.
- Optimized magnesium so boron's mineral-sparing effects had something to conserve.
- Kept vitamin D dosing steady to see whether boron shifted levels later.

Baseline labs:

- SHBG, free and total testosterone, estradiol ± metabolites, DHEA-S.
- 25-OH vitamin D.
- hs-CRP.
- Basic thyroid markers.

This created a snapshot of her hormonal voltage and inflammatory noise before touching boron.

Phase 2 (Weeks 4-6): Add boron cautiously

Then:

- Boron: 3-6 mg/day, usually as boron glycinate or citrate, with food.
- Foods: more avocados, nuts, legumes, dried fruit, and moderate red wine where appropriate.

Within several weeks, she noticed:

- Mood swings softened.
- Fewer 2 am awakenings.
- Energy felt smoother instead of jerking from hyper to hypo.

Around week 6, repeat labs showed:

- SHBG trending down.
- Free testosterone slightly higher.
- hs-CRP lower.
- 25-OH vitamin D modestly higher without changing dose.

These were subtle shifts, but they paralleled her experience of being "more even."

Phase 3 (Weeks 7-10): Integrate with life

With early improvement, they layered in:

- Resistance training 2- 3×/week to leverage better hormone availability.
- Continued magnesium and vitamin D for neuromuscular and bone support.
- Sleep and stress scaffolding: consistent bedtime, morning light, device curfew, brief daily relaxation practices.

By week 10:

- Her energy curve was a gentle arc instead of a roller coaster.
- Focus in high-stakes meetings returned.
- Abdominal weight gain slowed and began to reverse with training and nutrition.
- She described feeling "more like myself again."

Boron did not do this alone. But by nudging SHBG, vitamin D half-life, mineral handling, and inflammation, it allowed the rest of her efforts to land.

Important cautions

Boron is powerful at small doses.

- Typical diets: roughly 1-3 mg/day.
- Common supplemental bands in adults:
- 3-6 mg/day for general endocrine/mineral support.
- Up to 10 mg/day in short, supervised trials in select cases.

Use with care:

- In hormone-sensitive cancers or in patients on complex hormone regimens.

- In significant kidney disease or mineral-handling disorders, only under medical supervision.
- Avoid chronic high-dose use without monitoring.

Best viewed as a fine-tuning tool, not something to push aggressively without context.

Why boron belongs in this book

Boron is less famous than magnesium, zinc, or vitamin D, but it sits where several systems meet:

- Hormone availability, especially via SHBG.
- Vitamin D and mineral metabolism.
- Inflammatory tone.
- Neuromuscular and cognitive function.

In the language of earlier chapters,

if mitochondria are the processors,

magnesium is the conductor,

phosphorus/creatine forms the energy grid,

zinc is the immune security processor, then boron is a voltage controller on endocrine and inflammatory lines. It does not create power or signals, but shapes how they are delivered and buffered.

Sarah's story highlights a recurring theme:

- Lab values inside broad "normal" ranges can hide unstable control systems.
- Small changes in regulators like SHBG, vitamin D half-life, and inflammatory tone reshape daily experience.
- Targeted nutrition at these control nodes can stabilize entire networks.

You can have "normal" labs and still feel very abnormal, until someone checks the regulators, not just the outputs.

Boron in women: a clinical snapshot

For women in peri- and postmenopause, boron behaves less like a blunt hormone and more like a stability amplifier across endocrine, bone, brain axes.

Signals from human and mechanistic data suggest:

- Supports estrogen signaling and balance

- In postmenopausal women, ≈3 mg/day boron increased estradiol and 25-OH vitamin D and improved calcium retention in metabolic studies.
- This may mimic some protective estrogenic effects without acting as a drug-level hormone replacement.
- Improves bone and joint resilience
- Higher boron intake is associated with better bone markers and mineral status, especially when combined with vitamin D, calcium, and magnesium.
- Enhances cognitive and neuromuscular performance
- Adequate boron (~3 mg/day) improves reaction time, memory, dexterity, and attention compared with low-boron intake.
- Calms inflammatory background noise
- Supplementation reduces hs-CRP and certain cytokines, shifting the system away from chronic low-grade inflammation that worsens pain and fatigue.

In practice, boron often gives women a steadier hormonal signal to work with so that sleep, exercise, nutrition, and, when used, HRT have more predictable effects.

How boron affects free hormone levels

Boron's most consistent endocrine effect is on binding and availability, not brute-force overproduction.

- In men, 6-10 mg/day short-term lowered SHBG and raised free testosterone by roughly 20-25% in small studies, with concurrent drops in inflammatory markers.
- Mechanistically, by reducing SHBG and inflammatory drag, boron increases the fraction of testosterone and estradiol circulating as free, receptor-active hormone, even when totals shift only modestly.

For women, similar SHBG and inflammation effects likely explain:

- Why some perimenopausal patients feel more "present" and less volatile on modest boron doses.
- Why small changes in free fractions can translate into disproportionate improvements in mood stability, libido, energy, and mental sharpness, especially when SHBG is

elevated by stress, low-protein intake, oral contraceptives, or under-eating.

One line summary for readers:

Boron does not flood the system with new hormones; it frees and stabilizes what is already there while lowering inflammatory noise that distorts signaling.

Boron and future delivery systems

Beyond its micronutrient role, boron chemistry is being explored in experimental drug-delivery platforms, especially in the gut.

Preclinical work shows:

- Boron compounds can support intestinal epithelial health and increase villus height, improving nutrient transport.
- Boronate and boronic-acid-based materials can bind cell-surface sugars and form reversible complexes used in nanoparticles and hydrogels that release drugs in response to pH or oxidative stress.

In the coming decade, boron-based complexes are likely to be used as intestinal delivery scaffolds, leveraging boron's tolerance to gut pH and its ability to interact with glycocalyx sugars to deliver hormones, peptides, and micronutrients more predictably across the gut wall.

The next Chip: Copper, neural bandwidth

In the next chapter, attention turns to copper, the metal that underlies neural bandwidth, myelin integrity, and antioxidant defenses that keep fast, complex signaling in the brain and nervous system running smoothly.

SIDEBAR: What a 7-Day boron trial actually showed

A frequently cited human trial helps explain why boron gets attention in hormone conversations.

Study design:

- Participants: Healthy men
- Intervention: 10 mg/day boron for 7 days
- Measurements: Sex hormones, SHBG, vitamin D, inflammatory markers

Key findings after just 7 days:

- Free testosterone increased

- Estradiol decreased
- SHBG decreased
- DHT increased
- 25-OH vitamin D increased
- hs-CRP and TNF-α decreased (inflammation markers)

This is a short trial; it doesn't prove long-term outcomes or effects in women. But it demonstrates two important points:

- Boron can move hormone-binding and inflammatory markers in humans, not just in theory.
- These changes can happen quickly, which is why some people feel shifts in a matter of weeks.

Future work requires longer, larger trials, but this study earned boron a place in discussions of functional endocrinology.

SIDEBAR: Boron, vitamin D, and bones

Vitamin D, calcium, magnesium, and boron form a quiet alliance around bone and mineral health.

Boron's contributions:

- Improves calcium retention and reduces urinary losses
- Reduces magnesium excretion, conserving a mineral critical for ATP use and enzyme function
- Helps raise or maintain 25-OH vitamin D levels, likely by slowing its breakdown

In postmenopausal women, where bone loss accelerates due to declining estrogen, this cluster matters.

Small trials and reviews suggest that boron supplementation can improve bone markers and may support bone density when combined with adequate vitamin D, calcium, and magnesium.

Boron isn't a replacement for foundational bone strategies, but it plugs into the same control panel and helps the system waste less.

SIDEBAR: Boron and brain performance

Boron's cognitive effects are subtle but repeatable in controlled settings.

In classic diet-controlled experiments, researchers compared low boron intake (~0.25 mg/day) versus adequate intake (~3 mg/day) in healthy adults:

Under low boron intake, subjects showed:

- Slower reaction times
- Poorer short-term and long-term memory
- Lower manual dexterity
- Reduced attention and vigilance
- More sluggish eye-hand coordination

When boron intake was increased to adequate levels, these measures improved.

These aren't dramatic, overnight changes. But day after day, they add up, resulting in:

- Fewer "What was I about to do?" moments
- Less fumbling in motor tasks
- Slightly sharper attention and tracking

For people who live on the edge of their cognitive capacity, attorneys, programmers, clinicians, pilots, that small shift in baseline can matter.

CHAPTER 8: Copper: Neural Bandwidth and Repair

When the wires start to fray

High-speed internet is not just about a fast modem. It depends on the physical cables, bundles of insulated wires or fiber that carry huge amounts of information without interference. When those cables degrade, insulation cracks, conductors corrode, you get lag, dropped connections, and corrupted data, no matter how good the server is.

The nervous system has similar requirements.

Nerve impulses travel along axons that are insulated by myelin, a fatty sheath that increases conduction speed and reduces signal loss. Copper is critical for enzymes that help build and maintain this insulation, for mitochondrial energy production in neurons, and for antioxidant defenses that protect these high-demand cells from oxidative stress.

When copper is too low, myelin can deteriorate and certain antioxidant defenses weaken. When copper is excessive or poorly regulated, it can become pro-oxidant. Either imbalance can impair "neural bandwidth", the speed, clarity, and reliability of your nervous system.

This is Marcus's story.

Marcus's slow, subtle unraveling

Marcus was 52, an IT consultant who had spent decades troubleshooting complex systems. He prided himself on being able to "hold multiple threads" in his mind, the mental parallel processing his work demanded.

Over several years, he noticed changes that did not fit simple aging.

- Walking felt slightly unsteady, especially in the dark or on uneven surfaces. He began using railings he'd never needed before.
- His hands felt clumsier. Typing accuracy dropped. Buttoning shirts and threading cables took effort.
- He had numbness and tingling in his feet and hands, a vague sense that his legs were not fully "online."

- His thinking felt slower. He could still do his job, but tasks that once felt effortless left him mentally drained. He would re-read technical documentation and lose the thread.

Brain and spine MRI were reported as "normal for age." Routine labs were "acceptable." He was told this might be early neuropathy or a nonspecific age-related change.

Marcus disagreed. The pattern felt progressive, not random.

An integrative, neurologically-savvy clinician added something most workups had skipped: a careful look at copper status and zinc-copper balance.

Copper in the nervous system

Copper sits in several critical positions in neural biology.

Myelin formation and maintenance

Myelin is produced by oligodendrocytes in the CNS and Schwann cells in the PNS. Copper-containing enzymes and copper-dependent mitochondrial function support the synthesis and maintenance of this insulation.

Copper deficiency has been associated with demyelinating syndromes and neuropathies that can mimic subacute combined degeneration (classic B12 deficiency), multiple sclerosis, or even motor neuron disease.

Typical features include:

- Gait disturbance (ataxia, spasticity, wide-based gait).
- Sensory changes (paresthesias, numbness, loss of vibration and proprioception).
- Myelopathy (spinal cord involvement), often affecting dorsal columns.

Spinal MRI:

- About 47-50% of reported copper-deficiency myelopathy cases show dorsal column T2 hyperintensities.
- Roughly half have normal cord MRI, so normal imaging does not rule out copper-related myelopathy.

Marcus's normal MRI, therefore, did not exclude copper insufficiency as a contributor to his symptoms.

Energy production in neurons

Copper is a key component of cytochrome c oxidase (Complex IV), the final enzyme in the mitochondrial electron transport chain. Neurons are among the most energy-dependent cells; sustained signaling requires robust ATP generation.

Copper is delivered to mitochondria via dedicated transport and chaperone systems. When copper is inadequate:

- Complex IV function declines.
- Mitochondrial copper content can fall significantly, even as cytosolic copper may rise due to impaired utilization.

In Marcus's case, neurons could be structurally intact on MRI yet running on a constrained power supply.

Antioxidant defense

Copper is part of Cu/Zn superoxide dismutase (SOD1), which converts superoxide radicals into less reactive species, limiting oxidative injury generated during normal metabolism.

- Too little copper: SOD1 activity drops, weakening defenses.
- Too much poorly bound copper: can catalyze harmful redox reactions, especially if ceruloplasmin and other binding proteins are low.

Neurotransmitter synthesis

Copper-dependent enzymes such as dopamine β-hydroxylase convert dopamine to norepinephrine. Copper insufficiency can therefore alter catecholamine balance and contribute to mood, attention, and autonomic symptoms.

What happens when copper is inadequate

Low or imbalanced copper can produce a characteristic cluster:

- Impaired myelin maintenance and spinal cord tracts.
- Reduced neuronal ATP output (Complex IV dysfunction).
- Greater susceptibility to oxidative damage.
- Altered neurotransmitter synthesis.

Excess unbound copper, by contrast, can drive oxidative stress and neurotoxicity. Balance is critical.

As Marcus's clinician put it: "You can have fraying insulation (myelin), dimmed power (mitochondria), and weakened surge protection (SOD), all from the same deficiency. That's why your symptoms feel like a system-wide slowdown."

Marcus's copper status

His workup included:

- Serum copper.
- Ceruloplasmin (≈95% of serum copper is bound here).
- Zinc (to calculate zinc:copper or copper:zinc ratio).
- Standard neurologic labs to exclude other causes.

Findings:

- Copper and ceruloplasmin at the low-normal edge.
- Zinc mildly elevated relative to copper, consistent with relative copper insufficiency.
- No clear alternative explanation on imaging or other labs.

The clinician reviewed that adult copper deficiency can present with gait difficulty, sensory changes, and a myelopathy that:

- Often mimics B12 deficiency ("B12 deficiency without low B12").
- Sometimes mimics MS or motor neuron disease (ALS-like presentations).

Risk factors include:

- Prior gastric surgery (especially Roux-en-Y bypass).
- Malabsorption (celiac disease, IBD).
- Chronic high-dose zinc intake.
- Rare genetic disorders (Menkes, Wilson's, though Wilson's is usually associated with excess copper).
- Very low copper intake in restrictive diets.

Marcus had no profound deficiency, but his pattern, symptoms, and copper ratio suggested that optimizing copper and its cofactors could matter in a high-demand nervous system.

The bandwidth analogy

Think of his nervous system as a high-speed network.

- Myelin = insulation around cables that allows fast, clean transmission.

- Axons = the conductors inside those cables.
- Mitochondria in neurons = power supplies driving signal propagation.
- Copper-dependent enzymes = maintenance crews keeping both insulation and power conversion intact.

When copper is insufficient:

- Insulation thins or becomes patchy.
- Signal speed slows and jitter increases.
- Some signals never arrive, or arrive degraded.
- More "effort" is required to transmit the same information.

Marcus's nervous system felt like an office with aging, partly frayed wiring, everything technically connected, but glitches emerging under load.

Copper, zinc, and balance

Zinc and copper share absorption and transport pathways and coexist in enzymes like Cu/Zn SOD1.

The relationship

- Both are absorbed in the proximal small intestine.
- Excess zinc induces metallothionein in enterocytes.
- Metallothionein binds copper with higher affinity than zinc, trapping copper in intestinal cells, which are sloughed every few days.
- Net effect: chronic high-dose zinc can cause progressive copper depletion, even when dietary copper is adequate.

Too much copper relative to zinc, on the other hand, can promote oxidative stress and inflammatory signaling.

Typical intakes

- Copper: ~0.9-1.5 mg/day in most adults.
- Zinc: ~8-11 mg/day, higher in some therapeutic contexts but usually with monitoring.

Copper-rich foods:

- Organ meats (liver), shellfish, nuts/seeds, whole grains, dark chocolate, legumes.

People who:

- Take high-dose zinc (>40-50 mg/day) for months.
- Use zinc-containing denture adhesives heavily.
- Avoid copper-rich foods or have malabsorption.

...are at particular risk of drifting into functional copper deficiency.

Ratios

Functional clinicians often look at:

- Serum/plasma copper:zinc ratio: ~0.7, 1.0 is commonly considered balanced; higher values often track with inflammation and relatively higher copper, lower values with relative copper deficiency or zinc excess.
- Some instead express a zinc:copper ratio; in that case, ≈1.0, 1.3 zinc:copper is often targeted.

Marcus's pattern suggested slightly too much zinc relative to copper, consistent with his symptoms.

Marcus's copper restoration plan

The plan was cautious and iterative.

Step 1: Remove excess zinc load

- Reviewed all supplements and fortified products.
- Stopped unnecessary zinc, especially any doses >25 mg/day.
- Re-evaluated diet for hidden zinc sources.

Step 2: Reintroduce copper-rich foods

Gradual addition of:

- Small portions of liver (~1×/week).
- Shellfish if tolerated.
- Nuts, seeds, dark chocolate.
- Legumes.

This food-first approach provided a gentle increase in copper with other supportive nutrients.

Step 3: Targeted copper supplementation (when appropriate)

Given his symptoms, labs, and absence of contraindications (notably no Wilson's disease):

- Low-dose copper at 1-2 mg/day as a chelated form (e.g., copper bisglycinate) was added under supervision.

- Copper, ceruloplasmin, and zinc were rechecked periodically to avoid overshooting and to maintain balance.
- Any signs of intolerance or unexpected lab shifts prompted reassessment.

Step 4: Supportive measures

- Continued magnesium and B-complex to support neuronal energy and repair.
- Antioxidants (including vitamin C) to help balance oxidative stress as copper-dependent systems recovered.
- Movement and balance training to leverage neuroplasticity as the metabolic environment improved.

Marcus's recovery timeline

Over several months:

- Weeks 1-6
- Little subjective change; labs showed copper and ceruloplasmin edging upward.
- His diary still recorded missteps and re-reads.
- Weeks 6-12
- Walking felt steadier, especially in low light.
- Tingling and numbness diminished.
- Cognitive "snap" improved; typing errors dropped.
- Months 3-6
- Sustained mental work felt less draining.
- Fine motor tasks, buttons, cables, felt more automatic.
- Gait continued to steady; sensory symptoms largely resolved.

By month 6, he said, "It feels like my reflexes came back", both physically and mentally.

Important note on recovery

Neurological recovery from copper deficiency or insufficiency is often slow and incomplete if damage is advanced.

- Hematologic abnormalities (anemia, neutropenia) usually improve quickly.
- Spinal cord and nerve changes may take months and may not fully reverse, especially if treatment is delayed.

Marcus's relatively early intervention and moderate deficits gave him a better chance at meaningful recovery.

Why copper belongs in this book

Earlier chapters established:

- Mitochondria as processors.
- Magnesium as the conductor.
- Phosphorus and creatine as the energy grid.
- Zinc as the immune security processor.
- Boron as the voltage controller on endocrine and inflammatory lines.

Copper is the maintenance engineer for neural bandwidth and power conversion.

Copper helps ensure:

- Myelin stays intact so signals travel fast and clean.
- Mitochondria in neurons can produce ATP efficiently.
- Antioxidant defenses protect neurons from metabolic stress.
- Neurotransmitter synthesis runs smoothly.

Marcus's story underscores:

- "Normal" ranges can miss functional copper insufficiency, especially when zinc is high.
- Copper deficiency can masquerade as B12 deficiency, MS, or motor neuron disease.
- Early detection and correction can halt or reverse decline in many cases.
- Both copper deficiency and excess are harmful; balance is the goal.

Cuproptosis: Copper-Driven mitochondrial cell death

Copper has long been known as a critical cofactor for mitochondrial enzymes such as cytochrome c oxidase (Complex IV). Recent work adds a new layer: cuproptosis, a regulated cell-death pathway triggered by excess copper binding to lipoylated TCA cycle enzymes.

Mechanistically, cuproptosis involves:

- Copper accumulation in the mitochondrial matrix

- Binding of copper to lipoylated enzymes (e.g., dihydrolipoamide S-acetyltransferase)
- Aggregation of these proteins and loss of Fe-S cluster proteins
- Proteotoxic stress, loss of mitochondrial function, and cell death

This relationship links copper status directly to mitochondrial viability, beyond "deficiency vs. toxicity." Both too little and too much copper can drive pathology:

- Copper deficiency → impaired Complex IV activity, myelopathy, neuropathy
- Copper overload → cuproptosis, particularly in rapidly dividing or metabolically active cells

Clinically, this reinforces your existing emphasis on balanced copper and zinc:

- Avoid chronic high-dose zinc without copper monitoring.
- In patients with neurodegenerative disease, unexplained cytopenias, or severe fatigue, consider checking copper, ceruloplasmin, and Cu:Zn ratio before aggressive supplementation.

In the next chapter, attention turns to vitamin C, not just as an antioxidant but also as a structural and signaling molecule that underlies collagen integrity, neurotransmitter synthesis, and the resilience of vascular and connective tissues.

SIDEBAR: Copper deficiency Myelopathy—The great mimic

Copper deficiency myelopathy is an under-recognized cause of progressive neurological decline.

Clinical presentation

- Gait disturbance (ataxia, spasticity, wide-based gait).
- Sensory changes (paresthesias, numbness, loss of vibration and position sense).
- Weakness (usually legs > arms).
- Cognitive changes in some cases.
- Anemia, leukopenia, thrombocytopenia in many patients.

What it mimics

- Subacute combined degeneration (B12 deficiency), so closely that CDM is sometimes called "B12 deficiency without the B12 deficiency."
- Multiple sclerosis.
- Motor neuron disease (ALS-like presentations reported).

Labs

- Low serum copper.
- Low ceruloplasmin.
- Cytopenias on CBC.

MRI

- Dorsal column T2 hyperintensities are classic, but up to ~40-50% of cases have normal MRI.

Treatment

- Oral copper (typically 2-6 mg/day) and IV copper in severe malabsorption.
- Stop excess zinc.
- Address underlying surgery- or disease-related malabsorption.

Prognosis

- Early treatment → good recovery in many patients.
- Delayed treatment → incomplete recovery and residual deficits.

Key takeaway: In patients with progressive gait/sensory changes, normal B12, cytopenias, and a history of gastric surgery or zinc use, check copper and ceruloplasmin.

SIDEBAR: Copper and zinc, the balancing act

Copper and zinc are both essential trace minerals, but they exist in a delicate balance.

Why balance matters

- Shared absorption pathways in the small intestine.
- High zinc intake induces metallothionein, which preferentially binds copper and traps it in enterocytes.
- Trapped copper is lost when enterocytes slough off, reducing systemic copper.
- Cu/Zn SOD1 needs both metals; imbalance impairs antioxidant defenses.

Imbalance consequences

- Too much zinc, not enough copper:
- Copper deficiency → myelopathy, neuropathy, anemia.
- Impaired mitochondrial Complex IV.
- Weakened SOD1.
- Too much copper, not enough zinc:
- Copper overload → oxidative stress, tissue injury (as in Wilson's disease).

Practical ranges

- Copper: ~0.9-1.5 mg/day in most adults.
- Zinc: ~8-11 mg/day in diet, higher if supplemented with monitoring.
- When supplementing both, many clinicians use ~8-15 mg zinc per 1 mg copper, adjusting to labs.

Serum ratios

- Copper:zinc ≈0.7-1.0 or zinc:copper ≈1.0-1.3 are commonly used functional targets; deviations can flag imbalance.

Clinical guidance

- If using zinc >25-30 mg/day long-term: monitor copper and consider adding 1-2 mg copper.
- If supplementing copper: monitor zinc and avoid >2-3 mg/day chronically without clear indication and labs.
- Favor whole-food sources for maintenance.

Interactions between zinc supplementation and copper status

Mechanism

- Zinc and copper share intestinal transport.
- High zinc → metallothionein induction → preferential copper binding → copper loss with enterocyte turnover.

Clinical consequences

- Copper deficiency causing:
- Anemia, neutropenia, thrombocytopenia (can mimic MDS).
- Myelopathy, peripheral neuropathy, proprioceptive loss.
- Skin/hair changes.

Post-COVID spike

- Increased zinc use for "immune support" has led to more zinc-induced copper deficiency cases.
- Some patients initially worked up for MDS or ALS before zinc/copper imbalance was recognized.

Prevention

- Keep chronic zinc intake moderate unless monitored.
- Add copper when zinc is high.
- Check copper, ceruloplasmin, and zinc in unexplained cytopenias or myelopathy.

CHAPTER 9: Vitamin C: Surge Protection and Structural Repair

The surge protector and repair crew

Every serious electronics setup uses surge protectors and grounding to handle power spikes and electrical "noise." Without them, sudden surges can damage sensitive components and shorten the lifespan of the whole system.

The body runs complex, high-energy processes all day: metabolism, immune responses, exercise, stress reactions, detoxification. All of these generate biochemical "sparks" in the form of reactive oxygen species (ROS) and other free radicals.

You need a system that can both:

- Absorb and neutralize those surges.
- Repair the structural damage they cause.

Vitamin C sits at a central point in that system. It works as:

- A water-soluble antioxidant that neutralizes ROS.
- A cofactor for enzymes that build strong collagen in joints, skin, blood vessels, gums, and other tissues.
- A supporter of immune cell function, movement, and clean resolution after infection.

When vitamin C status is marginal or low, full scurvy is rare in modern settings, but the system loses surge protection and repair capacity. Over time, the effects can be significant.

This is Elena's story.

Elena's slow leak

Elena was 39, a recreational endurance athlete and single mother of two. She ran half-marathons, juggled a demanding job, and prided herself on "pushing through" anything.

Over several years, a slow erosion in resilience appeared:

- Joints ached more after runs; soreness felt more tendinous and lingered.
- Bruises appeared easily and faded slowly.

- Cuts and scrapes that once healed in days now took one to two weeks.
- She caught every cold her children brought home, and each illness lingered.
- Skin looked dull and tired despite fitness and healthy weight.

Her response was to train harder. The extra load only made her feel more worn down.

Basic labs (CBC, metabolic panel, thyroid) were unremarkable. She was told she was healthy, "probably overdoing it," and should rest more.

A nutritionally oriented clinician saw a different pattern: high physical stress, frequent minor infections, and constant demand, all of which require robust antioxidant and repair systems. Vitamin C stood out as a likely weak point.

What vitamin C actually does

Vitamin C (ascorbic acid) is best known for "colds," but its roles span structural biology, redox control, and immune regulation.

Collagen synthesis and structural integrity

Vitamin C is required for the enzymes prolyl hydroxylase and lysyl hydroxylase, which hydroxylate proline and lysine residues in collagen.

These iron-dependent dioxygenases require:

- 2-oxoglutarate.
- Fe^{2+}.
- Molecular oxygen.
- Ascorbic acid to maintain iron in the reduced state.

Hydroxylation allows collagen chains to:

- Form stable triple helices.
- Cross-link properly.
- Achieve full tensile strength.

Without enough vitamin C:

- Collagen is under-hydroxylated and structurally weak.
- Procollagen accumulates and is not fully converted to mature collagen.

This affects:

- Blood vessels: increased fragility, easy bruising, subcutaneous bleeding.
- Skin: reduced strength, elasticity, wound tensile strength, and barrier function.
- Joints and tendons: weaker connective tissue, higher injury risk, slower repair.
- Gums: bleeding, gingival swelling, poor healing.

Full vitamin C deficiency (scurvy) causes bleeding gums, petechiae, poor wound healing, fatigue, and ultimately organ failure if untreated. Long-term marginal intake does not cause classic scurvy but can yield suboptimal collagen function and chronic "slow leak" symptoms.

Modern reviews confirm that 4-hydroxyproline residues are essential for the thermal stability of the collagen triple helix at body temperature and that inadequate hydroxylation leads to denaturation and loss of structural support.

Elena's easy bruising, lingering soreness, and slow wound healing were not random; they were signs that her collagen repair crew was understaffed.

Antioxidant and "surge protector"

Vitamin C is a water-soluble electron donor. It:

- Directly neutralizes ROS and reactive nitrogen species in aqueous compartments.
- Regenerates other antioxidants, such as vitamin E and glutathione, restoring them to active form.
- Helps protect lipids, proteins, and DNA from oxidative damage, particularly during and after intense exercise or illness.

In exercise and physical stress:

- Vitamin C can reduce markers of lipid peroxidation, such as MDA after intense activity.
- Combined vitamin C and E has reduced muscle damage, inflammatory response, and hemolysis in some athletic trials.

A 2025 review of oxidative stress biomarkers notes that elevated MDA, 8-OHdG, and F2-isoprostanes reflect systemic oxidative stress and correlate with disease severity in conditions from hypertension to diabetic complications. These markers provide objective evidence of oxidative burden that vitamin C and other antioxidants help control.

This antioxidant "surge protection" is especially relevant for endurance athletes like Elena, who experience repeated high oxygen demand, which generates substantial oxidative stress.

However, some ROS signaling is needed for training adaptation. The goal is adequate protection without blunting beneficial signals, a balance, not a blockade.

Immune function

Vitamin C accumulates to millimolar concentrations inside certain immune cells, especially neutrophils.

It supports:

- Chemotaxis: movement of neutrophils to infection sites.
- Phagocytosis: engulfing and killing pathogens.
- Oxidative burst: ROS generation to kill microbes, while helping shield the cells themselves.
- Resolution: promoting neutrophil apoptosis and clearance by macrophages, reducing prolonged tissue damage and excessive NETosis.

A comprehensive review concluded:

"Vitamin C stimulates neutrophil migration to the site of infection, enhances phagocytosis and oxidant generation, and microbial killing. At the same time, it protects host tissue from excessive damage by enhancing neutrophil apoptosis and clearance by macrophages, and decreasing neutrophil necrosis and NETosis."

The NIH Office of Dietary Supplements likewise notes that vitamin C accumulates in phagocytic cells and can enhance chemotaxis, phagocytosis, and microbial killing, while also supporting wound healing via effects on immune and inflammatory cells.

Buffered vitamin C has increased NK-cell cytotoxicity in toxin-exposed individuals, and supplementation in stressed or athletic populations can improve neutrophil function and reduce infection severity or duration.

Elena's pattern, catching every cold, prolonged recovery, matched what happens when neutrophils do not have enough vitamin C to do their job efficiently.

Neurotransmitter and hormone synthesis

Vitamin C is a cofactor for:

- Dopamine β-hydroxylase, which converts dopamine to norepinephrine.
- Enzymes in adrenal steroid and catecholamine metabolism.

Adrenal glands accumulate high levels of vitamin C and release it during stress. This ties ascorbate into mood, alertness, and stress handling, and helps explain why Elena felt not only physically worn but mentally "flat" in her worst stretches.

Assessing vitamin C status

Vitamin C is rarely measured in routine practice, but it can be assessed directly.

Plasma ascorbic acid (most common)

- Method: HPLC or LC, MS/MS.
- Specimen: plasma (protected from light, processed and frozen quickly).
- Interpretation (typical ranges):
- <11 µmol/L (<0.2 mg/dL): deficiency (scurvy risk).
- 11-28 µmol/L (0.2, 0.5 mg/dL): marginal/inadequate tissue stores.
- 28-40 µmol/L (0.5, 0.7 mg/dL): low-normal; may be suboptimal under high demand.
- *40 µmol/L (>0.7 mg/dL): generally adequate; saturation ≈70-80 µmol/L.*

Leukocyte ascorbic acid (specialty)

- More closely reflects tissue stores and body pools in research.
- Technically challenging, influenced by cell counts, and not widely available.
- Less reliable in acute illness, when leukocytes rapidly consume vitamin C.

When to consider testing:

- Symptoms: easy bruising, poor wound healing, gum bleeding, fatigue.
- High-demand states: heavy training, chronic disease, smoking, malabsorption, very low fresh produce intake.
- Clinical suspicion of scurvy or marginal status.

Assessing oxidative stress load

Because vitamin C is a key antioxidant, oxidative stress markers help gauge whether surge protection is adequate.

Common biomarkers:

- 8-OHdG: oxidative DNA damage (urine or plasma).
- F2-isoprostanes: lipid peroxidation; considered highly reliable in vivo.
- MDA: lipid peroxidation; less specific but widely available.
- Protein carbonyls: oxidative protein damage.
- Total antioxidant capacity: overall reserve.

Interpretation:

- Elevated 8-OHdG and F2-isoprostanes suggest increased oxidative damage; the system is generating more "sparks" than it can neutralize.
- Elevated oxidative markers plus low-normal plasma vitamin C strongly support the need for enhanced antioxidant support.

Serial measurements can track response to diet, supplementation, and lifestyle changes.

Elena's testing pattern

Elena's clinician combined:

- History: easy bruising, slow wound healing, frequent infections, long illness duration.
- Lifestyle: high training volume, single-parent stress, high overall demand.
- Diet: irregular fresh produce, reliance on convenience foods.

Targeted labs (when available):

- Plasma ascorbic acid: low-normal (≈25-30 μmol/L), marginal under her demand.
- Oxidative stress:

- 8-OHdG: elevated, indicating oxidative DNA damage.
- F2-isoprostanes: elevated, reflecting lipid peroxidation from training and stress.
- MDA: elevated, consistent with high oxidative turnover.

Interpretation:

- High oxidative load with borderline antioxidant reserve, the biochemical equivalent of running a data center with inadequate surge protection and an overworked repair crew.

Her clinician summarized: "You're generating sparks faster than you're putting them out. And your repair crew, the collagen team, is under-resourced. We need to fix both."

Elena's 16-week surge protection and repair plan

Step 1: Baseline support (Weeks 1-4)

Goals: raise vitamin C intake and shore up collagen and antioxidant systems.

Diet:

- Daily vitamin C, rich foods: citrus, berries, kiwi, bell peppers, broccoli, Brussels sprouts, kale.
- Emphasis on colorful plants for polyphenols and additional antioxidants.

Supplemental vitamin C:

- 500-1000 mg/day, split into 1 or 2 doses with food.
- Buffered or liposomal forms if GI sensitivity appeared.

Structural support:

- Optional collagen peptides.
- Adequate total protein, especially glycine, proline, and lysine.

Within a few weeks:

- Soreness after runs eased slightly.
- Bruises faded faster.
- Cuts and scrapes healed more quickly.

Step 2: Higher demand support (Weeks 5-8)

Once tolerance was clear:

- Vitamin C increased to 1500-3000 mg/day in divided doses, titrated to bowel tolerance.

- Upper range used on very heavy training or high-stress days.

Other supports:

- Continued collagen and high-protein intake.
- Magnesium, zinc, and foundational nutrients maintained.
- Attention to sleep and hydration.

By Week 8:

- Fewer "post-viral" crashes.
- Shorter, milder minor illnesses.
- Faster resolution of soreness and small injuries.
- Improved skin appearance and less gum sensitivity.

Follow-up oxidative markers trended downward from clearly elevated baseline values.

Step 3: Integration and fine-tuning (Weeks 9-16)

With better surge protection and repair:

- Vitamin C maintained at 1000-2000 mg/day, with flexible increases during:
- Heavy training blocks.
- Acute illness.
- Intense stress periods.

Her training plan incorporated rest days and periodization. Diet remained rich in whole plant foods.

By Week 16:

- Training cycles produced far less cumulative wear.
- Bruising, gum bleeding, and slow wound healing largely resolved.
- Infection frequency dropped; recovery was faster.
- She felt more robust and less on the edge of breakdown.

Vitamin C was not the only factor, but it restored a missing layer of surge protection and structural repair, enabling everything else to work better.

Why people respond differently to supplementation

Not everyone notices a dramatic change from vitamin C, especially if:

- Baseline intake of fruits and vegetables is strong.

- Stress, training, and infection loads are moderate.

Demand for vitamin C rises sharply in:

- High training loads.
- Chronic psychological stress.
- Frequent infections.
- Pollution and toxin exposure.
- Smoking.
- Chronic inflammatory conditions.
- Major wounds, surgery, or trauma.

In these states, "normal" intake may not suffice to maintain optimal collagen integrity, wound healing, immune function, and antioxidant balance, even if classic scurvy never appears.

Elena's story shows how chronic demand exceeding supply produces not a dramatic collapse but a slow leak of resilience.

Practical considerations and safety

Vitamin C is water-soluble and generally safe at common supplemental doses.

Typical intakes:

- RDA: ~75-90 mg/day, sufficient to prevent scurvy, not necessarily to optimize performance.
- Common clinical bands: 500-2000 mg/day in higher-demand individuals.

Higher oral doses:

- 3000-6000 mg/day are sometimes used short-term under supervision.
- Main side effect is GI upset or loose stools (bowel tolerance), guiding dose reduction or division.

Cautions:

- History of certain kidney stones (e.g., calcium oxalate) or specific metabolic disorders → discuss high-dose vitamin C with a clinician.
- Very high doses in iron overload disorders may theoretically enhance iron absorption.

- Intravenous vitamin C is a distinct modality and requires medical supervision.

The NIH notes that plasma vitamin C is the standard clinical status measure; leukocyte vitamin C may better reflect stores but is more difficult to measure and is not routinely used.

How vitamin C fits with the other "chips"

Vitamin C interacts with many systems in this book:

- With vitamin E, glutathione, and lipoic acid: it forms a regeneration network covering different cellular compartments.
- With collagen and structure: supports connective tissue so magnesium-driven muscle and vascular function have a strong frame.
- With mitochondria: helps protect mitochondrial membranes and DNA from oxidative damage while magnesium and phosphorus drive ATP production.
- With immune function and zinc: supports neutrophil and lymphocyte function and modulates resolution of inflammation.
- With vascular integrity: maintains blood vessel strength, improving nutrient delivery without leakiness.

In the "chip" analogy:

Vitamin C is the surge protector and repair crew, ensuring that peaks in oxidative stress and physical wear do not burn out the components you have optimized elsewhere.

Elena's story underlines that:

- You can be "fit" yet structurally and oxidatively under-supported.
- Long-term marginal deficits in repair and protection quietly erode performance and resilience.
- Bringing this layer online allows mitochondrial, mineral, hormonal, and immune upgrades to operate in a safer, more durable environment.

In the next chapter, the focus shifts to integration: how all the chips and systems combine into a coordinated architecture, and how to think about optimizing them as a whole rather than as isolated parts.

SIDEBAR: Vitamin C and Collagen—The molecular details

Key points:

- Vitamin C is a cofactor for prolyl and lysyl hydroxylases.
- These enzymes hydroxylate proline and lysine residues in procollagen, forming hydroxyproline and hydroxylysine.
- The reaction requires 2-oxoglutarate, Fe^{2+}, O_2, and ascorbate.
- Hydroxylation stabilizes the triple helix and permits proper cross-linking.

Without adequate vitamin C:

- Hydroxylation falters.
- Collagen triple helices are unstable.
- Cross-linking is impaired.
- Connective tissue becomes fragile, and wounds heal poorly.

Experimental work shows vitamin C can increase collagen synthesis and improve connective tissue healing in tendons, ligaments, and skin, especially when paired with sufficient amino acid substrate and mechanical loading.

SIDEBAR: Vitamin C, exercise, and oxidative stress

Intense exercise increases oxygen consumption and ROS production.

Studies show:

- Vitamin C (often 500-1000 mg/day, sometimes with vitamin E) can:
- Reduce MDA and other lipid peroxidation markers post-exercise.
- Lower some muscle damage and soreness markers.
- Attenuate inflammatory responses and red blood cell hemolysis in repeated high-intensity bouts.

A key nuance:

- Antioxidant strategies can blunt excessive oxidative stress but should not entirely eliminate ROS signals, which are part of training adaptation.
- In ultra-endurance contexts, some very high-dose antioxidant protocols have paradoxically been associated with higher

oxidative markers post-race, underscoring that more is not always better.

Practical takeaway: Use vitamin C to support recovery and protect from excessive oxidative damage, especially during heavy blocks, while preserving smart training design.

SIDEBAR: Vitamin C and wound healing

Vitamin C participates in all phases of wound healing:

- Inflammatory phase: supports neutrophil function, controls ROS generation, and promotes resolution.
- Proliferative phase: promotes fibroblast proliferation, collagen synthesis, and angiogenesis.
- Remodeling phase: supports collagen maturation and cross-linking, improving tensile strength.

Deficiency slows wound closure and reduces scar strength; supplementation improves healing in people with low status, high inflammation, or trauma.

For someone like Elena, constant microtrauma from running and daily minor injuries, vitamin C is a quiet but essential foreman on the repair crew.

SIDEBAR: Vitamin C and Neutrophil Function—The evidence

A 2019 systematic review of randomized trials found that:

- Neutrophils actively accumulate vitamin C to millimolar levels.
- Supplementation can improve chemotaxis, phagocytosis, oxidative burst, and appropriate apoptosis.
- Populations that benefit most include:
- Athletes under heavy training.
- Post-MI patients.
- Older adults with weakened immunity.
- People under chronic stress or with recurrent infections.

For patients like Elena, adequate vitamin C does not guarantee immunity, but it equips neutrophils to respond, kill, and clean up efficiently.

GLOSSARY: Key terms for Chapter 9

- **Vitamin C (ascorbic acid):** Water-soluble vitamin functioning as an antioxidant and enzyme cofactor, essential for collagen synthesis, immune function, and oxidative protection.
- **Collagen:** Main structural protein in skin, tendons, ligaments, bone, vessels, and gums; stability depends on vitamin C, dependent hydroxylation.
- **Prolyl/lysyl hydroxylase:** Vitamin C-dependent enzymes that hydroxylate proline and lysine in procollagen.
- **Hydroxyproline/hydroxylysine:** Modified amino acids critical for collagen triple-helix stability.
- **Scurvy:** Clinical vitamin C deficiency state with fatigue, bleeding gums, petechiae, poor wound healing, and possible organ failure.
- **Reactive oxygen species (ROS):** Highly reactive oxygen-containing molecules produced by metabolism; excess causes oxidative damage.
- **8-OhdG**: Marker of oxidative DNA damage.
- **F2-isoprostanes:** Products of lipid peroxidation; reliable in vivo oxidative stress biomarkers.
- **MDA (malondialdehyde):** Lipid peroxidation product used as a common oxidative stress marker.
- **Neutrophils:** First-responder white blood cells; vitamin C supports their migration, killing, and resolution.
- **Chemotaxis:** Directed movement of immune cells toward injury or infection signals.
- **Oxidative burst:** Rapid ROS generation by neutrophils to kill pathogens.
- **NETosis:** Neutrophil cell death that releases DNA nets to trap pathogens; excessive NETosis can cause tissue damage.
- **Bowel tolerance:** Highest oral vitamin C dose tolerated before loose stools occur.
- **Liposomal vitamin C:** Vitamin C encapsulated in phospholipids for improved absorption and GI tolerance.

- **RDA:** Recommended Dietary Allowance; average daily intake sufficient for most healthy individuals.
- **Plasma ascorbic acid:** Standard clinical measure of vitamin C status; ≤11 μmol/L indicates deficiency.
- **Leukocyte ascorbic acid:** Vitamin C in white cells; research index of tissue stores, less available clinically.

CHAPTER 10: Integration: The Complete System

From individual chips to a living architecture

By now, you have met each of the major "chips" in your biological computer: mitochondria, magnesium, B12 and folate, zinc, phosphorus and creatine, boron, copper, and vitamin C.

Each chapter focused on one chip in the system. In reality, your body is not running these chips one at a time. It is running all of them simultaneously, and they are constantly talking to each other.

This chapter is about stepping back to see how they work together as a whole and how to think about your own optimization without getting lost in the details.

Three levels of optimization

It helps to think in three tiers. Most people live somewhere along this spectrum, and knowing where you are matters.

Survival level is what medicine traditionally aims for: keeping you alive and preventing obvious disease. It is why your doctor checks your labs and treats high blood pressure or diabetic crisis. Standard lab ranges are built around this level; they catch people sick enough to diagnose, but they are wide bands that include everyone "not sick enough to treat right now."

Functional level is where you feel and perform "normal" for your age. You get up, you work, you live. Many people never quite reach this; they drift in a gray zone of fatigue, brain fog, poor sleep, pain, and constant minor infections. They are technically alive and not diagnosed with disease, but something is clearly off.

Optimization level is your personal best: stable energy throughout the day without crashes, sleep that is actually restorative, thinking that is clear and sustained, mood that is resilient, immunity that works. Your body recovers from exercise, from stress, from life.

Most of the people in this book, Jake, Sarah, Marcus, Elena, started somewhere between survival and functional. They were alive, they were "fine" on basic testing, but they were nowhere near their actual potential. The work you have seen was moving them toward optimization.

Why magnesium matters first

Think of magnesium this way: ATP is the energy currency of every cell in your body. But ATP does not work alone. ATP only becomes usable when it is bound to magnesium, when it becomes Mg-ATP.

Every system that uses energy depends on this: your mitochondria burning fuel, your muscles contracting, your immune cells mounting a response, your brain firing thoughts, your hormones being synthesized. All of them are burning Mg-ATP.

Without enough magnesium, you cannot activate the enzymes that run the electron transport chain. Without those enzymes working, your mitochondria cannot produce ATP efficiently, no matter how many calories you eat or how well you sleep. You have the raw materials, but the power plant is running on the emergency generator.

This is why magnesium deficiency is so insidious. It does not cause one symptom, it erodes everything. Your muscles feel weak and crampy. Your heart skips. Your brain gets foggy. Your mood dips. Your sleep fragments. Your immune system falters. All because the energy currency is essentially stuck in traffic.

This is why addressing magnesium is one of the first and most cost-effective steps you can take. Get this right, and everything else works better.

Methylation: The master dimmer switch for your genes

B12 and folate sit at the center of methylation, a biochemical process that determines whether genes are turned on or off.

Every day, your cells are adding or removing methyl groups (tiny chemical tags) from your DNA. These tags control which genes are expressed and which are silenced. They affect how your myelin gets built, how your neurotransmitters get made, how your DNA repairs itself.

When methylation works well, your genes are stable, your neurotransmitters are balanced, and your brain tissue holds together. When methylation falters, when B12 or folate is low, homocysteine starts to climb. This is not just a number on a lab. Elevated homocysteine is a sign that something upstream is broken.

Homocysteine damages your brain and blood vessels in multiple ways at once. It oxidizes your mitochondria. It overstimulates your NMDA receptors, killing neurons. It damages the inside of blood vessels, promoting small strokes and white matter lesions. It disrupts methylation itself, creating a vicious cycle.

People with mild cognitive impairment or early dementia often have elevated homocysteine. So do people who have strokes. So do people with depression.

The best functional medicine clinicians check homocysteine early because it is a modifiable risk factor. Getting it down to 8-10 μmol/L (much lower than standard "normal") can slow or stop some of these processes if you catch it early.

Immunity as a security system

Your immune system is not separate from everything else. It is like a security system running 24/7, checking for intruders, clearing away damage, and managing inflammation.

Zinc is your immune security processor. Vitamin C is both the surge protector and the cleanup crew.

When either one is low, the system stutters. You catch more infections. When you do get sick, your immune response is blunt; it overheats the whole building instead of neutralizing the intruder. The inflammation lingers. You have persistently elevated hs-CRP, which stresses your mitochondria, disrupts your hormones, and impairs your methylation.

Chronic low-grade inflammation is like running with the "check engine" light on all the time. Your mitochondria work harder. Your hormones swing more. Your collagen breaks down faster. Your brain fog gets worse. Everything decays a little faster.

Fix your security system, optimize zinc, vitamin C, and vitamin D, and you often stabilize many downstream problems.

The energy distribution grid

Phosphorus and creatine are your energy distribution system. They act like a backup generator and power grid, buffering ATP and allowing rapid energy regeneration when you need it.

Copper sits downstream, supporting Complex IV in your mitochondria and maintaining myelin so signals travel fast.

If your phosphorus and creatine are low, you cannot handle peak demands. You can cruise along at baseline, but the moment you hit a heavy workout or a stressful week or a big cognitive push, you crash. Your system has no buffer.

If your copper is off, too low or too high, myelin thins and signal speed slows. Neural bandwidth narrows. You think a bit slower, you react a bit slower, you recover a bit slower.

If you are someone who can handle moderate stress but crashes under high load, the problem is often in this system: phosphorus, creatine, copper, and the overall energy distribution architecture.

Exercise as a Mitophagy signal: The FUNDC1 mechanism

Exercise is universally recognized as one of the most powerful longevity interventions, but the mechanisms underlying its benefits extend far beyond cardiovascular conditioning or calorie burn. At the cellular level, exercise is a mitochondrial quality-control signal that simultaneously triggers mitochondrial biogenesis (the formation of new mitochondria) and mitophagy (the removal of old, damaged mitochondria).

This "turnover cycle" is essential for maintaining mitochondrial health, and its decline with sedentary aging is a major driver of metabolic disease, sarcopenia, and functional decline.

FUNDC1: The exercise-responsive mitophagy receptor

FUNDC1 (FUN14 domain-containing 1) is a mitophagy receptor embedded in the outer mitochondrial membrane. Unlike PINK1/Parkin, which responds primarily to mitochondrial membrane potential collapse, FUNDC1 responds to hypoxia, metabolic stress, and exercise-induced signals.

During exercise, multiple stressors activate FUNDC1:

1. Transient hypoxia: High-intensity or endurance exercise creates localized oxygen deficits in working muscle, triggering HIF-1α (hypoxia-inducible factor 1-alpha), which upregulates FUNDC1 expression.
2. Metabolic stress: ATP depletion and AMP accumulation activate AMPK, which phosphorylates and activates FUNDC1 and other mitophagy machinery.
3. Calcium signaling: Exercise-induced calcium release from the sarcoplasmic reticulum activates phosphatases (e.g., PGAM5)

that dephosphorylate FUNDC1 at Ser13, dramatically increasing its affinity for LC3 and triggering mitophagy.

4. ROS signaling: Controlled ROS bursts during exercise act as signaling molecules, promoting both mitochondrial biogenesis (via PGC-1α) and mitophagy (via FUNDC1 and PINK1/Parkin).

The result: Exercise-damaged mitochondria are tagged by FUNDC1, engulfed by autophagosomes, and degraded, making room for newly synthesized mitochondria via PGC-1α signaling.

Evidence: Exercise upregulates FUNDC1 by 60-80%

Animal and human studies consistently demonstrate that exercise training increases FUNDC1 expression and activity:

- Mice: Voluntary wheel running for 4 weeks increased skeletal muscle FUNDC1 protein levels by 60-80%, with parallel increases in LC3-II (autophagosome marker) and decreases in damaged mitochondrial content.
- Humans: Acute exercise (single bout of resistance or endurance training) increases FUNDC1 mRNA and protein expression within 3-6 hours post-exercise, peaking at 12-24 hours.
- Chronic training: 12 weeks of combined aerobic and resistance training in older adults (age 65-80) significantly increased muscle FUNDC1, PINK1, and LC3-II, with corresponding improvements in mitochondrial respiratory capacity and reductions in oxidative stress markers.

Importantly, sedentary aging is associated with downregulation of FUNDC1, contributing to the accumulation of dysfunctional mitochondria in aged muscle.

Exercise modality matters

Different types of exercise activate mitophagy through different mechanisms:

Exercise type	**Primary mitophagy trigger**	**Optimal protocol**

Aerobic/endurance	Hypoxia, AMPK, sustained ATP demand	30-60 min moderate-vigorous intensity, 3-5×/week
High-intensity interval training (HIIT)	Severe transient hypoxia, maximal AMPK activation, ROS bursts	20-30 min (e.g., 4×4 min hard / 3 min easy), 2-3×/week
Resistance training	Mechanical tension, calcium signaling, localized metabolic stress	3-5 sets, 6-12 reps, progressive overload, 2-4×/week
Combination (concurrent training)	Additive effects from aerobic + resistance	Aerobic 3×/week + resistance 2-3×/week (ideal for aging populations)

Clinical pearl: For mitochondrial health specifically, moderate-to-vigorous aerobic exercise and HIIT appear most effective at upregulating FUNDC1 and mitophagy markers, while resistance training is essential for maintaining muscle mass and mTOR signaling.

The ideal program combines both aerobic work for mitophagy and metabolic health, resistance work for anabolism and functional strength.

Exercise is the only intervention that does all three

What makes exercise unique is that it simultaneously:

1. Signals mitochondrial biogenesis via PGC-1α, NRF1, and TFAM, telling cells to build new mitochondria
2. Activates mitophagy via FUNDC1, PINK1/Parkin, and AMPK, telling cells to remove old mitochondria
3. Provides hormetic stress via controlled ROS and metabolic challenge, strengthening stress-response pathways without causing net damage

No drug, supplement, or fasting protocol can replicate all three effects simultaneously.

Why sedentary aging accelerates mitochondrial dysfunction

In the absence of exercise:

- FUNDC1 expression declines by 30-50% in aged muscle

- PINK1/Parkin activity decreases, allowing damaged mitochondria to accumulate
- PGC-1α signaling weakens, reducing mitochondrial biogenesis
- The turnover cycle stalls: old mitochondria are not removed, new mitochondria are not built, and the mitochondrial network becomes increasingly dysfunctional

This creates a feedforward loop:

- Mitochondrial dysfunction → reduced ATP → exercise intolerance → further sedentary behavior → more mitochondrial dysfunction

Breaking the cycle: Even small amounts of structured exercise can reactivate FUNDC1, restore mitophagy, and initiate mitochondrial turnover. The earlier the intervention, the faster the response.

Clinical protocols: Exercise as a mitophagy prescription

For deconditioned or elderly patients (restore baseline function)

- Start: 10-15 min walking daily, gradually increasing to 30 min
- Progress to: 3-4×/week moderate-intensity aerobic (brisk walking, cycling, swimming) at 60-70% max heart rate
- Add: 2×/week resistance training (bodyweight, bands, or light weights), focusing on major muscle groups
- Timeline: Mitochondrial markers (FUNDC1, PGC-1α) begin improving within 2-4 weeks; functional improvements (endurance, strength) within 6-8 weeks

For active adults (optimize mitochondrial health)

- Aerobic base: 3-5×/week, 30-60 min, mix of moderate (Zone 2, conversational pace) and vigorous (Zone 3-4, hard but sustainable)
- HIIT: 1-2×/week, e.g., 4×4 min intervals at 85-95% max HR with 3 min active recovery
- Resistance: 3-4×/week, full-body or split routine, progressive overload, 6-12 rep range
- Recovery: 1-2 rest or active recovery days (yoga, walking, stretching)

For athletes or advanced trainees (periodize for mitophagy)

- Base phase (8-12 weeks): High volume, moderate intensity → maximize mitochondrial density via PGC-1α and FUNDC1 upregulation
- Build phase (6-8 weeks): Add intensity (HIIT, tempo work) → enhance mitochondrial efficiency and turnover
- Peak/taper: Reduce volume, maintain intensity → allow supercompensation and mitochondrial remodeling
- Off-season: Active recovery with maintenance training → sustain FUNDC1 and PGC-1α expression

UCOS + Exercise Synergy

Exercise-induced mitophagy is amplified when combined with UCOS:

UCOS Component	Synergy with Exercise-Induced Mitophagy
---	---
Magnesium	Required for ATP synthesis and muscle contraction; deficiency blunts exercise adaptation
NAD^+ precursors	Fuel SIRT1/3 activation post-exercise, enhancing both mitophagy and mitochondrial biogenesis
Creatine	Maintains ATP during high-intensity work, allowing greater training stimulus for mitophagy signaling
Leucine + protein	Post-workout mTOR activation ensures that mitochondrial biogenesis matches mitophagy (turnover, not depletion)
Omega-3 fatty acids	Reduce post-exercise inflammation, improve mitochondrial membrane composition, enhance FUNDC1 signaling
Spermidine	Enhances general autophagy; combined with exercise-induced mitophagy creates comprehensive cellular cleanup

Urolithin A	Amplifies PINK1/Parkin and likely receptor-mediated pathways; stacks with exercise FUNDC1 activation

Bottom line: Exercise + UCOS produces multiplicative, not merely additive, effects on mitochondrial quality.

Patient language: Why exercise is the best mitochondrial medicine

"Exercise is the only thing that tells your body to both build new mitochondria and throw out the old, broken ones at the same time. It's not just about burning calories or getting your heart rate up; it's about triggering a complete mitochondrial upgrade.

When you exercise, especially when you push into that uncomfortable but sustainable zone, your muscles experience controlled stress: low oxygen, rising lactate, a flood of calcium. Your cells recognize this and activate a cleanup protein called FUNDC1, which grabs damaged mitochondria and sends them to the recycling bin.

At the same time, exercise activates PGC-1α, the master switch for building brand-new, efficient mitochondria to replace the ones you just cleared.

No pill can do both at once. That's why people who exercise regularly have mitochondria that look 10-20 years younger than their chronological age. And it's why we prescribe exercise as precisely as we prescribe supplements: the right dose, the right intensity, the right frequency.

You're not 'just working out.' You're giving your 37 trillion cells the signal to rebuild themselves."

Hormonal voltage and stability

Boron is a voltage controller for your hormonal system. It can lower SHBG, increase free testosterone, support vitamin D metabolism, and shift inflammatory signals downward.

Your hormones, testosterone, estrogen, cortisol, thyroid, insulin, create your "voltage environment." When they swing wildly or sit chronically low, everything feels unstable. Your energy dips. Your mood swings. Your body composition shifts. Your brain feels foggy.

Stable hormonal control does not mean "normal" levels. It means clean control, responsive to what you need, without the wild peaks and crashes.

When boron is optimized and your hormonal system stabilizes, people often describe it this way: "I finally feel like myself again."

A Practical Map for Getting Started

Real life is messy, and everyone is different. But most people benefit from thinking in layers.

Start with the foundation. Sleep matters. Nutrition matters, real food, adequate protein, lots of plants. Move your body daily. Learn to down-shift your nervous system. These are non-negotiable.

Then address the core biochemical chips. Check your magnesium status (or at least assess your symptoms and diet). Get your vitamin D, B12, and homocysteine tested. Look at zinc status and the zinc:copper balance. Make sure you are eating enough vitamin C-rich foods, or supplementing if your demand is high.

Assess your systems. Do you have steady energy, or do you crash? Is your brain clear or foggy? Do you get sick often, or do you recover quickly? Do your hormones feel stable? Do your joints stay healthy, or do you get hurt easily? These patterns tell you where the bottlenecks are.

Then optimize. Based on what you find, layer in targeted support. CoQ10 and NAD+ for mitochondria. Methylfolate and methylcobalamin for methylation. Zinc and vitamin C for immunity. Boron for hormones. Copper balance for neural function. And always, always make sure magnesium is solid underneath it all.

Once the obvious bottlenecks are handled, you can refine everything else, how you train, how you eat, whether certain hormetic stressors (cold, heat, fasting) are right for you.

Why people feel so different when systems are restored

The stories in this book, Jake recovering his muscle function, Sarah finding stable energy, Marcus getting his coordination back, Elena healing from chronic overuse, all follow the same pattern.

The person was not sick in a diagnosable way. They were just depleted, stuck between survival and functionality. But the depletion was in systems that matter: energy, methylation, immunity, hormonal control.

When you find and fix the right bottleneck, you do not feel "a bit better." You feel transformed. Energy that was flat becomes flowing. Thinking that was slow becomes quick. Mood that was reactive becomes resilient. Recovery that was slow becomes fast.

This is not because of a magic supplement. It is because you took an engineering approach to a biological system: you identified what was missing, you restored it, and the whole architecture got better.

The role of your genes

No two people are identical. Your genes shape how sensitive you are to nutritional imbalances.

Some people have an MTHFR variant that makes it harder to convert regular folate into the active form. They accumulate homocysteine more easily and benefit more from 5-methylfolate and B12 support.

Some people have a COMT variant that makes them metabolize dopamine slowly. They are naturally focused, but they are also more vulnerable to stress. They benefit from magnesium, SAMe, and careful antioxidant support.

Some people have FUT2 variants that alter their gut bacteria and how they absorb B12. They may need more targeted probiotic or B12 support to optimize.

This is why two people with the same symptoms and the same basic labs can respond differently to the same intervention.

This book is a map, not a protocol. It tells you what systems exist and what to look for. You and your clinician still decide where to start, how fast to move, and which levers matter most for you.

What optimization actually feels like

When all the systems are tuned, people describe a common experience:

Your energy is steady. You wake up without an alarm and feel ready. You work or train or create, and you feel capable. You do not have the dramatic 2 pm crash or the evening slump. You have normal variation, but no crashes.

Your sleep is deep. You fall asleep without racing thoughts. You stay asleep. You wake up rested.

Your thinking is clear. You can focus on hard things. You can hold complex ideas. You are creative. You bounce back from mistakes.

Your mood is stable. Stress does not derail you. Small frustrations do not trigger outsized reactions. You feel resilient.

Your body works. You can train and recover. Injuries heal cleanly. Random pains do not appear. Your immune system handles minor infections quickly.

Your aging feels different. People with optimized systems do not feel old. They feel capable. They feel like their system can actually adapt and recover, rather than just slowly declining.

This is not perfection. Life still brings crises and losses and hard seasons. But your system's ability to respond, absorb, and recover is fundamentally different when the chips are powered.

The core argument

This book is not an argument for a specific diet, supplement, or technology.

It is an argument that your body is engineered with remarkable logic and clarity. Many of the vague, chronic, life-limiting symptoms people live with are not random. They are the predictable result of specific missing inputs.

There is immense value in taking an engineering approach: measuring, testing, identifying what is broken, and deliberately fixing it. Not guessing. Not hoping. Actually looking and then addressing what you find.

Your biology is alive and responsive. How you fuel it, protect it, and tune it determines not just how long you live, but how you live.

In the final chapter, the lens widens. We step back from individual biology and ask bigger questions: How could this systems thinking reshape medicine itself? What becomes possible when we stop treating symptoms and start thinking about optimization? What does it mean to be human when both AI and human performance are changing so rapidly?

SIDEBAR: The Mg-ATP foundation

Magnesium is not just one mineral among many. It is foundational in a way that few nutrients are.

ATP, the energy molecule, only becomes usable when magnesium binds to it. This Mg-ATP complex is what actually powers your cells.

Every enzyme that runs on ATP needs magnesium.

Your electron transport chain needs magnesium. Your muscles need magnesium to contract. Your neurons need magnesium to fire. Your immune cells need magnesium to activate. Your hormones need magnesium to be synthesized.

When magnesium is low, everything slows. Your mitochondria are less efficient. Your DNA repair falters. Your immune response is blunt. Your hormones swing. Your brain gets foggy.

This is why addressing magnesium is often the single highest-impact move. It does not cure everything, but it creates the foundation on which everything else can work better.

SIDEBAR: The Homocysteine story

Homocysteine is a marker that tells you something is wrong upstream in methylation.

When B12, folate, or B6 is low, or when you have genetic variants that slow these pathways, homocysteine rises. This is not just a number. Elevated homocysteine damages your brain and blood vessels.

It promotes small strokes. It disrupts blood flow to the brain. It kills neurons. It disrupts methylation itself, creating a vicious cycle. People with early dementia often have elevated homocysteine. So do people with depression and cardiovascular disease.

The solution is straightforward but requires early action: methylfolate, methylcobalamin, B6, and sometimes betaine. Getting homocysteine down to 8-10 μmol/L (much lower than the standard "normal") can slow or reverse early cognitive changes if you catch it early.

The point is not just to lower a number. It is to restore the methylation system so your genes can regulate properly, your neurotransmitters can balance, and your neurons can stay healthy.

SIDEBAR: When your genes matter

Your genetic variants are not your destiny, but they do shape how sensitive you are to imbalances.

An MTHFR variant means you need active folate, not regular folic acid. A COMT variant means you are naturally focused but need more stress support. A FUT2 variant means you need more targeted B12 and probiotic support.

Understanding this does not require expensive genetic testing. But if you know that certain systems are struggling, you can ask: "Do I have a variant in this gene?" and adjust your approach accordingly.

The goal is personalization: not a one-size-fits-all protocol, but a clear framework that lets you and your clinician dial in what actually works for you.

GLOSSARY: Key Terms for Chapter 10

Mg-ATP (Magnesium-ATP Complex): The biologically active form of ATP, in which magnesium ions bind to stabilize the molecule and enable energy transfer in cellular reactions.

Methylation: The addition of a methyl group to DNA, proteins, or other molecules. Controls gene expression, neurotransmitter balance, and DNA repair.

Homocysteine (Hcy): An amino acid produced during methionine metabolism. Elevated levels are linked to brain and vascular damage.

MTHFR (Methylenetetrahydrofolate Reductase): An enzyme that converts folate to 5-MTHF. Genetic variants reduce enzyme activity and elevate homocysteine.

COMT (Catechol-O-Methyltransferase): An enzyme that breaks down dopamine and estrogen. The Val158Met variant affects the clearance rate and stress resilience.

FUT2 (Fucosyltransferase 2): An enzyme affecting gut microbiota and B12 absorption. Variants alter immune function and nutrient absorption.

5-MTHF (5-Methyltetrahydrofolate): The active form of folate, used directly in methylation reactions.

SAMe (S-Adenosylmethionine): A methyl donor involved in neurotransmitter synthesis, detoxification, and gene regulation.

Epigenetics: Changes in gene expression that do not alter the DNA sequence itself.

Hyperhomocysteinemia (HHcy): Elevated blood homocysteine levels, linked to vascular and cognitive decline.

Leukoaraiosis: White matter lesions in the brain, associated with small-vessel disease and cognitive decline.

Nutrigenetics: The study of how genetic variants influence response to nutrients.

Personalized Nutrition: Tailoring dietary and supplement interventions based on genetics, metabolism, and individual patterns.

Energy system

(Mitochondria, Magnesium, Phosphorus/Creatine, Copper, Vitamin C)

- **Magnesium:** ATP: Most intracellular ATP is bound to magnesium as Mg-ATP, and this complex is what actually powers ATP-dependent enzymes. Magnesium is required for every kinase reaction and for the proper function of Complexes I and V, so low Mg impairs ATP generation even if caloric intake is adequate.
- Phosphocreatine buffer: Creatine and phosphocreatine act as a "rapid-response battery," shuttling high-energy phosphates between mitochondria and sites of demand (myofibrils, ion pumps, synapses), especially during high-intensity or rapidly changing loads.
- Copper at Complex IV: Copper is essential for cytochrome c oxidase (Complex IV); copper deficiency reduces Complex IV activity and mitochondrial respiratory capacity, particularly in high-energy tissues like the brain and spinal cord.
- Vitamin C as mitochondrial shield: Vitamin C scavenges ROS in aqueous compartments and helps protect mitochondrial membranes and mtDNA from oxidative damage, especially under stress or heavy exercise.

Clinical cues: "Can do baseline but crashes with peaks" (big workout, call schedule, deadline week) → think Mg + creatine + copper status + vitamin C sufficiency.

2. Structural System

(Collagen, Myelin, Vascular Integrity)

- Collagen and vitamin C: Prolyl and lysyl hydroxylases require ascorbate to produce hydroxyproline and hydroxylysine; these residues stabilize the triple helix and allow proper crosslinking. Subclinical C deficiency shows up as easy bruising, slow wound healing, tendon pain, and fragile gums long before frank scurvy.

- Myelin and copper: Copper is crucial for oligodendrocyte and Schwann-cell myelin maintenance via its roles in mitochondrial ATP production (Complex IV) and antioxidant defense (Cu/Zn SOD). Copper deficiency myelopathy presents with dorsal column dysfunction, gait ataxia, and proprioceptive loss, often mimicking B12 deficiency or MS.
- Vessels and ECM: Vitamin C, dependent collagen and elastin crosslinking, plus adequate copper and lysyl oxidase, maintain vascular tensile strength and prevent micro-hemorrhage and leukoaraiosis.

Clinical cues: "Bruises and tendons that don't make sense" or "slow, subtle gait and balance changes" → structural system; think vitamin C + copper + protein/aa sufficiency.

3. Information System

(Methylation, Homocysteine, Neurotransmitters, Epigenetics)

- Methylation core: B12, folate (5-MTHF), and B6 maintain one-carbon metabolism and remethylate homocysteine to methionine, generating SAMe for DNA, RNA, phospholipid, and neurotransmitter methylation.
- Homocysteine toxicity: Elevated tHcy drives oxidative stress, endothelial dysfunction, NMDA-mediated excitotoxicity, white matter damage, and accelerates medial temporal lobe atrophy. It also alters amyloid and tau biology epigenetically.
- Cognition and mood: Hyperhomocysteinemia is independently associated with vascular cognitive impairment: Alzheimer's disease, depression, and gait instability. Intervention trials using B12/folate/B6 lowering homocysteine have slowed brain atrophy and cognitive decline in MCI subgroups.
- Magnesium cross-talk: Mg is required for methionine adenosyltransferase (SAMe synthesis) and for DNA/RNA polymerases, linking Mg status to methylation efficiency and genome maintenance.

Clinical cues: "Brain fog + mood shift + elevated homocysteine (even if B12 'normal')" → information system bottleneck.

4. Security / Immune, Inflammatory System

(Zinc, Vitamin C, Magnesium, Boron)

- **Zinc: Essential for thymic function:** T-cell maturation, NK and cytotoxic T activity, and over 300 zinc-dependent enzymes. Zinc deficiency increases infection risk, impairs barrier integrity, and promotes a pro-inflammatory cytokine pattern.
- Vitamin C: Accumulates in neutrophils at millimolar concentrations; enhances chemotaxis, phagocytosis, oxidative burst, and then orderly apoptosis and efferocytosis, limiting collateral tissue damage and excessive NETosis.
- Magnesium: Emerging data show Mg modulates T-cell activation, cytokine production, and inflammasome activity; low Mg is associated with higher CRP, IL-6, and impaired immune regulation.
- Boron: Human work suggests boron lowers hs-CRP and TNF-α and may upregulate antioxidant enzymes, shifting the basal inflammatory set point downward.

Clinical cues: "Always a cold, always a little inflamed (hs-CRP >1, 2) with joint aches and brain fog" → prioritize zinc, vitamin C, Mg, + consider boron as an inflammatory 'voltage' modulator.

5. Hormonal Voltage System

(Boron, Zinc, Mg, Vitamin D, Copper, COMT/MTHFR Context)

- Boron and sex hormones: Small trials (6-10 mg/day) show boron can lower SHBG and increase free testosterone in men, modulate estradiol, and raise 25-OH vitamin D while lowering inflammatory markers. Mechanistically, boron appears to influence steroid hormone metabolism, vitamin D activation, and membrane transport.
- Zinc and steroidogenesis: Zinc is required for LH-driven testosterone synthesis and modulates 5α-reductase and aromatase activity; zinc deficiency lowers testosterone and impairs androgen receptor signaling.
- Magnesium and hormone signaling: Mg influences insulin receptor signaling, HPA axis tone, and sex steroid receptor function; hypomagnesemia is associated with insulin resistance, hypertension, and higher stress reactivity.

- Vitamin D and immune, endocrine cross-talk: Vitamin D modulates innate and adaptive immunity, HPT/HPA axes, and interacts with Mg and boron in calcium, phosphate and bone, hormone networks.
- Copper and neuroendocrine function: Copper is needed for dopamine β-hydroxylase (dopamine → norepinephrine) and for hypothalamic, pituitary neurotransmitter balance; both deficiency and excess can dysregulate mood, autonomic tone, and reproductive hormones.
- Genetic sensitivity (COMT/MTHFR): COMT Val158Met variants alter catecholamine and estrogen clearance; MTHFR variants alter methylation of steroid receptors and estrogen metabolism, changing how "voltage" (catecholamines, estrogens) is tolerated.

Clinical cues: "Hormones 'technically normal' but patient feels unstable, PMS, perimenopause chaos, low libido, flat mood" → think free hormone availability (SHBG), zinc/boron status, Mg for stress buffering, and COMT/MTHFR-driven sensitivity.

Five-system clinical summary

1. **Energy System** (Mitochondria, Mg, Phosphorus/Creatine, Copper, Vitamin C)

Generates and buffers cellular ATP, enabling you to handle both baseline and peak demands.

Symptoms when it fails: can do "normal days" but crash with hard weeks or workouts. Heavy legs, post-exertional fatigue, prolonged DOMS. Need caffeine to function; wired-tired at night.

Key molecules/nutrients: Magnesium (Mg-ATP), Creatine/phosphocreatine, Copper (Complex IV), Vitamin C (mitochondrial ROS control).

Useful labs: RBC magnesium, CMP (creatinine, liver, glucose), Creatine kinase (if overreaching), Copper, ceruloplasmin. Optional: lactate, urinary organic acids.

2. **Structural System** (Collagen, Myelin, Vessels)

Maintains physical integrity of tendons, joints, skin, vessels, and myelin.

Symptoms when it fails: easy bruising, slow wound healing. "Tendinous" pain, recurrent sprains. Subtle gait/balance changes, proprioceptive loss. Gum bleeding or sensitivity.

Key molecules/nutrients: Vitamin C (collagen hydroxylation), Copper (myelin, lysyl oxidase), Protein/amino acids (glycine, proline, lysine), Zinc (repair enzymes).

Useful labs: Plasma vitamin C, Copper, ceruloplasmin, CBC (anemia, cytopenias in copper issues), MRI (if myelopathy suspected), CRP (background inflammation).

3. **Information System** (Methylation, Homocysteine, Neurotransmitters, Epigenetics)

Regulates gene expression, neurotransmitter balance, and neural integrity.

Symptoms when it fails: Brain fog, slowed processing, word-finding issues. Mood lability, depression, anxiety. Headaches, sensory sensitivity. Family history of dementia or early strokes.

Key molecules/nutrients: B12, folate (5-MTHF), B6, choline, betaine, homocysteine, magnesium (SAMe synthesis, DNA repair).

Useful labs: Serum B12, folate, homocysteine (goal ~8-10 umol/L), MMA, holo-TC (if B12 borderline), RBC magnesium. Optional: genetic panel (MTHFR, COMT).

4. **Security / Immune-Inflammatory System** (Zinc, Vitamin C, Magnesium, Boron)

Detects and clears threats, manages inflammation, and resolves damage.

Symptoms when it fails: "I catch everything," frequent colds/URIs. Prolonged post-viral fatigue. Achy, puffy, low-grade inflammatory pain. hs-CRP mildly elevated; "inflammaging" pattern.

Key molecules/nutrients: Zinc (T-cell, NK function), Vitamin C (neutrophils, resolution), Magnesium (T-cell, cytokine modulation), Boron (CRP, TNF-α modulation).

Useful labs: CBC with diff, Zinc, copper, Zn:Cu ratio, Plasma vitamin C, hs-CRP, ESR. Optional: 8-OHdG, F2-isoprostanes (oxidative load).

5. **Hormonal Voltage System** (Boron, Zinc, Mg, Vitamin D, Copper, COMT/MTHFR Context)

Sets hormonal "voltage" and responsiveness (sex steroids, stress hormones, thyroid).

Symptoms when it fails: "Normal" labs but feel hormonally off: low libido, PMS/PMDD, perimenopause chaos. Energy and mood swings, mid-afternoon crash. Poor stress tolerance, wired-tired pattern. Body composition shifts despite similar inputs.

Key molecules/nutrients: Boron (SHBG, free T, vitamin D, inflammation), Zinc (steroidogenesis), Magnesium (receptor signaling, HPA axis), Vitamin D, Copper (dopamine to norepinephrine, neuroendocrine), COMT/MTHFR variants (estrogen/catechol clearance, receptor methylation).

Useful labs: SHBG, total and free testosterone, estradiol (plus progesterone in women), 25-OH vitamin D, TSH, free T4, free T3, Zinc, copper, Zn:Cu ratio. Optional: DUTCH or 24-hr urine hormones, genetic panel (COMT, MTHFR, FUT2).

CHAPTER 11: When the Current Fails

The Electrical Cascade of Cellular Dysfunction

Introduction: The sixty-eight minute cascade

August 14, 2003, 3:05 pm. A single power transmission line in northern Ohio sagged into an overgrown tree and failed. System operators, their alarm software already compromised by an earlier bug, remained unaware as electricity sought alternate paths through neighboring lines. Within three minutes, those lines became overloaded. By 3:30 pm, multiple transmission failures cascaded through Ohio and Michigan. The grid operator's computerized safeguards, designed to prevent exactly this scenario, had been silenced by a software failure 90 minutes earlier.

At 4:10 pm, voltage fluctuations propagated into Pennsylvania and New York. Plant operators watched helplessly as the wave of instability reached their facilities. One by one, protective relays, circuit breakers on a massive scale, detected the dangerous conditions and automatically disconnected their generators from the failing grid. This was supposed to save the system. Instead, it accelerated the collapse.

By 4:13 pm, just 68 minutes after that first tree contact, 265 power plants had gone offline. Fifty-five million people across eight US states and Ontario sat in darkness. The cascade was complete.

Now, imagine a different scenario.

You're sitting at your desk on a Tuesday afternoon when suddenly, a blood clot no larger than a grain of rice lodges in the middle cerebral artery supplying your left motor cortex. Blood flow drops to zero in the vessels downstream. Within 30 seconds, ATP production in those neurons falls by 50%. Within 2 minutes, the neurons begin to depolarize as their ion pumps slow. Within five minutes, calcium floods into cells at concentrations 100 to 1,000 times normal. Within 10 minutes, mitochondria become overloaded with calcium and begin producing massive amounts of reactive oxygen species instead of ATP.

By the 20-minute mark, the mitochondrial permeability transition pore, a molecular point of no return, has opened in millions of neurons. They are committed to death. By 30 minutes, if no intervention has occurred, an area of your motor cortex the size of a quarter has progressed from functioning tissue to irreversibly damaged necrotic core.

The pattern is identical to the 2003 blackout: one failure, cascade amplification, safety mechanisms overwhelmed, system collapse. The timescale is different, minutes instead of hours, but the principle is the same. In your brain right now, 86 billion "power plants" are generating electrical signals 100 times per second. Each one depends on thousands of mitochondria continuously producing ATP. When one critical neuron's mitochondria fail, a cascade can begin that you might recognize as a stroke, a seizure, or simply the gradual dimming of memory and cognition we call aging.

This is the story of how the living chip fails when its electrical system overloads and its power supply depletes. More importantly, it's the story of how to prevent that cascade before it reaches the point of no return.

Part 1: The electrical circuit of consciousness

Your Neuron Is a Battery-Powered Circuit

Consider a simple electrical circuit in your home: a light switch, copper wires, a light bulb, and a circuit breaker. When you flip the switch, voltage pushes electrons through the wire toward the bulb. The electrons encounter resistance from the wire material, which opposes their flow but allows enough current through to illuminate the bulb. If too many appliances draw power simultaneously, the current exceeds the wire's capacity. The wire heats up. The circuit breaker, sensing dangerous conditions, trips and disconnects the power before the wire can melt or catch fire.

Your neurons operate on strikingly similar principles, with one critical difference: they are battery-powered circuits that can never fully recharge.

The voltage in a neuron is called the membrane potential, measured not in volts but in millivolts (mV). At rest, your neurons maintain a charge difference of approximately -70 mV across their cell membrane, negative inside, positive outside. This is equivalent to about 10 million volts per meter of membrane thickness, making the neuron membrane one of the strongest electric fields in biology.

The current consists not of electrons flowing through copper, but ions, electrically charged atoms, flowing through channels in the cell membrane. The three primary ions are sodium (Na^+), potassium (K^+), and calcium (Ca^{2+}). During an action potential, approximately one billion sodium ions rush into a typical neuron, driven by both the electrical gradient and their concentration difference across the membrane (10 times higher outside than inside).

The resistance comes from multiple sources: the cell membrane itself acts as an insulator with resistance values of 1,000 to 10,000 $\Omega{\cdot}cm^2$, ion channels provide variable resistance depending on whether they're open or closed, and the cytoplasm inside the axon creates axial resistance that limits how fast signals can propagate. Input resistance, the total resistance "seen" at the neuron's cell body, varies considerably by cell type: pyramidal neurons show approximately 82 megaohms (MΩ), while granule cells can exceed 249 MΩ.

The circuit breaker is the refractory period. After a neuron fires an action potential, it enters an absolute refractory period lasting about 1 millisecond, during which it physically cannot fire again. The sodium channels are inactivated and require time to reset. This is followed by a relative refractory period of 3-4 milliseconds, during which the neuron can fire but requires stronger stimulation than usual. These refractory periods serve the same purpose as your home's circuit breaker: they prevent continuous, uncontrolled firing that would damage the system.

The power supply is the ATP continuously produced by mitochondria, which is immediately consumed by the Na^+/K^+-ATPase pumps. These molecular machines use ATP to export three sodium ions and import two potassium ions with each cycle. This restores the ion gradients that the action potential depleted.

📓 SIDEBAR: Neurons for 6th Graders

Your Brain Runs on Electricity!

Your neurons are like tiny batteries in your brain. Just like a TV remote needs batteries to send signals, your neurons need to be "charged up" to send messages.

Here's how it works:

- Your neuron keeps more of certain atoms (called ions) on the outside than on the inside

- When it's time to send a message, little doors (called channels) open
- The atoms rush inside like kids rushing into school when the bell rings
- This creates an electrical signal that zooms down the neuron
- Then tiny pumps work really hard to push those atoms back outside
- These pumps need energy (called ATP) from your cell's power plants (mitochondria)

The problem: Those pumps use up most of your neuron's energy just keeping it ready to fire! It's like your phone battery draining even when you're not using it, just keeping the screen ready to turn on.

What can go wrong:

- Too many signals at once = Overload (like plugging too many things into one outlet)
- Power runs out = The pumps stop working
- Without the pumps = Your neuron can't send messages anymore
- If this happens to lots of neurons = Stroke, seizure, or brain damage

When Circuits Overload: Excitotoxicity

Return to that household electrical circuit, but now imagine connecting ten high-power appliances to a circuit designed for five. Current surges through the wires, exceeding their rated capacity. Voltage begins to sag as the electrical system struggles to maintain the flow. The wires heat up from the excess current (a phenomenon called Joule heating, where heat = I^2R, current squared times resistance). Temperature rises. Insulation begins to degrade. If the circuit breaker fails to trip, the wire can melt, creating an open circuit, or short against other wires, creating a closed circuit to ground. In the worst case, the wire ignites nearby flammable materials. The overload has caused catastrophic failure.

Neurons experience a remarkably similar phenomenon called excitotoxicity, literally "toxic excitation." It occurs most dramatically during stroke, traumatic brain injury, and status epilepticus (prolonged seizure), but contributes to neurodegeneration in Alzheimer's, Parkinson's, and ALS as well.

The mechanism begins with excessive release of glutamate, the brain's primary excitatory neurotransmitter. Glutamate normally signals neurons to fire by opening ion channels, particularly NMDA receptors, specialized channels that are permeable to calcium when opened. Under normal conditions, a brief pulse of glutamate opens NMDA receptors, allowing a controlled influx of calcium that triggers downstream signaling cascades essential for learning and memory.

During excitotoxicity, glutamate concentrations in the synaptic space increase 10 to 100-fold. This occurs when energy failure prevents astrocytes (support cells) from clearing glutamate from the extracellular space, or when massive depolarization triggers uncontrolled glutamate release from neurons. The result: NMDA receptors and other glutamate receptors remain open for prolonged periods. Calcium pours into neurons.

Normal intracellular calcium concentration hovers around 100 nanomolar (nM). During excitotoxicity, this can increase to 100-1,000 micromolar (μM), a 1,000 to 10,000-fold increase. This calcium overload triggers a cascade of destructive processes:

Protease activation: Calcium activates calpains, enzymes that cleave structural proteins and break down the cytoskeleton. The neuron's internal scaffolding literally disassembles.

Phospholipase activation: These enzymes break down membrane phospholipids, destroying the integrity of both the plasma membrane and internal organelle membranes. The neuron becomes leaky.

Nitric oxide synthase activation: Excessive nitric oxide production leads to peroxynitrite formation, a reactive nitrogen species that damages proteins, lipids, and DNA through nitrosylation reactions.

Mitochondrial calcium overload: Mitochondria attempt to buffer the calcium surge by importing it through the mitochondrial calcium uniporter (MCU). But mitochondria can only handle so much. When mitochondrial matrix calcium exceeds a critical threshold, approximately 50-100 μM, the mitochondrial permeability transition pore (mPTP) opens.

This is the molecular point of no return.

The Overheating Effect: Metabolic Crisis

When an electrical circuit carries excess current, temperature rises. The increased thermal energy causes atoms in the metal lattice to vibrate more vigorously, which paradoxically increases resistance (positive temperature coefficient). More resistance generates more heat (I^2R), creating a positive feedback loop. If the system cannot dissipate heat faster than it's generated, temperature continues to climb until something breaks, insulation melts, solder joints fail, semiconductor junctions destroy themselves.

Neurons don't experience thermal overheating in the literal sense (brain temperature rises only about 1-2°C during intense activity). Instead, they experience metabolic overheating, a crisis of energy supply and demand.

Consider the energetics: a single action potential requires the Na^+/K^+-ATPase pump to restore gradients by exporting approximately 300-400 million sodium ions. Since the pump exchanges 3 sodium ions for 2 potassium ions per ATP molecule, each action potential requires roughly 100-130 million ATP molecules. For a neuron firing at 100 Hz (100 action potentials per second), this represents 10-13 billion ATP molecules per second just for the pumps, not counting the energy required for synaptic vesicle recycling, protein synthesis, axonal transport, and maintaining other ion gradients.

The numbers are staggering: the human brain, comprising only 2% of body weight, consumes 20% of resting metabolic energy. Of this energy, 30-70% goes directly to the Na^+/K^+-ATPase pumps. Neurons are operating near their energetic capacity under baseline conditions.

When the firing rate increases, as during a seizure, when neurons may fire at 500+ Hz, energy demand can increase 5 to 10-fold. Mitochondria attempt to compensate by increasing ATP production. The electron transport chain runs faster. Proton pumping accelerates. ATP synthase spins at maximum velocity.

But there are limits. Oxygen delivery may be insufficient (particularly during a stroke). Glucose supply may be inadequate (during hypoglycemia). The electron transport chain itself may be damaged or deficient (in mitochondrial diseases or aging). When demand exceeds supply, several pathological processes begin:

ATP depletion: Cellular ATP drops from 3-5 millimolar (mM) toward zero. Studies in cultured proximal tubule cells demonstrated that ATP depletion to 70% of normal levels triggers compensatory mechanisms (increased glycolysis and mobilization of phosphocreatine). Below 50%, ion gradient dissipation begins. Below

25%, apoptotic pathways activate. Below 15%, necrosis becomes inevitable.

Ion gradient collapse: As ATP levels fall, the Na^+/K^+ pumps slow proportionally. The ion gradients that normally require constant energy to maintain begin to dissipate. Sodium accumulates intracellularly; potassium leaks out. The resting membrane potential depolarizes from -70 mV toward -50 mV or even -40 mV.

Paradoxical hyperexcitability: Counterintuitively, neurons become more excitable as they depolarize. The membrane potential is closer to the threshold for firing action potentials (-55 mV), so smaller stimuli can trigger firing. This increases firing rate, which increases energy demand, which accelerates ATP depletion, a vicious cycle.

Cellular swelling: Sodium accumulation draws water into the cell osmotically, causing cytotoxic edema. The cell swells. In the confined space of the skull, this swelling compresses blood vessels, further reducing oxygen and glucose delivery, another vicious cycle.

Depolarization block: Eventually, the membrane becomes so depolarized that sodium channels remain inactivated. The neuron can no longer fire action potentials despite receiving stimulation. It has entered electrical silence, not because it's healthy and resting, but because it's so energy-depleted it cannot generate the voltages required for signaling.

Like an overheated circuit that has triggered its thermal shutdown, the neuron has ceased to function. Unlike a circuit that cools and resumes operation, if the energy crisis persists, the neuron will not recover.

Part 2: The battery that can't be recharged

The Fundamental Energy Storage Problem

Electrical circuits can store energy in capacitors and batteries. A capacitor, made of two conductive plates separated by an insulator, stores charge directly as separated positive and negative charges. Discharge is nearly instantaneous, microseconds to milliseconds. A battery stores energy chemically, with discharge times of minutes to hours depending on capacity and load. Both provide buffer capacity when the main power supply fails.

Your neurons lack this luxury. They cannot store ATP in meaningful quantities.

The reason is thermodynamic and evolutionary. ATP is an extraordinarily unstable molecule; its three phosphate groups are negatively charged and repel each other with considerable force. The phosphoanhydride bonds between these phosphates are "high-energy" bonds, meaning they release substantial free energy (approximately 30.5 kJ/mol under standard conditions, 50-60 kJ/mol under cellular conditions) when hydrolyzed to ADP or AMP. This instability makes ATP an excellent energy currency; it readily donates its phosphate group to drive otherwise unfavorable reactions, but it is a terrible energy storage molecule.

Cells maintain ATP concentrations of only 3-5 mM. For a typical neuron with a volume of approximately 4,000 cubic micrometers (μm^3), this represents roughly 10 million ATP molecules. If the neuron fires a single action potential requiring 100-130 million ATP just for the Na^+/K^+ pumps, and we account for synaptic transmission (which is even more energy-intensive), a single action potential can consume the entire ATP content of a small segment of axon.

Neurons compensate by producing ATP continuously. Mitochondria, particularly enriched at synapses (where energy demand is highest) and at the axon initial segment (where action potentials initiate), generate ATP at remarkable rates. The human body produces and consumes approximately 70 kilograms of ATP per day, nearly equal to body weight. This ATP is not stored; it is synthesized and consumed in a continuous cycle with an average lifetime of less than one minute.

There is one small buffer: phosphocreatine. This high-energy compound can transfer its phosphate group to ADP, regenerating ATP rapidly via the creatine kinase reaction. Muscle cells contain substantial phosphocreatine reserves (20-30 mM). The brain contains approximately 5-10 mM. This provides perhaps 5-10 seconds of buffer during an energy crisis, enough to buy time for mitochondria to ramp up production, but not enough to survive prolonged energy failure.

The clinical implications are profound. In cardiac arrest, when blood flow to the brain ceases, neurons have:

- 5-10 seconds of phosphocreatine buffer
- 10-30 seconds of residual ATP

- 1-2 minutes of glycolysis (anaerobic glucose metabolism, which produces only 2 ATP per glucose versus 32-36 ATP from oxidative phosphorylation)
- After 3-5 minutes: ion gradients collapse, calcium overload begins, mitochondrial damage initiates
- After 5-10 minutes: irreversible neuronal damage

This is why the window for successful resuscitation is so narrow. This is why "time is brain" during stroke, when every minute of delayed treatment results in loss of 1.9 million neurons, 14 billion synapses, and 12 kilometers of myelinated nerve fibers.

📓 SIDEBAR: Energy Crisis for 6th Graders

Why Your Brain Can't Store Energy Like a Battery

Imagine if your phone battery could only hold enough power for 5 seconds of use, and it had to make new electricity every single second while you were using it. That's how your brain works!

The Energy Problem:

- Your neurons make energy (ATP) constantly, like a factory that never stops
- They can't make big piles of ATP to save for later (it's too unstable)
- It's like trying to save lightning in a bottle; it just doesn't work
- Your body makes 70 kilograms (155 pounds!) of ATP every day
- That's almost as much as you weigh!
- But you don't get heavier because you use it up as fast as you make it

What happens when power runs out:

- **0-10 seconds**: Your brain uses its tiny backup supply (like the last bit of battery)
- **10-60 seconds**: Your brain switches to emergency power (makes energy without oxygen, but very slowly)
- **1-5 minutes**: The pumps that keep your neurons working start to slow down
- **5-10 minutes**: Your neurons start to break and can't be fixed

Why this matters:

- If your heart stops = brain has only 5-10 minutes before permanent damage
- If you have a stroke = every minute, millions of brain cells die
- This is why ambulances rush to the hospital!
- Doctors say "time is brain" because the faster you get help, the more brain cells survive

The Energy Depletion Cascade: A Timeline

The progression from normal function to irreversible damage follows a predictable timeline that has been characterized in multiple experimental models and clinical contexts.

T = 0 seconds: Insult begins

The trigger varies: arterial occlusion (stroke), cardiac arrest, hypoglycemia, mitochondrial toxin exposure, severe traumatic brain injury. Blood flow to a brain region drops to zero, or glucose delivery ceases, or oxidative phosphorylation stops. ATP production falls dramatically or stops entirely.

T = 30 seconds: ATP falls to 50%

Neurons detect the energy crisis via AMP-activated protein kinase (AMPK), a cellular energy sensor that is activated when the ATP/ADP ratio drops. AMPK triggers compensatory responses: glycolysis increases (attempting to generate ATP anaerobically), protein synthesis decreases (reducing energy consumption), autophagy activates (attempting to recycle damaged organelles for their components).

Phosphocreatine buffers are mobilized. The creatine kinase reaction accelerates, converting phosphocreatine to ATP. This provides perhaps 10-15 seconds of temporary support.

T = 2 minutes: ATP falls to 70%

Glycolysis is now running at maximum capacity, converting glucose to pyruvate and generating 2 ATP per glucose molecule (compared to 32-36 ATP when mitochondria are functioning). But glycolysis produces lactate as a byproduct. Lactate accumulates, decreasing pH. The intracellular environment becomes acidic, pH drops from 7.2 to 6.5 or lower.

Acidosis inhibits many enzymes. Ironically, it also inhibits some of the calcium-activated proteases that cause damage, providing a small protective effect initially. But the acidosis also indicates that the energy crisis is deepening.

The Na^+/K^+-ATPase pumps begin to slow. They're still working, but at perhaps 70-80% of normal capacity. Ion gradients start to weaken. The sodium gradient, normally 10:1 (outside:inside), might decrease to 8:1. The potassium gradient shifts similarly.

T = 5 minutes: ATP falls to 50%

Ion gradients have weakened substantially. Membrane potential depolarizes from -70 mV toward -55 to -60 mV. Neurons become hyperexcitable; as they approach the firing threshold, they discharge spontaneously or in response to minimal stimuli.

This creates a catastrophic increase in energy demand. Action potentials consume ATP. Synaptic transmission consumes even more ATP (vesicle recycling is one of the most energy-intensive neuronal processes). The neurons most affected by energy depletion fire more, further depleting their energy, creating a positive feedback loop.

Glutamate begins to accumulate in the extracellular space. Astrocytes normally take up glutamate via sodium-dependent transporters, but these transporters are ATP-dependent and slow as energy levels decline. Additionally, depolarized neurons release glutamate spontaneously.

T = 10 minutes: ATP falls to 25-30%

This represents a critical threshold. Multiple studies have identified that 25-30% of normal ATP levels mark the point at which apoptotic pathways activate irreversibly. The cell is committed to death, even if ATP levels subsequently recover.

Calcium has been entering neurons through voltage-gated channels (opened by depolarization) and NMDA receptors (opened by glutamate). Cytoplasmic calcium, normally 100 nM, has increased to 1-10 μM. Mitochondria attempt to buffer this calcium by importing it through the mitochondrial calcium uniporter.

Mitochondrial matrix calcium increases. When it exceeds approximately 50-100 μM, the mitochondrial permeability transition pore begins to open.

T = 15-20 minutes: ATP falls to 15% or below

The mPTP has opened. This creates a non-selective pore in the inner mitochondrial membrane with a diameter of approximately 3 nanometers, large enough for molecules up to 1,500 Daltons to pass through.

Consequences of mPTP opening:

- Proton gradient collapses (protons leak back into the matrix)
- ATP synthase reverses direction, consuming ATP instead of producing it
- ATP levels plummet further (positive feedback)
- Cytochrome c is released from the intermembrane space
- Reactive oxygen species production increases dramatically

Cytochrome c in the cytoplasm binds to Apaf-1 (apoptotic protease-activating factor-1), forming the apoptosome. The apoptosome activates caspase-9, which in turn activates executioner caspases (caspase-3, -6, -7). These caspases cleave hundreds of cellular proteins, systematically disassembling the cell. Even if ATP levels were somehow restored at this point, the apoptotic cascade proceeds to completion.

Simultaneously, necrotic processes accelerate. Without ATP, the plasma membrane Na^+/K^+ pumps have stopped. Sodium has accumulated intracellularly to near-equal concentrations inside and out. Water follows sodium osmotically. The cell swells dramatically, cytotoxic edema. The plasma membrane, stretched beyond its elastic limit, ruptures. Intracellular contents spill into the extracellular space, triggering inflammatory responses that damage adjacent cells.

T = 30 minutes: Complete failure

If no intervention has occurred, restoration of blood flow in stroke, return of spontaneous circulation after cardiac arrest, or glucose administration in hypoglycemia, the affected neurons are dead or dying irreversibly.

In stroke, this represents the "core" of the infarct: tissue that will definitely die. Surrounding it is the "penumbra": tissue with marginally adequate blood flow from collateral vessels, functioning abnormally but not yet committed to death. The penumbra can be saved if blood flow is restored quickly, but with every passing minute, more penumbral tissue transitions to the core.

The oft-cited statistic bears repeating: in a typical ischemic stroke affecting the middle cerebral artery territory, 1.9 million neurons die per minute. Over a 4.5-hour window (the maximum time for tissue plasminogen activator administration), 513 million neurons die, along with 14 billion synapses and 12 kilometers of myelinated axons. The brain ages 3.6 years each hour a stroke goes untreated.

Part 3: Resistance, interference, and the corruption of information

The Multiple Layers of Biological Resistance

Electrical engineers calculate circuit behavior using Ohm's Law: $V = IR$ (voltage equals current times resistance). Current flows in direct proportion to voltage and in inverse proportion to resistance. A wire with high resistance impedes current flow; low resistance allows current to flow freely.

Neurons obey the same physics, but with far more complexity. Rather than a single resistance value, neurons possess multiple, dynamic, and interacting resistances:

Membrane resistance (Rm): The lipid bilayer of the cell membrane is an excellent insulator. Its resistance, typically 1,000-10,000 $\Omega \cdot cm^2$, prevents ions from freely diffusing across. This is essential; without this resistance, ion gradients would dissipate instantly and neurons could not function. However, membrane resistance varies with ion channel density and activity. A membrane densely packed with open channels has lower resistance than one with few channels.

Channel resistance: Individual ion channels, when open, have conductance (the inverse of resistance) measured in picosiemens (pS). A typical sodium channel might have 10-20 pS conductance; potassium channels, 20-30 pS. While this may seem minuscule, a neuron might have millions of channels, and when many open simultaneously during an action potential, the total conductance becomes substantial.

Axial resistance (Ra): The cytoplasm inside the axon is not a perfect conductor. It has resistance that impedes the flow of ionic current longitudinally down the axon. Axial resistance, typically 50-200 $\Omega \cdot cm$, depends primarily on axon diameter. Wider axons have lower axial resistance (more cross-sectional area for current to flow), enabling faster signal propagation. This is why giant axons in squid can reach 1 millimeter in diameter: evolution's solution for rapid conduction before myelin evolved.

Input resistance (Rin): This is the total resistance "seen" at the soma (cell body) and represents the combination of membrane resistance and axial resistance throughout the dendritic tree. Input resistance determines how much the membrane potential changes in response to a given synaptic current. Studies using whole-cell patch clamp recordings demonstrate remarkable variability: pyramidal neurons exhibit approximately 82 MΩ, parvalbumin-positive interneurons 149 MΩ, and granule cells 249 MΩ. Higher input resistance means greater voltage change for the same current input, increased excitability.

Capacitance: While not technically resistance, the membrane capacitance profoundly affects neuronal electrical behavior. The cell membrane acts as a capacitor: two conductors (intracellular and extracellular fluid) separated by an insulator (lipid bilayer). Membrane capacitance is remarkably constant across species at approximately 1 microfarad per square centimeter ($\mu F/cm^2$). Total capacitance increases with membrane area; larger neurons have more capacitance.

Capacitance creates a time delay in voltage changes. When current is injected into a neuron, voltage doesn't change instantaneously; rather, it rises exponentially with a time constant $\tau = Rm \times Cm$ (membrane resistance times membrane capacitance). Typical neuronal time constants range from 10-50 milliseconds. This means that neurons act as low-pass filters: rapidly changing inputs are averaged and smoothed, while slowly changing inputs can build up over time (temporal summation).

What Interferes with Current Flow: The Resistance Cascade

Just as electrical signals face interference from multiple sources, resistive losses, capacitive delays, electromagnetic interference, thermal noise, biological signals face numerous obstacles that progressively degrade information transmission:

1. Metabolic Resistance (ATP Depletion)

As ATP levels fall, the Na^+/K^+ pumps slow proportionally. Ion gradients weaken. The "driving force" for any ion, the electrochemical gradient that pushes it through open channels, equals the difference between the membrane potential and that ion's equilibrium potential (the Nernst potential).

For sodium at rest:

- Membrane potential: -70 mV
- Sodium Nernst potential: +60 mV
- Driving force: -70 - (+60) = -130 mV (strong inward)

When ATP depletion causes gradients to weaken:

- Sodium gradient decreases from 10:1 to perhaps 5:1
- Sodium Nernst potential drops from +60 mV to +42 mV
- Membrane potential depolarizes to -55 mV
- New driving force: -55 - (+42) = -97 mV (25% reduction)

This 25% reduction in driving force means 25% less sodium influx during action potentials. Peak voltage decreases from +30 mV to perhaps +10 mV. Smaller action potentials are more likely to fail at branch points or to attenuate over distance. Signal transmission becomes unreliable.

2. Ion Gradient Resistance (Electrochemical Interference)

The weakening of ion gradients has second-order effects. Action potential propagation depends on the local current flow ahead of the propagating wave, which brings the adjacent membrane to threshold. If the action potential amplitude is reduced (smaller sodium influx due to weaker gradient), the local current is weaker. The adjacent membrane may fail to reach the threshold. Propagation fails, particularly at impedance mismatches such as branch points where an axon splits into two daughter branches.

Computational models demonstrate that action potentials can propagate reliably through a uniform axon even with 30-40% reduced amplitude, but fail at branch points with as little as 20% amplitude reduction. This creates a spatial pattern of failure: propagation succeeds in unbranched segments but fails at decision points where the signal must choose a path.

3. Channel Resistance (Physical Obstruction)

Multiple factors can increase channel resistance or decrease the number of functional channels:

Inactivation: Voltage-gated sodium channels possess a ball-and-chain inactivation mechanism. After opening in response to depolarization, an intracellular domain swings into the pore and physically blocks it within 1 millisecond. The channel remains inactivated until the membrane potential repolarizes below approximately -60 mV. During energy depletion, when membrane potential remains partially depolarized (-55 to -50 mV), a greater fraction of sodium channels remains inactivated at rest. Fewer channels are available to open during the next action potential.

Pharmacological blockade: Local anesthetics (lidocaine, bupivacaine) preferentially bind to open or inactivated sodium channels, blocking sodium influx and preventing action potential propagation. This is precisely the goal in anesthesia: to block pain signal propagation. Similar effects occur with toxins: tetrodotoxin from pufferfish binds sodium channels with extraordinary affinity (Kd ~ 1 nM), causing paralysis and death.

Disease states: Channelopathies, genetic mutations affecting ion channel genes, can increase or decrease channel function. Epilepsy can result from gain-of-function sodium channel mutations, causing hyperexcitability. Conversely, loss-of-function mutations cause periodic paralysis. Multiple sclerosis involves demyelination that exposes normally hidden potassium channels, allowing current to leak out and preventing action potential propagation.

pH and ionic strength: Channel function is exquisitely sensitive to local conditions. Acidosis (low pH) inhibits sodium channels and many other channels, providing a small protective effect during ischemia when lactate accumulation lowers pH. Conversely, altered extracellular potassium (which increases during intense neuronal activity when neurons release potassium) depolarizes adjacent cells and alters channel kinetics.

4. Membrane Resistance Changes (Dynamic Interference)

Membrane resistance is not fixed. It varies dynamically with channel opening and closing, and pathologically with membrane damage:

Increased leak currents: When membranes are damaged by oxidative stress, lipid peroxidation creates holes and structural defects. Ions leak across the membrane, decreasing membrane resistance. This creates a futile cycle: ion pumps work harder to restore gradients, consuming more ATP, depleting energy faster, causing more membrane damage.

Gap junction coupling: Some neurons are electrically coupled through gap junctions, protein channels connecting adjacent cells that allow ions and small molecules to pass directly. Gap junctions can shunt current away from its intended target. During an energy crisis, gap junctions may allow calcium and other toxic signals to spread from damaged to healthy neurons.

Demyelination effects: Myelin insulation increases membrane resistance in the internodal regions (between nodes of Ranvier) by 100 to 1,000-fold. In multiple sclerosis, autoimmune destruction of myelin eliminates this insulation. Membrane resistance drops. The current that should flow longitudinally to the next node instead leaks out radially through the demyelinated membrane. Additionally, the exposed membrane contains potassium channels that allow outward potassium current, further impeding propagation. Conduction velocity drops from 100 meters per second to 1 meter per second or fails entirely.

■ SIDEBAR: Resistance and Interference for 6th Graders

Why Signals Get Weaker and Confused

Imagine trying to have a conversation with your friend, but there are lots of problems:

Problem 1: Weak Batteries (Metabolic Resistance)

- Your walkie-talkie batteries are dying
- Your voice gets quieter and quieter
- Your friend can barely hear you
- **In your brain**: When energy runs low, electrical signals get weaker

Problem 2: Static on the Line (Channel Problems)

- Some of your walkie-talkie buttons are stuck
- Others don't work at all
- You can only use a few channels
- **In your brain**: Ion channels can get blocked or broken

Problem 3: Holes in the Wire (Membrane Damage)

- Your walkie-talkie case is cracked
- Electricity leaks out through the cracks
- The signal gets lost before reaching your friend

- **In your brain**: Damaged cell membranes leak ions

Problem 4: Bad Insulation (Demyelination)

- The plastic coating on wires gets stripped off
- Electricity escapes into the wrong places
- Messages don't reach where they're supposed to go
- **In your brain**: Diseases like MS damage the insulation (myelin) around neurons

What Happens to Information:

- First: High-speed information is lost (like losing the high notes in music)
- Then: Medium-speed information gets corrupted (like a scratched CD)
- Finally: Even slow, simple information fails (like a phone call dropping completely)

This is why when your brain has problems, you might lose:

- Quick reactions first
- Then memory and attention
- Then basic functions last

Frequency-Dependent Failure: When Information Becomes Noise

Information in the nervous system is encoded in multiple ways, but two are predominant: **rate coding** (how frequently a neuron fires) and **temporal coding** (the precise timing of spikes). A neuron responding to a bright light might fire at 100 Hz; in darkness, perhaps 10 Hz. A neuron participating in memory retrieval might fire in precise temporal relationships with other neurons, with timing accuracy of 1-2 milliseconds.

Energy depletion and the resistance changes it causes systematically degrade both forms of coding:

Rate coding degradation: As ATP depletes and ion gradients weaken, the maximum sustainable firing rate decreases. A neuron that could fire at 100 Hz under normal conditions might manage only 50 Hz at 70% ATP, 20 Hz at 50% ATP, and become silent at 25% ATP. The dynamic range of the neuron, the difference between minimum and maximum firing rates, is compressed. A neuron that could encode 10 different stimulus intensities by varying firing rate between

10-100 Hz might be able to encode only 3 intensities (10-30 Hz) when energy-depleted.

Information theory quantifies this loss. If a neuron's firing rate can take on N distinguishable values, it encodes $\log_2(N)$ bits of information per spike. A neuron with 10 distinguishable rates (10, 20, 30... 100 Hz) encodes $\log_2(10) \approx 3.3$ bits per spike. Compressed to 3 rates, it encodes $\log_2(3) \approx 1.6$ bits per spike, a 52% information loss.

Temporal coding degradation: Precise spike timing degrades even more rapidly. Temporal precision depends on rapid, reliable action potential initiation and propagation. Multiple factors reduce precision during an energy crisis:

Increased spike jitter: The time from stimulus to spike becomes more variable. Normally, spike timing might vary by ±0.5 milliseconds across trials. During energy depletion, this increases to ±2-5 milliseconds. Information encoded in sub-millisecond timing relationships is lost.

Propagation velocity variability: Action potential conduction velocity depends on the amplitude and rate of rise of the action potential. As these decrease (due to weakened ion gradients), velocity becomes more variable. A signal that normally arrives at a synapse 5.0 milliseconds after initiation might arrive anywhere from 4.5 to 6.5 milliseconds. Neural networks that depend on precise temporal convergence fail to compute correctly.

Refractory period lengthening: Recovery from action potentials takes longer when ion gradients are weak and ion pumps are slow. The relative refractory period extends from 3-4 milliseconds to 10-20 milliseconds. Minimum inter-spike interval increases. High-frequency information is physically impossible to transmit.

Increased spontaneous firing: Energy-depleted, depolarized neurons fire spontaneously even without input. This "noise" firing increases the background rate. Signal-to-noise ratio degrades. Meaningful signals become difficult to distinguish from random activity.

The progressive information collapse:

At 90% ATP— Subtle: High-frequency rate coding (>100 Hz) fails first, sub-millisecond temporal precision degrades.

Clinically: No symptoms or subtle deficits in rapid processing.

At 70% ATP— Moderate: Maximum firing rate drops to 50 Hz, temporal precision to ±2 ms.

Clinically: Slowed reaction times, attention deficits, working memory impairment.

At 50% ATP —Severe: Maximum firing rate 20 Hz, temporal precision ±5 ms, significant spontaneous firing.

Clinically: Confusion, inability to form new memories, impaired consciousness.

At 25% ATP Critical: Most neurons fire irregularly at 5-10 Hz or are silent, no temporal precision.

Clinically: Loss of consciousness, with only brain stem reflexes remaining.

Below 15% ATP— Complete: Electrical silence, no information transmission.

Clinically: Brain death.

The living chip processes information through electrical signals transmitted across chemical synapses by billions of neurons firing in precise spatiotemporal patterns. When energy fails, the chip doesn't suddenly stop; it progressively loses computational capacity, first the highest-frequency information, then the mid-frequency, then the basic functions. Like a computer processor throttling down as it overheats, the brain throttles its information processing as it runs out of power. Unlike a computer that stabilizes at reduced performance, the brain's energy crisis, if not reversed, continues to worsen through positive feedback loops until complete system failure.

PART 4: REVERSE CURRENTS AND THE TOXIC BACKFLOW

The Electron Transport Chain: A One-Way Street That Can Run Backward

The electron transport chain (ETC) in mitochondria functions, under normal conditions, as a precisely orchestrated sequence of electron transfers coupled to proton pumping. Electrons enter at Complex I (from NADH) or Complex II (from $FADH_2$), flow through coenzyme Q, Complex III, cytochrome c, and finally Complex IV, where they reduce oxygen to water. At Complexes I, III, and IV, this electron flow drives proton pumping from the mitochondrial matrix to the intermembrane space, creating an electrochemical gradient: the mitochondrial membrane potential, typically -140 to -180 mV (negative inside).

This gradient powers ATP synthase, which uses the energy of protons flowing back into the matrix to drive the phosphorylation of ADP to ATP, approximately 2.5 ATP per pair of electrons entering at Complex I, 1.5 ATP per pair entering at Complex II.

The system is directional by design: electrons flow "downhill" energetically from NADH (high redox potential) to oxygen (low redox potential), releasing energy in controlled steps. The direction is thermodynamically favorable, spontaneous and irreversible under normal conditions.

But "normal conditions" is the critical qualifier.

Reverse Electron Transport (RET): Under specific pathological conditions, particularly high mitochondrial membrane potential combined with abundant succinate (the substrate for Complex II) and reduced coenzyme Q pool, electrons can flow *backward* through Complex I. Instead of NADH donating electrons to Complex I, Complex I forces electrons onto NAD^+, reducing it to NADH. This requires energy input (drawn from the proton gradient), making it thermodynamically unfavorable but possible when conditions are right.

The problem: RET at Complex I produces reactive oxygen species (ROS) at extraordinarily high rates, potentially converting 50% or more of consumed oxygen to superoxide rather than the 2-4% under normal forward transport. This superoxide production occurs at the flavin mononucleotide (FMN) site of Complex I, where partially reduced FMN can directly reduce oxygen to superoxide.

When does RET occur?

Ischemia-reperfusion injury: During ischemia (loss of blood flow), oxygen supply drops to zero but substrate-level phosphorylation continues. Succinate accumulates from several sources: reversal of succinate dehydrogenase (Complex II), breakdown of accumulated fumarate, and de novo synthesis from glutamate. When blood flow is restored (reperfusion), oxygen suddenly returns. Abundant succinate drives Complex II, reducing the coenzyme Q pool. If the membrane potential is high (because ATP synthase has been inhibited or damaged), electrons back up and force their way backward through

Complex I. Massive ROS production ensues, often called the "ROS burst" of reperfusion.

Studies using RET-specific inhibitors (metformin, rotenone at low doses) demonstrate that RET contributes significantly to reperfusion injury. Blocking RET during the first minutes of reperfusion reduces infarct size by 30-50% in animal models of stroke and myocardial infarction.

High fat oxidation states: Beta-oxidation of fatty acids produces abundant $FADH_2$ (which enters at Complex II) and acetyl-CoA (which feeds the TCA cycle, producing more $FADH_2$). If ATP demand is low (membrane potential is high) but fatty acid oxidation is high, as during a ketogenic diet with insufficient energy expenditure, the coenzyme Q pool becomes severely reduced. This creates conditions favoring RET and increased ROS production.

Mitochondrial dysfunction: In aging and neurodegenerative disease, damaged respiratory chain complexes may operate less efficiently, creating localized regions of over-reduction despite overall decreased ATP production. These dysfunctional mitochondria can produce disproportionate ROS through both forward and reverse electron transport.

The consequences of ROS overproduction:

Superoxide (O_2^-) is converted to hydrogen peroxide (H_2O_2) by superoxide dismutase. Hydrogen peroxide, while less reactive than superoxide, can diffuse through membranes and, in the presence of iron, undergo Fenton chemistry to produce hydroxyl radical (·OH), the most reactive ROS, capable of damaging virtually any biological molecule it contacts

Lipid peroxidation: Hydroxyl radical attacks polyunsaturated fatty acids in membranes, initiating chain reactions that propagate through the lipid bilayer. Lipid peroxidation products include 4-hydroxynonenal (4-HNE) and malondialdehyde (MDA), both of which covalently modify proteins, inactivating enzymes and transporters. The membrane becomes rigid, leaky, and dysfunctional.

Protein oxidation: ROS oxidize amino acid side chains, particularly cysteine, methionine, and tyrosine residues. Oxidized proteins often misfold and aggregate. Mitochondrial proteins, the very respiratory chain complexes producing ROS, are particularly vulnerable, creating a vicious cycle: ROS damage complexes → damaged complexes produce more ROS → more damage.

mtDNA damage: Mitochondrial DNA, located in the matrix with minimal protective histones and adjacent to the ROS-producing respiratory chain, accumulates damage at rates 10 to 20 times higher than nuclear DNA. mtDNA encodes 13 critical respiratory chain proteins. Mutations in these genes further impair respiratory function, producing more ROS, and creating another vicious cycle.

Calcium dysregulation: ROS enhance calcium influx through plasma membrane channels and promote calcium release from intracellular stores. Simultaneously, ROS inhibit calcium pumps that normally export calcium. The result: calcium overload, which triggers the opening of the mitochondrial permeability transition pore, further worsening mitochondrial function.

When Pumps Run Backward: The Na^+/Ca^{2+} Exchanger Reversal

Normally, the Na^+/Ca^{2+} exchanger (NCX) exports one calcium ion in exchange for importing three sodium ions, driven by the sodium gradient (maintained by the Na^+/K^+-ATPase). This is a critical mechanism for calcium homeostasis, accounting for approximately 20% of calcium removal from neurons.

But the NCX is electrogenic (net charge movement) and reversible. Its direction depends on both the sodium gradient and the membrane potential. The reversal potential, the voltage at which NCX changes direction, can be calculated from the Nernst-like equation:

ENCX = 3ENa - 2ECa

Under normal conditions (membrane at -70 mV, strong sodium gradient), the exchanger runs in "forward" mode: sodium in, calcium out. But when both the membrane potential depolarizes (approaching -40 mV) and intracellular sodium accumulates (under a weak gradient), the exchanger can reverse: sodium out, calcium in.

This reversal is catastrophic. Rather than helping to reduce calcium overload, the NCX becomes a calcium influx pathway, exacerbating the very problem it normally solves. Studies of cardiac ischemia (where NCX reversal is well-characterized) demonstrate that NCX reversal contributes significantly to calcium overload and cell death. Specific NCX inhibitors that preferentially block reverse mode (like

KB-R7943) provide protection in models of ischemia and excitotoxicity.

The broader principle: **ion transporters and exchangers evolved to operate within specific ranges of membrane potential and ion gradients. During an energy crisis, when these parameters move outside normal ranges, transporters can reverse, run futilely, or become pathologically active, converting from protective mechanisms to destructive forces.**

Part 5: The cascade Accelerates— positive feedback and system collapse

The Mitochondrial Permeability Transition Pore: Point of No Return

The mitochondrial permeability transition pore (mPTP) represents a molecular decision point between cellular life and death. Under normal conditions, the mPTP opens transiently, for milliseconds, to release calcium from mitochondria when matrix calcium becomes elevated. These brief openings are reversible and protective.

Under pathological conditions, sustained high matrix calcium (>50-100 μM), oxidative stress, low ATP, low pH (temporarily inhibits opening, but prolonged acidosis eventually promotes it), and high inorganic phosphate can cause the mPTP to open persistently. The pore, with a diameter of approximately 3 nanometers, allows the passage of molecules up to 1,500 Daltons.

Consequences of persistent mPTP opening:

Mitochondrial membrane potential collapse: The electrochemical gradient that powers ATP synthase dissipates. Protons leak back into the matrix through the open pore. $\Delta\Psi m$ decreases from -140 to -180 mV toward zero.

ATP synthase reversal: Without the proton gradient to drive it forward (synthesizing ATP), ATP synthase runs backward, hydrolyzing ATP to pump protons outward, attempting to restore the gradient. This is futile; the pore immediately leaks protons back. The net effect: ATP consumption rather than production, accelerating energy depletion.

Cytochrome c release: Collapse of the outer mitochondrial membrane integrity (through swelling and rupture) releases cytochrome c, normally confined to the intermembrane space, into the cytoplasm. Cytochrome c binds Apaf-1, forming the apoptosome, which activates caspase-9 and initiates the caspase cascade. Apoptosis proceeds to completion even if the initial insult is removed.

Mitochondrial swelling and rupture: Osmotic forces draw water into the matrix through the open pore. The mitochondrion swells. The outer membrane, less elastic than the inner membrane, ruptures. Additional pro-apoptotic factors (AIF, Smac/DIABLO, endonuclease G) are released, activating both caspase-dependent and caspase-independent cell death pathways.

The mPTP represents a point of no return because its opening triggers multiple irreversible processes simultaneously. Even if the mPTP opening is brief (10-30 seconds) and the pore then closes, sufficient cytochrome c may have been released to commit the cell to apoptosis. Experimental studies demonstrate that preventing mPTP opening with cyclosporine A (which inhibits cyclophilin D, a component of the mPTP complex) reduces infarct size by 30-40% in stroke models when administered during reperfusion.

The Positive Feedback Loops: Why Rescue Becomes Impossible

Multiple interconnected positive feedback loops accelerate neuronal energy crisis from a potentially recoverable insult to irreversible damage:

Loop 1: ATP depletion → Ion pump failure → Depolarization → Increased firing → More ATP depletion

As described earlier, ATP depletion slows the Na^+/K^+ pumps, causing partial depolarization. Depolarized neurons fire more readily (hyperexcitability). Increased firing consumes more ATP for pump restoration. A 10% decrease in ATP might increase firing by 20%, which in turn increases ATP consumption by 30%, creating a 50% decrease in ATP and exponential acceleration.

Loop 2: ATP depletion → Pump failure → Calcium accumulation → Mitochondrial damage → Less ATP production

Energy depletion prevents calcium pumps (plasma membrane PMCA, ER/SR SERCA) from functioning. Calcium accumulates. Mitochondria take up excess calcium, which triggers mPTP opening, which damages mitochondria, which reduces ATP production further. Each iteration through this loop amplifies the deficit.

Loop 3: Mitochondrial dysfunction → ROS production → Mitochondrial damage → More ROS

Damaged mitochondria produce ROS. ROS damage respiratory chain complexes and mtDNA. Damaged complexes produce more ROS. The cycle accelerates until mitochondria are producing almost entirely ROS and almost no ATP, resulting in complete functional failure.

Loop 4: Membrane depolarization → Glutamate release → NMDA activation → Calcium influx → More depolarization

Depolarized neurons release glutamate. Glutamate opens NMDA receptors on neighboring neurons. Calcium enters through NMDA receptors, causing depolarization. Depolarized neurons release more glutamate. The excitotoxic cascade spreads through neural networks.

Loop 5: Cellular swelling → Vascular compression → Reduced blood flow → Worsened ischemia

Ion pump failure causes sodium and water accumulation (cytotoxic edema). Cells swell. In the rigid confines of the skull, swelling compresses blood vessels, reducing blood flow to adjacent regions. Those regions become ischemic, triggering the same cascade. The infarct expands spatially.

The mathematical inevitability of cascade failure:

Positive feedback loops create exponential growth. A quantity growing by positive feedback follows the equation:

$dX/dt = k \cdot X$

Where X is the quantity (e.g., calcium concentration, ROS levels) and k is the rate constant. The solution is exponential growth:

$X(t) = X_0 \cdot e^{(kt)}$

For example, if ROS production doubles every 5 minutes ($k = 0.139$ min^{-1}), then:

- T=0: ROS = 1× baseline
- T=5 min: ROS = 2× baseline
- T=10 min: ROS = 4× baseline
- T=15 min: ROS = 8× baseline
- T=20 min: ROS = 16× baseline

By 20 minutes, ROS has overwhelmed all antioxidant defenses. Compare this to linear growth (adding a constant amount at each time step), which might take 80 minutes to reach 16× the baseline. Positive feedback collapses the system exponentially faster than linear processes can compensate.

This is why intervention windows are so narrow. There exists a critical threshold, around 25-30% of normal ATP, or 10-15 minutes into ischemia, beyond which positive feedback loops dominate and the cascade becomes irreversible. Before this threshold, restoring blood flow or providing energy substrates can rescue neurons. Beyond this threshold, restoration of blood flow may paradoxically worsen damage (reperfusion injury), as oxygen can drive massive ROS production from dysfunctional mitochondria.

📕 SIDEBAR: The Cascade for 6th Graders

Why Damage Gets Worse So Fast: The Feedback Loop

Imagine you're in a room with one candle for light. You're trying to read a book.

Step 1: The candle starts to go out → Room gets darker

Step 2: You lean closer to see → You accidentally blow on the candle

Step 3: Candle gets even dimmer → You lean even closer

Step 4: You knock the candle over → Now it's completely dark

Step 5: In the dark, you trip and hurt yourself → Makes everything worse

This is called a "positive feedback loop", but there's nothing positive about it!

In your brain during a stroke:

- **Step 1**: Energy starts running out → Neurons work harder to fix it
- **Step 2**: Working harder uses MORE energy → Energy runs out faster
- **Step 3**: Without energy → Toxic calcium floods in
- **Step 4**: Calcium damages the power plants (mitochondria) → Even less energy
- **Step 5**: Damaged power plants make poison (ROS) → Damages everything else

Why doctors rush:

- **0-10 minutes**: Problem starting, but fixable
- **10-20 minutes**: Getting worse fast, still might be fixable
- **20-30 minutes**: Approaching "point of no return"
- **After 30+ minutes**: Feedback loops too strong, permanent damage

The key lesson: The sooner you stop the first problem, the easier it is to prevent all the other problems that follow. Every minute counts!

From Single Cell to Network Collapse: Spatial Propagation

Thus far, we've focused on events within individual neurons. But neurons don't exist in isolation; they form networks. The energy crisis propagates spatially through these networks, much as the 2003 blackout cascaded from one power plant to the next.

Mechanisms of spatial propagation:

Vascular insufficiency: The primary infarct (dead tissue) is surrounded by penumbra, tissue with marginal blood flow from collateral vessels. Metabolically stressed but not yet dead, penumbral neurons function abnormally. As they become depolarized and release glutamate, they trigger spreading depolarization (also called cortical spreading depression), a wave of neuronal and glial depolarization that propagates at 2-5 mm/min across the cortex. Each spreading depolarization event causes a transient increase in energy demand (to restore ion gradients), worsening the already-tenuous energy supply. Repeated waves of spreading depolarization convert penumbra to core, salvageable tissue to dead tissue.

Cytotoxic edema and mechanical compression: Swollen neurons and glia compress local microvasculature, reducing blood flow in adjacent regions. Those regions then become ischemic and swell, compressing their neighboring regions. The infarct expands like a slow-motion explosion.

Inflammatory cascade: Dead and dying neurons release damage-associated molecular patterns (DAMPs), intracellular molecules like ATP, HMGB1, and heat shock proteins that, when released extracellularly, activate immune responses. Microglia (brain-resident immune cells) become activated, releasing cytokines (TNF-α, IL-1β, IL-6) and reactive oxygen and nitrogen species. These inflammatory mediators damage adjacent neurons. Activated microglia also become migratory, spreading inflammation to distant brain regions.

Network effects: In neural circuits, loss of 10% of neurons increases the computational and metabolic load on the remaining 90%. They must fire more frequently to maintain circuit function. Increased firing means increased energy consumption. Energy-stressed neurons are more vulnerable to damage. The remaining 90% begin to fail at accelerated rates. This is why neurodegeneration often follows sigmoid kinetics: slow initial progression (compensatory mechanisms maintaining function despite ongoing cell loss), followed by rapid acceleration (compensation failing), followed by plateau (extensive damage, little function remaining).

The network collapse parallels the power grid cascade:

In the 2003 blackout:

- Initial failure created a load imbalance
- Adjacent components took on excess load
- Those components became overloaded and failed
- Remaining grid components faced even more imbalance
- Cascade accelerated until protective systems disconnected generators
- System collapsed to zero output

In stroke:

- Initial infarct creates functional deficit
- Adjacent neurons increase activity to compensate
- Those neurons become metabolically stressed and fail
- Remaining neurons face even more demand
- Cascade accelerates until neurons enter depolarization block
- Network function collapses to zero

The parallel is not metaphorical; it is an identical underlying mathematics. Any system in which components are interdependent, failure of one component increases the load on the remaining components, and positive feedback exists, will exhibit cascade failure dynamics. Power grids, financial markets, immune responses, and neural networks follow the same principles.

The key insight for intervention: Cascade failures can be stopped by breaking the positive feedback loops or by increasing system resilience (spare capacity, redundancy, repair mechanisms) before the critical threshold is reached. In power grids, this means load shedding, redundant transmission paths, and rapid protective relay response. In the brain, this means restoring blood flow (thrombolysis, thrombectomy), providing alternative energy substrates (ketones, lactate), blocking excitotoxicity (NMDA antagonists, though clinical trials have been disappointing), and preventing ROS damage (antioxidants, mPTP inhibitors).

Part 6: Root causes, why the living Chip fails

We have described the cascade: how energy depletion and electrical dysfunction amplify each other through positive feedback, leading to system failure. But what initiates the cascade? Understanding root causes is essential for prevention.

Primary Energy Failure: When Generators Cannot Produce Power

Mitochondrial DNA mutations: The mitochondrial genome is a small (16,569 base pair) circular DNA encoding 13 respiratory chain proteins, 22 tRNAs, and 2 rRNAs. It is maternally inherited and present in multiple copies per cell (heteroplasmy). Mutations accumulate with age, approximately 0.5-1% increase per decade. Most cells tolerate substantial mtDNA mutation burden (up to 60-80%) before respiratory function fails, due to complementation between wild-type and mutant genomes. However, once the threshold is exceeded, ATP production plummets.

Inherited mitochondrial diseases (MELAS, MERRF, Leigh syndrome) typically involve higher mutation loads (70-90%) and present in childhood or young adulthood with neurological symptoms: seizures, stroke-like episodes, ataxia, cognitive decline, and manifestations of neuronal energy failure.

Acquired mtDNA mutations increase with age and in neurodegenerative diseases. Post-mortem studies of Alzheimer's disease patients show 3-5 fold increases in mtDNA mutations in affected brain regions compared to age-matched controls.

Respiratory chain complex deficiencies: Beyond mtDNA mutations, nuclear genes encoding most respiratory chain proteins (>1,500 genes involved in mitochondrial function) can be mutated or polymorphic variants with reduced function. Complex I deficiency is the most common (40% of mitochondrial diseases) and particularly devastating. Complex I is responsible for approximately 40% of proton pumping and is a major site of ROS production when deficient.

Fuel supply disruption: Even with normal mitochondria, inadequate substrate delivery causes energy failure:

Hypoglycemia (<50 mg/dL): Neurons depend almost exclusively on glucose as fuel. Below 50 mg/dL, cognitive symptoms appear, including confusion and difficulty concentrating. Below 30 mg/dL, loss of consciousness occurs. Below 20 mg/dL, seizures and permanent brain damage can result.

Ischemia/hypoxia: Oxygen is the final electron acceptor in the electron transport chain. Without oxygen, oxidative phosphorylation stops. Glycolysis can provide 2 ATP per glucose, but this is insufficient for neurons and unsustainable due to lactate accumulation and acidosis.

Thiamine (vitamin B1) deficiency: Thiamine pyrophosphate is a cofactor for pyruvate dehydrogenase (converts pyruvate to acetyl-CoA) and α-ketoglutarate dehydrogenase (TCA cycle enzyme). Thiamine deficiency, most common in alcoholics, causes Wernicke-Korsakoff syndrome: acute confusion, ataxia, eye movement abnormalities (Wernicke encephalopathy) followed by permanent memory deficits (Korsakoff syndrome). The pathology: neuronal energy failure in mammillary bodies, thalamus, and other diencephalic structures.

Primary Electrical Failure: When Circuits Malfunction

Channelopathies: Genetic mutations affecting ion channel genes cause diverse diseases. Sodium channelopathies (SCN genes) cause epilepsy (gain-of-function mutations increasing neuronal excitability) or periodic paralysis (loss-of-function mutations preventing muscle action potentials). Potassium channelopathies (KCNQ genes) cause cardiac arrhythmias (long QT syndrome) and episodic ataxia. Calcium channelopathies cause familial hemiplegic migraine and ataxia.

These are primary electrical failures; the power supply (mitochondria) is fine, but the circuit itself is miswired or has faulty components.

Demyelination: Multiple sclerosis, Guillain-Barré syndrome, and leukodystrophies involve the destruction of myelin, the insulation that enables rapid action potential propagation. Without myelin, conduction velocity drops 10 to 100-fold, action potentials fail to propagate, and, critically, energy consumption increases because more membrane must be depolarized per unit distance traveled.

Oxidative Stress: The Overheating That Damages Everything

Normal metabolism produces ROS as a byproduct; 2-4% of oxygen consumed is incompletely reduced to superoxide. Antioxidant systems (superoxide dismutase, catalase, glutathione peroxidase, vitamins E and C) normally neutralize this ROS. Damage occurs when ROS production exceeds antioxidant capacity.

Excessive ROS production: Mitochondrial dysfunction (damaged respiratory chain complexes, reverse electron transport), inflammation (microglial activation), and toxin exposure increase ROS production from 2-4% to 10-50%.

Antioxidant depletion: Aging, neurodegenerative disease, and chronic stress deplete antioxidants. Glutathione, the most abundant cellular antioxidant, decreases 20-40% with age and is further depleted in Alzheimer's and Parkinson's disease.

Calcium Dysregulation: The Short Circuit

Calcium, normally maintained at ~100 nM cytoplasmic concentration, serves as a ubiquitous second messenger. But concentrations above ~1-10 μM become toxic. Calcium dysregulation occurs through:

Excessive influx: NMDA receptor overactivation (excitotoxicity), voltage-gated calcium channel activation (from depolarization), reversed Na^+/Ca^{2+} exchanger operation (during energy failure), and store-operated calcium entry (when ER calcium stores deplete).

Impaired buffering: ATP-dependent calcium pumps (PMCA, SERCA) slow or fail during an energy crisis. Mitochondria, attempting to buffer excess calcium, become overloaded and undergo permeability transition.

The common pathway: Regardless of initial cause, energy failure, electrical dysfunction, oxidative stress, inflammation, and elevated intracellular calcium are the final common pathway to cell death. This is why calcium dysregulation represents the convergence point of diverse insults.

Aging, Inflammation, Toxins, and Neurodegeneration

Space precludes exhaustive discussion, but briefly:

Aging: Progressive accumulation of mtDNA mutations, declining mitochondrial function (20% decrease in respiratory capacity by age 70), impaired protein homeostasis, chronic low-grade inflammation ("inflammaging"), and decreased antioxidant capacity. Aging is not a disease per se, but rather a progressive decline in system resilience that makes other insults more likely to cascade into failure.

Inflammation: Microglial activation releases cytokines, chemokines, and ROS that can directly damage neurons and impair mitochondrial function. Chronic inflammation (from obesity, diabetes, chronic infections, autoimmune disease) contributes to neurodegeneration.

Toxins: Environmental toxins (heavy metals, pesticides, industrial chemicals) and pharmaceutical agents (certain antipsychotics, statins, chemotherapy) can directly inhibit mitochondrial function or increase oxidative stress.

Neurodegeneration: Alzheimer's, Parkinson's, Huntington's, and ALS all involve, as a core feature, mitochondrial dysfunction and bioenergetic failure. Whether this is primary (mitochondrial cascade hypothesis of Alzheimer's) or secondary (downstream of protein aggregation or other pathology) remains debated, but the end result is the same: neurons cannot generate sufficient ATP to maintain function, and the cascade begins.

Conclusion: Resilience of the living Chip

The living chip, your brain, with its 86 billion neurons firing 100 times per second, each powered by thousands of mitochondria producing 70 kilograms of ATP per day, is simultaneously robust and fragile.

Robust because of redundancy: multiple neurons encode the same information; multiple mitochondria per cell; multiple antioxidant systems; multiple repair mechanisms. Neural plasticity allows surviving neurons to take over the functions of damaged ones. Mitophagy (selective autophagy of damaged mitochondria) removes dysfunctional units before they poison the cell. DNA repair enzymes fix mutations before they accumulate. The system is engineered for resilience.

Fragile because of cascade dynamics: one failure can amplify through positive feedback loops to system collapse. The inability to store ATP means continuous dependence on mitochondrial function. The energy cost of maintaining ion gradients means neurons operate near maximum capacity with minimal spare energy. The confined space of the skull means swelling from injury directly compresses tissue, worsening ischemia. The blood-brain barrier, protective against toxins, also impedes immune responses and limits the delivery of some therapeutic agents.

Understanding the cascade reveals intervention opportunities:

Before the threshold (minutes to hours before irreversible damage):

- Restore blood flow: thrombolysis, thrombectomy
- Provide alternative fuels: ketones, lactate
- Support mitochondria: CoQ10, NAD^+ precursors, PQQ
- Reduce energy demand: therapeutic hypothermia, sedation
- Block excitotoxicity: NMDA antagonists (limited clinical success)
- Enhance antioxidants: N-acetylcysteine, vitamin E

At the threshold (minutes, during acute injury):

- Prevent mPTP opening: cyclosporine A (under investigation)
- Support calcium buffering: calcium channel blockers (limited efficacy)
- Reduce inflammation: corticosteroids (controversial, may worsen outcomes)

After the threshold (hours to days, secondary prevention):

- Prevent spreading depolarization: ketamine, magnesium
- Control edema: osmotic agents (mannitol), surgical decompression
- Modulate inflammation: balance pro- and anti-inflammatory responses
- Support repair: growth factors, rehabilitation

Long before the threshold (years, prevention):

- Maintain cardiovascular health: blood pressure, lipids, diabetes control
- Support mitochondrial health: exercise (most potent mitochondrial biogenesis stimulus), adequate sleep, avoid toxins
- Dietary factors: Mediterranean diet, omega-3 fatty acids, polyphenols
- Cognitive reserve: education, cognitive engagement, social connections
- Stress management: chronic stress depletes energy and increases inflammatory tone

The most profound insight from understanding the electrical and energy cascade of neuronal failure is this: **the brain is not a static organ that suddenly breaks**. It is a dynamic system that continuously balances energy supply and demand, constantly repairs damage, and operates with narrow margins of safety. Small chronic insults, poor sleep, chronic stress, poor diet, and a sedentary lifestyle erode those margins year after year. When an acute insult occurs, such as a stroke, traumatic injury, or severe infection, there is no reserve capacity. The cascade begins immediately and progresses rapidly.

Conversely, optimization of mitochondrial health, cardiovascular fitness, metabolic flexibility, and cognitive reserve builds resilience. The same acute insult that causes permanent disability in an individual with no reserve may be survived with minimal deficits in someone with optimized resilience.

The living chip can fail catastrophically when one mitochondrion's failure cascades through interconnected systems. But with understanding comes the power to intervene, to prevent the initial failure, to interrupt the cascade before the point of no return, and to build resilience that prevents minor insults from becoming catastrophic failures.

Your neurons are electrical circuits powered by molecular generators, operating with exquisite precision but minimal margin for error. Understanding their vulnerability is the first step toward protecting them. Understanding the cascade mechanisms is the first step toward intervention. Understanding resilience factors is the first step toward prevention.

The 2003 blackout taught power grid engineers valuable lessons about cascading failures: better monitoring, faster response, increased redundancy, and improved communication. The lessons translated into concrete improvements, and the North American grid is more resilient today than in 2003.

Your brain's "grid" can be made more resilient, too. The principles are the same: monitor health markers, respond quickly to warning signs, build redundancy through cognitive reserve and neural plasticity, and improve communication through education and awareness.

The living chip is vulnerable. But it need not fail.

AUTHOR'S NOTE

This chapter has synthesized electrical engineering principles, cellular bioenergetics, neuroscience, and clinical medicine to explain how neuronal energy and electrical failure cascade from single-cell dysfunction to catastrophic network collapse. The analogies to electrical circuits and power grids are not mere metaphors; they reflect genuine parallels in the underlying physics and mathematics of interconnected systems that are vulnerable to cascading failures.

For the clinician, the key takeaways are:

1. Time-to-intervention windows are physiologically determined by ATP depletion kinetics and positive feedback loops
2. Mitochondrial health is foundational to neuroprotection
3. Cascade failures can be prevented by early intervention before critical thresholds
4. Long-term brain health requires continuous attention to modifiable risk factors

For the patient and health-conscious individual:

1. Brain health is inseparable from metabolic and mitochondrial health
2. Prevention is exponentially more effective than treatment after damage occurs
3. Lifestyle factors (exercise, sleep, diet, stress management) directly affect neuronal resilience
4. Early warning signs (cognitive changes, movement disorders) should prompt immediate evaluation

The living chip, your brain, is the most complex and remarkable system in the known universe. Understanding how it fails illuminates how to protect it. May this knowledge translate into longer, healthier cognitive lives for all who read it.

CHAPTER 12: The Future of Optimization

Your Blueprint for a Life Beyond "Not Sick"

The moment of reckoning

This chapter is written from concrete experience in exam rooms, not ivory towers. It is based on decades of watching people slowly lose energy, clarity, and resilience while being told their labs are "normal." Patients who have sat across the desk, describing lives that feel like they are shrinking, while the printout says everything is fine.

"Fine" can become a prison.

You now understand magnesium as the master conductor of ATP, B12 and folate as methylation code-writers, zinc as an immune security processor, phosphorus and creatine as your energy grid, boron as a hormonal voltage controller, copper as neural bandwidth, and vitamin C as surge protection and structural repair. These are not just nutrients; they are infrastructure.

But knowledge alone does not change outcomes. The gap between understanding and action is where most health journeys fail, not from lack of information, but from lack of urgency and structure.

The cost of waiting

David was 42, a high-performing executive who had been running on fumes for years.

He knew his sleep was poor. He knew his brain fog was worsening. He knew his sex drive had disappeared and his joints ached in the morning. On paper, he was "fine": fasting glucose in range, lipids "acceptable," thyroid "normal." His primary care doctor told him, "You're getting older. This is what 40 feels like."

He believed that, for three more years.

By 45, when he finally walked into an optimization clinic:

- He was prediabetic.
- Testosterone sat in the bottom few percentiles for his age.
- RBC magnesium was low.
- Homocysteine was in the range associated with vascular and cognitive risk.

- His heart-rate variability looked like someone living in permanent fight-or-flight.

The work itself was straightforward: restore magnesium and vitamin D, repair methylation with B12/folate/B6, correct zinc, copper balance, stabilize sleep and circadian rhythm, support mitochondria with CoQ10 and an NAD^+ precursor, and then address hormones and peptides where appropriate.

Within 12 weeks, he said, "I forgot what it felt like to be alive."

While David regained health, the one thing that cannot be fixed is time. He lost three high-stakes years of cognition, connection, and presence while damage accumulated below the threshold of "overt disease."

The key question is not "Can optimization help?" but "How early are you willing to move?"

Why your doctor will not tell you this

Most physicians work inside a system designed to identify and code disease, not optimize function.

- Fasting glucose of 99 mg/dL is "normal," even though risk curves for cardiovascular and cognitive disease rise well before the diabetic cutoff.
- Vitamin D at 30-32 ng/mL is "in range," even though immune, skeletal, and endocrine benefits are stronger in the 40-60 ng/mL band for many people.
- Homocysteine at 14 µmol/L is often ignored, despite evidence that much lower levels are associated with less vascular and brain injury.

The system is not hiding optimization. It was simply never built for that level of care. Fifteen-minute visits, reimbursement that rewards throughput, and guidelines anchored to "avoid catastrophe" rather than "support best possible function" all steer care toward survival, not performance.

The medical system's job is to keep you from dying today.

No one in that system is paid to ask whether you will still recognize your spouse and children twenty years from now. That question now belongs to you.

Why now matters more than ever

You are living in the most biochemically hostile environment humans have faced:

- Ultra-processed, nutrient-poor food and mineral-depleted soils.
- Persistent pollutants, endocrine disruptors, and microplastics.
- Chronic psychological stress with few physiological "off-ramps."
- Light at night and circadian chaos.
- Sedentary routines punctuated by sporadic over-exertion.

Against that backdrop, the "chips" in this book, magnesium, B12/folate, zinc, phosphorus/creatine, boron, copper, vitamin C, are no longer minor upgrades. They are the minimum viable requirements for the system to operate as designed.

When you run low on multiple chips at once:

- Mitochondria fragment and lose efficiency.
- Methylation patterns drift: homocysteine rises, DNA repair falters, neurotransmitters skew.
- Immune networks slide into chronic, low-grade inflammation.
- Hormonal "signal-to-noise" worsens.
- Structural repair slows and remains incomplete.

Waiting for overt disease before intervening is like ignoring cracks in a bridge until the deck falls into the river.

How you actually experience the five systems

The previous chapter reframed the biochemistry into five interacting systems. This is how they present in real life:

- Energy system, "Can I handle a hard week?"
- Mg-ATP, creatine/phosphocreatine, copper at Complex IV, vitamin C as mitochondrial shield.
- When underpowered: baseline days are tolerable, but heavy weeks or workouts cause disproportionate crashes.
- Structural system, "Do I hold together?"
- Vitamin C, dependent collagen, copper-dependent myelin and cross-linking, protein and amino acids, zinc for repair enzymes.

- When compromised: bruises that do not match trauma, stubborn tendon pain, slow wound healing, subtle gait or balance changes.
- Information system, "Is my code stable?"
- B12, folate, B6, methylation, homocysteine, magnesium, neurotransmitter metabolism.
- When strained: brain fog, mood shifts, word-finding issues, early executive dysfunction, "not quite myself."
- Security / immune, inflammatory system, "Can I defend and resolve?"
- Zinc and vitamin C for frontline immunity, magnesium for T-cell and cytokine modulation, boron for inflammatory tone.
- When dysregulated: frequent infections, prolonged recovery, mildly elevated hs-CRP, vague joint and vascular "smoldering."
- Hormonal voltage system, "Is the signal clean?"
- Boron (SHBG and free hormones, vitamin D handling), zinc (steroidogenesis), magnesium (receptor signaling, HPA tone), vitamin D, copper and COMT/MTHFR-linked sensitivity.
- When noisy: "normal" hormone labs but unstable energy, PMS/perimenopause chaos, low libido, poor stress tolerance.

When you feel "off," those sensations are the system-level expression of multi-chip under-provisioning and overload.

The 12 hallmarks of aging: Where mitochondria sit in the network

In 2013, López-Otín and colleagues proposed nine "hallmarks of aging." In 2023, this model was expanded to twelve hallmarks, reflecting a decade of new data. These hallmarks:

- Appear with aging
- Accelerate aging when experimentally worsened
- Can delay or reverse aging when therapeutically targeted

The updated 12 are:

1. Genomic instability
2. Telomere attrition

3. Epigenetic alterations
4. Loss of proteostasis
5. Disabled macroautophagy
6. Deregulated nutrient sensing
7. Mitochondrial dysfunction
8. Cellular senescence
9. Stem cell exhaustion
10. Altered intercellular communication
11. Chronic inflammation
12. Dysbiosis

These hallmarks are not separate silos. They form a tightly knit network:

- Mitochondrial dysfunction drives chronic inflammation and senescence via mtDNA leakage, NLRP3 activation, and SASP.
- Disabled macroautophagy prevents the removal of damaged mitochondria and proteins, worsening mitochondrial and proteostasis hallmarks.
- Dysbiosis alters nutrient signaling, redox balance, and mitochondrial metabolites (e.g., urolithin A, SCFAs).

A SRW/TruAge clinical trial is a concrete example of this network in action. In that 12-month study of SRW's Cel System formulas with TruDiagnostic/TruAge epigenetic analysis, participants showed:

- Mean biological age reduction of ~5.7 years on a SystemsAge clock
- Changes in methylation at >1,600 CpG sites linked to oxidative stress, protein biosynthesis, mitochondrial function, and inflammatory regulation
- Shifts in immune cell composition and reduced epiTOC2-estimated stem-cell division rates, suggesting lower replicative stress on proliferative systems

Those findings map directly onto several hallmarks: epigenetic alterations, mitochondrial dysfunction, chronic inflammation, and stem-cell exhaustion.

Hallmarks of aging and where they are located in this book

Hallmark	Plain language	Where you cover it
Genomic instability	DNA damage and repair problems	Appendix C (oxidative DNA damage, 8-OHdG, PARP), NAD^+/sirtuin sections
Telomere attrition	Chromosome end-caps wearing down	Briefly mentioned in Chapter 12 (future directions); mention with HBOT and exercise effects
Epigenetic alterations	Methylation/acetylation "software" drift	B12/folate/methylation chapter; NAD^+/sirtuin sections; SRW/TruAge study in Chapter 12
Loss of proteostasis	Protein misfolding, clumping	Autophagy sections (spermidine, fisetin, mitophagy), Appendix C (UPRmt, proteostasis)
Disabled macroautophagy	Broken cleanup/recycling	Autophagy/mitophagy chapters; spermidine, UA, fasting, exercise; "Goldilocks autophagy" warning
Deregulated nutrient sensing	mTOR/AMPK/insulin/IGF1 off balance	Leucine & BCAAs, metformin/berberine, AMPK, mTOR seesaw table, fasting windows
Mitochondrial dysfunction	Energy failure and redox chaos	Core of the book: Chapters 1, 10, Appendix C; NAD^+, CoQ10, PQQ, MB, UA, ALCAR, exercise
Cellular senescence	"Zombie" non-dividing cells	Fisetin section (senolytic), SASP and inflammaging, mitochondrial damage→mtDNA→SASP
Stem cell exhaustion	Repair/regeneration cells wearing out	Stem cell banking/expansion appendix; SRW/TruAge data on

		epiTOC2/stem-cell division
Altered intercellular communication	Distorted signaling between cells	Hormonal voltage section; SASP; exosomes, peptides, mitochondrial DAMPs
Chronic inflammation	"Inflammaging"	Zinc, vitamin D, omega-3, mitochondrial DAMPs, cGAS-STING, NLRP3, senolytics
Dysbiosis	Microbiome imbalance	Nutrition/UCOS terrain: fiber, polyphenols, UA production; SRW/microbiome tie-ins

Scientists now talk about twelve main ways our cells age. Think of them as twelve "failure modes" that gradually push us away from health.

1. DNA damage: Your genetic hardware gets nicked and broken faster than it's repaired.
2. Shortening telomeres: The protective caps on your chromosomes wear down with each cell division.
3. Epigenetic drift: The software that controls which genes are on or off becomes scrambled.
4. Protein junk: Misfolded and damaged proteins pile up because your cleanup systems can't keep up.
5. Broken self-cleaning (autophagy): Cells lose their ability to recycle old parts, including damaged mitochondria.
6. Wrong nutrient signals: Growth and starvation switches (like mTOR and AMPK) get stuck in the wrong positions.
7. Mitochondrial failure: Your power plants rust, leak, and misfire, making less ATP and more toxic byproducts.
8. Zombie cells (senescence): Old, damaged cells refuse to die and instead pump out inflammatory signals.
9. Stem-cell burnout: Your repair crews (stem cells) become exhausted and can't rebuild tissues effectively.

10. Garbled communication: Hormones, nerve signals, and cell-to-cell messages become noisy and distorted.
11. Smoldering inflammation: A low-grade, chronic "fire" burns in the background (inflammaging).
12. Gut microbiome imbalance: The ecosystem of microbes in your gut shifts toward species that promote inflammation and metabolic dysfunction.

Proteostasis: Keeping your proteins young

Your DNA is the blueprint, but proteins are the tools that actually do the work in your body. They run your enzymes, receptors, ion channels, hormones, and structural scaffolding. All of those proteins together are called your proteome. Every day, that proteome is being damaged and repaired, folded and refolded, recycled and rebuilt.

When you are young, your cells handle this easily. They:

- Fold new proteins correctly
- Refold proteins that got bent out of shape
- Break down proteins that are too damaged to save

As you age, that system slows down. Damaged proteins start to pile up. Some of them clump together into sticky aggregates that cells cannot easily clear. Aging researchers call this loss of proteostasis, the loss of the ability to keep your protein network stable and clean.

Your protocol was designed to help restore that balance. It does not just "raise energy" or "boost testosterone." It quietly supports protein quality control in four big ways.

1. Less Damage to Your Proteins Each Day

The first step in protecting your proteins is to cause less damage.

Two of the biggest sources of protein damage are:

- Oxidative stress (too many reactive oxygen species, or ROS)
- Glycation (sugar sticking to proteins and crosslinking them)

Your protocol lowers those upstream hits by:

- Improving mitochondrial efficiency with NAD+, PQQ, and other mitochondrial helpers. When mitochondria run more cleanly, they produce fewer damaging free radicals that leak onto nearby proteins.

- Providing vitamin C throughout the day in small doses. This shapes the redox environment so you still get normal ROS signals, but fewer big spikes that burn your proteins.
- Stabilizing sleep, hormones, and energy so you have fewer wild swings in blood sugar, stress hormones, and inflammation, all of which drive protein damage and glycation.

Think of this as lowering the number of new "dents and scratches" your proteins get every 24 hours.

2. Better Cleanup of Damaged Proteins and Organelles

The second step is to clear away the junk before it builds up.

Your cells use two main cleanup systems for proteins:

- The proteasome, a "shredder" that digests individual damaged proteins
- Autophagy and mitophagy, bulk recycling systems that engulf protein clumps and damaged organelles (like broken mitochondria)

Your protocol helps these systems in several ways:

- Morning autophagy signaling helps cells start the day in cleanup mode. Autophagy is how cells recycle damaged proteins and organelles.
- Improved NAD+ status supports autophagy and mitophagy through sirtuin and AMPK pathways, helping the cell tag and remove damaged parts.
- Better mitochondrial quality reduces "toxic leak" from failing mitochondria, which otherwise release signals that drive inflammation and more protein damage.

At night, deeper, more coherent sleep, helped by GABA and physiological-dose melatonin, extends the natural cleanup window when the brain's glymphatic system and cell-level autophagy are most active.

In plain language, you are giving your body more time and more signals each day to take out the trash.

3. More Energy and Support for Repair and Refolding

Proteins are not always thrown away. Often they are fixed.

To refold and repair damaged proteins, your cells need:

- Chaperone proteins (especially heat shock proteins)

- A stable energy supply (ATP)
- A healthy redox environment

Your protocol supports this layer by:

- Increasing ATP production in mitochondria, so chaperones and the proteasome have the energy they need to refold or shred damaged proteins.
- Providing copper peptide repair signals, which help rebuild collagen and other structural proteins in connective tissue, the "scaffolding" where long-lived protein damage often shows up.
- Keeping redox stress under control so chaperones are not working in a constant storm of new damage.

When you reduce damage and supply enough ATP and cofactors, the existing repair machinery starts to catch up.

4. A Clear Build Signal for Healthy Protein Synthesis

The last piece is what you tell the system to build.

If you only clear and repair but never give an anabolic instruction, the default in aging is to drift toward sarcopenia and frailty. That is a proteome problem too: fewer contractile proteins, fewer receptors, fewer enzymes in key tissues.

By supporting endogenous testosterone production through non-suppressive stimulation of the HPG axis, and by increasing free testosterone through effects on SHBG and estradiol balance, you give the body a strong, physiologic signal to build and maintain muscle, structural proteins, and many hormone-sensitive enzymes.

From a proteostasis angle, that means:

- The junk is cleared more effectively.
- The environment is cleaner and less oxidized.
- The energy and cofactors for repair are present.
- And the instruction is: use this capacity to build healthy, functional proteins, not just limp along.

That is what it means, in practical terms, for this protocol to support proteostasis.

Precision Longevity: AI, Multi-omics, and Biological Age Clocks

As longevity medicine matures, the field is moving from single biomarkers to integrated, AI-driven risk profiles built from multi-omics data and wearables.

Key components:

- Epigenetic clocks (e.g., Horvath, GrimAge, DunedinPACE, SystemsAge) estimating biological age and pace of aging from methylation patterns
- Proteomic and metabolomic signatures reflecting inflammation, mitochondrial function, and organ-specific aging
- Microbiome profiles linked to dysbiosis, inflammation, and mitochondrial metabolites
- Wearable data (HRV, sleep architecture, activity patterns) as continuous functional aging readouts

AI models can combine these inputs to refine:

- Who is aging fast vs. slow
- Which hallmarks are most active in a given patient (e.g., inflammation-dominant vs. mitochondrial vs. stem-cell exhaustion)
- Which interventions are most likely to help (nutritional, pharmacologic, behavioral)

The SRW/TruAge study is an early example of this approach, showing coherent improvements across multiple epigenetic clocks and immune markers with a targeted supplement regimen.

In practice, a three-layered monitoring strategy is realistic today:

1. Clinical aging measures
- Gait speed, grip strength, chair stand tests
- Cognitive screening, frailty scales
2. Core labs and surrogates
- hs-CRP, IL-6 (inflammation)
- Homocysteine, methylmalonic acid (methylation/mitochondrial links)
- GDF-15, NT-proBNP, cystatin C as "aging signals" for specific organs
3. Optional biological age tests (where available and affordable)

- Epigenetic clocks (TruAge, etc.) for baseline and 12-month comparisons
- Specialty mitochondrial/oxidative stress panels in selected patients

The UCOS framework can sit on top of this: you still treat energy, structure, information, security, and hormonal voltage, but you use clocks and AI-refined markers to track whether your interventions are actually slowing the biological aging curve.

UCOS: a framework, not a magic stack

UCOS, the Ultimate Cellular Optimization System, is simply a way to organize what you have learned. It is not a brand or a single protocol; it is an operating framework:

1. Stabilize terrain
- Sleep, food quality, movement, stress tools.
- No intervention outperforms a chaotic terrain.

2. Measure what matters
- A minimal optimization panel might include: RBC magnesium; B12, folate, homocysteine; zinc and copper; vitamin C; 25-OH vitamin D; hs-CRP; fasting insulin and glucose; lipids; and, when indicated, SHBG and free hormones.

3. Identify primary system bottlenecks
- Use patterns from Chapter 10 to connect symptoms plus labs to specific systems.

4. Correct core chips first
- Magnesium → methylation → zinc/vitamin C/immune support → boron/hormonal stability → copper/structural repair.

5. Add higher-order tools later
- NAD^+ precursors, peptides, senotherapeutics, and other advanced tools only after the foundations are stable and responsive.

In practice, this moves you from random supplementation to closed-loop engineering: test → intervene → retest → refine.

Detailed UCOS lab targets and step-by-step clinical checklists are provided in Appendix A and Appendix B so that Chapter 12 can stay focused on the "why" rather than the "how-to spreadsheet."

Emerging tools on top of foundations

Once foundations are in place: sleep, nutrition, movement, and core chips, there is a second tier of interventions with growing but still evolving evidence.

- NAD^+ precursors (such as NMN, NR, or appropriately dosed niacin) raise intracellular NAD^+, support mitochondrial function, and influence sirtuin/DNA repair pathways.
- Peptides (e.g., BPC-157, thymosin-derived fragments, GHK-Cu, tissue-specific bioregulators) are short signaling chains that appear to enhance repair, modulate immunity, and normalize gene expression in targeted tissues in early human and preclinical work.
- Senotherapeutics such as fisetin are being studied as senolytics, agents that help clear senescent cells and reduce inflammaging; early human trials are underway.

The Autophagy Goldilocks zone: Why more isn't always better

Mitochondrial autophagy (mitophagy) is essential for cellular health, but it operates within a narrow therapeutic window. Too little allows damaged mitochondria to accumulate and poison the cell with reactive oxygen species; too much removes functional mitochondria, triggering energy collapse.

This "double-edged sword" effect has been demonstrated across multiple model systems and represents one of the most important safety considerations in longevity medicine.

The danger of over-activation

In *Drosophila melanogaster* mtDNA mutant models, researchers found that PINK1 overexpression, intended to enhance mitochondrial quality control, triggered excessive mitophagy, removing more than 90% of total mitochondrial mass. The result was catastrophic: ATP synthesis collapsed, larval development arrested, and the organisms failed to reach adulthood despite having "better autophagy."

Similarly, sustained AMPK activation in mammalian cells initially improves mitochondrial function but eventually leads to:

- Excessive mitochondrial clearance and energy deficit
- Dysregulated mitochondrial quality control

- Aberrant decreases in mtDNA copy number
- Loss of mitochondrial stress adaptation capacity

The relationship between AMPK activity and mitochondrial health follows a classic inverted U-shaped curve: moderate activation is beneficial, but both chronic suppression and chronic overactivation are harmful.

Clinical implications

When designing autophagy-enhancing protocols, care should be taken not to combine too many activators simultaneously without appropriate monitoring. Stacking interventions such as spermidine (10 mg/day), rapamycin (pulse dosing), prolonged fasting (>3 days), high-dose metformin (if prescribed), and aggressive caloric restriction (<1,200 kcal/day) may push the response beyond the therapeutic window, particularly in older adults and in individuals with pre-existing mitochondrial dysfunction.

Warning signs of excessive mitophagy:

- Paradoxical worsening of fatigue despite "clean eating" and fasting
- Unexplained muscle weakness or loss (beyond expected caloric deficit)
- Exercise intolerance (inability to recover, worsening performance)
- Cold intolerance and metabolic slowdown
- Brain fog worsening rather than improving

If these emerge during aggressive autophagy protocols, pull back: reduce fasting frequency, add back calories (especially protein and carbohydrates around training), and consider pulsing autophagy enhancers (e.g., spermidine 5 days on / 2 days off) rather than continuous dosing.

The safe approach: Pulsed activation

Nature designed autophagy as a pulsed system: high during fasting/sleep, low during feeding/activity. Mimicking this pattern is safer than chronic activation:

- Autophagy pulse: Overnight fast (12-16 hours) + morning exercise + spermidine or urolithin A
- mTOR pulse: Post-workout nutrition with leucine-rich protein

- Daily rhythm: AMPK dominant (fasted morning) → mTOR dominant (fed afternoon) → AMPK dominant (overnight)

This approach removes damaged mitochondria during the cleanup phase and builds new, functional mitochondria during the growth phase, optimizing turnover without depleting the mitochondrial network.

Bottom line

Mitochondrial autophagy is both a shield (removing damage) and a spear (causing harm when dysregulated). The goal is not maximal autophagy but optimized autophagy, enough to clear damage, not so much that you remove functional organelles. Precision, monitoring, and pulsed activation are key.

All of these are powerful and should be used with clinical oversight, high-quality sourcing, and an understanding that the evidence base is still developing. They work best on top of a stable nutrient and systems foundation, not instead of it.

What an optimized life actually looks like

An optimized life is not perfect. It is simply different from the default trajectory.

A typical day might look like:

- Waking without an alarm most mornings, with HRV and sleep metrics trending more favorably over months.
- A stable base of magnesium, a methylated B-complex, vitamin D, omega-3s, zinc in balance with copper, vitamin C, and creatine, where appropriate.
- Morning sunlight and some movement to align circadian rhythms and improve glycemic control.
- Protein-anchored meals with minimal ultra-processed food and fewer large glucose swings.
- Resistance training two to three times per week, plus daily walking, to build muscle and mitochondrial capacity.
- Periodic, well-justified use of more advanced tools (NAD^+ support, specific peptides, senotherapeutic cycles) under supervision when injuries, cognitive projects, or recovery demands truly warrant them.

- Quarterly or semiannual labs to confirm that homocysteine, hs-CRP, vitamin D, zinc:copper, and hormonal markers are trending toward optimized ranges rather than just "in normal."

There are still bad nights and stressful weeks. Infections still happen. But the recovery curve becomes shorter, cleaner, and less damaging.

The hard truth

For many, Chapter 12 will be a compelling story that fades. Modern life is structured around convenience, not coherence.

The main barrier is not information, nor even time and finances.

The main barrier is belief.

If you have been told for decades that fatigue, pain, reduced libido, weight gain, and brain fog are "just getting older," the nervous system eventually accepts that story as reality. Under that story, it stops looking for alternatives.

Yet you have now seen that:

- Magnesium deficiency is common and profoundly multi-systemic.
- Hyperhomocysteinemia is a modifiable risk factor for vascular dementia and brain atrophy.
- Zinc, copper, vitamin C, and boron measurably alter immune and inflammatory behavior.
- Copper-deficiency myelopathy, once often disabling, can frequently improve when identified early.

These are not fringe concepts; they are documented in peer-reviewed literature and consensus statements. The gap is not evidence. The gap is between translation and execution.

Beyond "not sick"

Optimization is not about living forever or never getting sick. It is about changing the slope of the curve.

It is about:

- Having enough energy to participate fully in work and relationships.
- Preserving cognitive capacity so that learning and contribution remain possible.

- Maintaining muscle and bone so that falls and illnesses remain setbacks, not catastrophes.
- Extending healthspan, the years of independent mobility, intact cognition, and emotional presence.

Longevity science increasingly describes aging as a partly modifiable process driven by mitochondrial decline, chronic inflammation, hormonal drift, proteostasis loss, epigenetic noise, and the accumulation of senescent cells.

The "chips" in this book are levers on those processes:

- Magnesium and NAD^+ support for mitochondrial resilience.
- B12/folate/B6 and homocysteine control for vascular and brain integrity.
- Zinc, vitamin C, boron, and magnesium for immune and inflammatory balance.
- Vitamin C, copper, protein, and collagen substrates for structural repair.
- Boron, zinc, vitamin D, magnesium, and carefully managed hormone strategies for clean hormonal voltage.

Small, consistent corrections in these domains compound into large differences in lived trajectory.

Your 90-day inflection point

The exact protocol will vary, but the logic is stable. The first 90 days are about turning ideas into measurable change:

- Weeks 1-2: Terrain and testing
- Sleep hygiene, real food, daily movement.
- Order a core optimization panel (detailed in Appendix B).
- Weeks 3-4: Chip foundations
- Initiate magnesium, a methylated B-complex, vitamin D3/K2, omega-3s, zinc with copper balance, and vitamin C, at doses matched to you.
- Start simple resistance training and morning light exposure.
- Weeks 5-8: Energy and security systems
- Add creatine and, if appropriate, an NAD^+ precursor when energy and recovery still lag.

- Focus on stress de-loading and assess infections, soreness, bruise/repair patterns.
- Weeks 9-12: Fine-tuning and, when appropriate, advanced tools
- Re-check key labs; adjust B12/folate to bring homocysteine toward the single-digit range if safe.
- Consider advanced tools (e.g., peptides, senotherapeutic cycles) only if foundations are solid and under supervision.

After 90 days, you transition from "catch-up" to maintenance and strategic upgrade: labs every 6-12 months, periodic review of systems, and targeted additions as life stage and goals evolve. The detailed checklists and lab targets you saw sketched here are in the Appendices, so you or your clinician can turn them into action.

The legacy question

From this moment, two different futures are available.

In one, you recognize yourself in these pages, feel the tug of possibility, and then drift back to the default trajectory. The next twenty years follow the average of your genetics, your habits, and your zip code.

In the other, you treat this as an inflection point.

You do not do everything at once. You choose one system, one lab panel, one supplement, one sleep change, one training block, and then another. You iterate, like any good engineer. You treat your biology as a living architecture worth maintaining.

Your mitochondria, methylation patterns, immune networks, hormones, and connective tissues will faithfully reflect your inputs. They are not moral. They are not sentimental. They are programmable, within limits, by what you do next.

The blueprint is in your hands.

Now you decide what you build.

Dr. Steve

About the Author

Steven Warren, MD, DPA, is a physician and public health scholar specializing in longevity medicine, mitochondrial health, and systems-based optimization. He holds a medical degree from The George Washington University School of Medicine and a Doctorate in Public Administration, along with a BA in Chemistry, an MSCM (Master of Science in Community Medicine), and a Master's in Exercise Physiology.

Dr. Warren is triple board-certified in Family Medicine and Preventive Medicine, Addiction Medicine, and Hospice and Palliative Medicine, and is certified as an independent medical examiner. He is also a Certified Functional Medicine Practitioner and is completing advanced certification in Nutrition.

In his private practice in Salt Lake City, Utah, Dr. Warren integrates cutting-edge mitochondrial science, peptide therapy, and precision nutrient optimization to help patients restore cellular function and extend healthspan. His colleagues call him "The Mitochondrial Whisperer" for his ability to identify and correct the upstream cellular dysfunctions that manifest as chronic disease.

Dr. Warren is one of the creators of the UCOS (Ultimate Cellular Optimization System) framework and is affiliated with Best 365 Labs, which produces UCOS-aligned formulations. He lectures nationally on mitochondrial medicine, longevity protocols, and systems-based clinical practice. He loves spending time with his family and pursuing his passion for medicine, health optimization, and living the principles he teaches.

About the Co-Author

Darren Lopez, MBA, is a seasoned entrepreneur with over 23 years of experience in the nutraceutical, cosmeceutical, and anti-aging wellness industries. He holds a Bachelor of Science in Communications from the University of Utah and a Master of Business Administration from the University of Phoenix, where he graduated with a perfect 4.0 GPA. Throughout his career, Darren has designed over 50 health and wellness products — several of which have remained top sellers for more than a decade — including pioneering innovations in Methylene Blue and Vitamin C cellular health formulations, the patent-pending RECHARGE formula, and the MODS MAX™ absorption technology platform.

As CEO, Director, and Co-Founder of Best 365 Labs, a wholly owned subsidiary of BioScience Health Innovations Corp. (OTC: BHIC), Darren has built a publicly traded company rooted in longevity science and next-generation supplement delivery. He co-founded Lion's Fuel, a performance nutrition brand, and has spent his career working with athletes of all ages and abilities — from world champions and elite competitors to weekend warriors, high school and junior high athletes, and retirees determined to live their best lives. His formulations and protocols are designed to meet people where they are and help them reach the next level.

Darren lives in Riverton, Utah, with his family. He remains deeply committed to bringing affordable, science-backed cellular health products to market and believes that the best is always ahead.

APPENDIX X: The Mitochondrial Optimization Framework

When the Power Fails: Mitochondria as the Missing Link in Surgery, PRP, Cancer, and Post-Viral Disease

The engine beneath every protocol

Modern medicine quietly assumes that if the right drug, the right scalpel, or the right protocol is applied, the body will "take care of the rest." Hidden in that assumption is something dangerous: that the body *can* still take care of the rest—that the engine still runs.

That engine is the mitochondrion.

For decades, surgery, regenerative injections, cancer, and "long-COVID" have been treated as separate problems. When you zoom out and ask a simpler question, "What do all these failures have in common?", you repeatedly find the same underlying structure: cells that have lost the ability to make energy, clear debris, and coordinate repair.

This appendix brings The Living Chip together. Surgical Bio-energetic Failure, PRP failure, cancer as a metabolic disease, and post-viral syndromes are not separate mysteries. They are variations on one theme: mitochondria that cannot keep up with demand.

Surgical Bio-energetic Failure: the "perfect" operation that never recovers

In the OR, attention is on mechanics: alignment, decompression, margins. Almost no one asks, "Does this patient have the energetic reserve to heal what I am about to do to them?"

That is Surgical Bio-energetic Failure (SBF):

A state in which a patient's mitochondria cannot produce enough ATP to meet the metabolic demands of surgical trauma, wound repair, and immune defense.

When SBF is present, typical "complications" become predictable:

- Swelling that never fully settles.
- Wounds that look chronically "angry" rather than quietly knitting.

- Infections despite reasonable technique.
- Delayed or non-union, hardware that never feels fully integrated.
- Chronic pain long after structural healing should be complete.

At the cellular level, surgery demands:

- Hemostasis and clot organization.
- Rapid immune cell recruitment and debris clearance.
- ECM synthesis and remodeling.
- Axonal regeneration and synaptic rewiring.

Every step is ATP-intensive and redox-sensitive.

Operating on a patient in SBF is like trying to run a disaster-recovery operation with empty fuel tanks. The scalpel causes the acute injury, but mitochondria determine whether that injury resolves or becomes a chronic disability.

Professional note: perioperative mitochondrial disruption

Perioperative studies show that surgery and anesthesia can acutely impair mitochondrial respiration, reduce ATP production, alter calcium handling, promote fission, impair mitophagy, and increase oxidative stress in brain and peripheral tissues, contributing to postoperative neurocognitive dysfunction and poor recovery. Chronic pain is disproportionately common in primary mitochondrial disease and mitochondrial dysfunction, reinforcing mitochondria as a major driver of transition from acute to chronic pain states.

PRP: perfect seeds in dead soil

Platelet-rich plasma (PRP) looks ideal on paper: concentrated platelets rich in growth factors and cytokines, targeted to damaged tissues. Clinically, results are heterogeneous: some patients do extremely well; others feel little change.

The missing question is, "What did those growth factors land on?"

Growth factors are instructions, not building blocks. They only work when they land in living soil, cells with mitochondria capable of receiving and executing the signal. In tissue filled with senescent cells, chronic oxidative stress, and starved mitochondria, growth factors are like shouting detailed orders into a room of exhausted workers.

In that terrain, "PRP failure" is often a bio-energetic terrain problem, not a centrifuge problem.

Pre-habilitation logic applies here:

- Raise NAD^+ so cells can actually run repair programs.
- Support electron transport and reduce ROS noise so inflammatory signals can resolve.
- Nudge autophagy/mitophagy to clear damaged organelles and proteins before asking for new construction.

Only then are PRP "seeds" landing in a field with workers awake, energized, and ready to respond.

Professional note: PRP and mitochondria

Beyond growth factors, PRP appears to modulate oxidative stress and mitochondrial function directly. Preclinical work in impaired-healing models shows that PRP reduces ROS, improves antioxidant defenses, and, in some settings, transfers functional mitochondria from platelets to damaged cells, restoring bioenergetics and favoring epithelial-mesenchymal transitions favorable to repair. This places mitochondrial recovery and redox homeostasis at the center of PRP's benefits.

Cancer: when failed engines rewrite the code

Cancer is classically framed as an accumulation of nuclear DNA mutations. That framing is incomplete.

Decades ago, Warburg observed that cancer cells ferment glucose into lactate even in the presence of oxygen (aerobic glycolysis). Modern studies show that many tumors exhibit fragmented, abnormal mitochondrial networks, reduced oxidative phosphorylation, increased ROS, and altered mitochondrial signaling.

As mitochondria fail, they send retrograde distress signals to the nucleus:

- Upregulate glycolysis and glutaminolysis to compensate for lost respiration.
- Downregulate differentiation and apoptosis to keep cells alive under stress.
- Rewire growth and survival pathways.

Nuclear mutations may, in part, be a record of that metabolic crisis rather than its sole initiating cause.

This does not mean mitochondrial support alone treats cancer. It does mean:

- Maintaining mitochondrial integrity, redox balance, and quality control may reduce the likelihood of cells being forced into malignant survival programs.
- Targeting mitochondrial metabolism can modulate tumor behavior and response to standard therapies.

Professional note: cancer as a metabolic disease

Metabolic and mitochondrial models of cancer emphasize defects in oxidative phosphorylation, mtDNA mutations, altered dynamics, and chronic activation of glycolytic/hypoxic programs as upstream drivers. Experimental work shows that replacing dysfunctional mitochondria with healthy ones can partially reverse malignant phenotypes, supporting a model where mitochondrial integrity heavily influences nuclear expression and cell fate.

Long-COVID and post-viral syndromes: when cleanup stalls

After infections, especially COVID, a subset of patients are left with crushing fatigue, post-exertional crashes, dysautonomia, and brain fog, despite "normal" standard testing.

Multiple reviews now converge on the same picture:

- Reduced oxidative phosphorylation and reserve capacity in PBMCs and skeletal muscle.
- Abnormal mitochondrial morphology and impaired fusion/fission balance.
- Evidence of ongoing oxidative stress and disrupted mitophagy.

Long-COVID and related post-viral states look less like mysterious new diseases and more like chronic mitochondrial and clearance failure: power plants damaged, trash cans overflowing, cells stuck in a half-on, half-off metabolic limbo.

In that context, it is more useful to tell patients:

"We are going to help your cells take out the trash and turn the power back on"

than to promise unmeasurable "spike protein eradication."

Professional note: long-COVID and mitochondrial respiration

Long-COVID cohorts show impaired mitochondrial respiration in PBMCs and reduced muscle oxidative capacity, correlating with symptom severity years after acute infection. Reviews highlight mitochondrial health as central to pathophysiology and as a therapeutic target via pharmacologic agents, graded exercise, diet, and mito-nutraceuticals.

Chronic pain: when neurons cannot reset

Inflammation is meant to be a phase, not a lifestyle. After injury, pain and inflammation should resolve as tissue heals. In many patients, especially after surgery or repetitive strain, pain persists long after structural healing.

Sensory neurons are among the most energy-hungry cells:

- They constantly maintain ionic gradients, fire action potentials, and remodel synapses.
- All of this depends on dense, healthy mitochondrial networks.

When chronic inflammation and oxidative stress disrupt those networks, via sustained ROS, mtDNA damage, calcium overload, and impaired mitophagy, neurons become hyper-excitable and unable to reset. Pain signaling remains elevated even when tissue integrity is intact.

Supporting mitochondrial respiration, restoring NAD^+, rebalancing ROS, and restarting mitophagy/biogenesis are concrete ways to help the nervous system exit that stuck "on" state.

The evidence: mitochondria as infrastructure, not niche

If "mitochondria" sounds niche, it is only because medicine has normalized talking in organ silos. The literature increasingly treats mitochondrial dysfunction as a hallmark of aging and a shared mechanism across age-related diseases.

Patterns recur:

- ME/CFS and post-exertional states, impaired bioenergetics, redox imbalance, and abnormal mitochondrial signaling are repeatedly implicated.

- Mood disorders, mitochondrial ATP/redox shifts and inflammatory-mitochondrial loops intersect with depression and anxiety.
- Metabolic syndrome/diabetes, mitochondrial ROS, impaired oxidative capacity, and quality-control failure contribute to insulin resistance.
- Autoimmunity/chronic inflammation, damaged mitochondria release mtDNA and other DAMPs, driving cGAS, STING, TLR9, and inflammasomes.
- Cardiovascular disease, failing hearts show mitochondrial energetic and redox failure, not just pump mechanics.
- Neurodegeneration, Parkinson's and Alzheimer's repeatedly show complex I defects, mitophagy failure, and mitochondrial network disruption.
- Aging itself, mitochondrial dysfunction interlocks with all other hallmarks (senescence, inflammation, epigenetic drift, stem-cell exhaustion).

Mitochondria are not a specialty; they are infrastructure.

Mitochondrial-first medicine: a practical stance

When mitochondrial function is restored:

- Energy returns and post-exertional symptoms lessen.
- Inflammatory markers and symptoms often improve without heavy immunosuppression.
- Mood stabilizes because neurotransmitter systems now have energetic and redox stability.
- Insulin sensitivity and metabolic flexibility improve.
- Recovery from stress, training, and procedures accelerates.

Almost every effective intervention in longevity and regenerative medicine, exercise, sleep, fasting, circadian alignment, certain nutraceuticals, even many peptides, works by improving mitochondrial output, quality control, or both.

A mitochondrial hierarchy emerges:

1. Healthy mitochondria and basic terrain (sleep, light, movement, food).

2. Cofactors and core chips (magnesium, B vitamins, zinc/copper, vitamin C, D, creatine).
3. More targeted nutraceuticals and lifestyle hormesis (NAD^+ precursors, polyphenols, fasting, heat/cold).
4. Peptides, hormones, and advanced therapeutics.
5. Highly experimental longevity drugs.

You cannot safely or consistently build higher levels on a failing level 1.

From supplements to system repair

Across surgery, PRP, cancer, long-COVID, and chronic pain, the same story repeats:

- High-demand events are imposed on low-charge, high-debris cells.
- Mitochondria are too underpowered to coordinate effective repair.
- The system adapts by lowering capacity and raising alarms.

The practical implication:

The work is not to keep adding "one more supplement." The work is system repair.

Key levers:

- Restore electron flow through the respiratory chain.
- Preserve and replenish NAD^+ so repair enzymes, sirtuins, and mitochondria can function.
- Enhance autophagy and mitophagy so damaged components and post-infectious debris are cleared instead of accumulated.
- Calm retrograde "panic" signals from mitochondria to nucleus before they crystallize into chronic disease programs.

The tools, methylene blue, NAD^+ precursors, spermidine, exercise, circadian alignment, targeted probiotics, micronutrient repletion are chapter-specific.

The principle is this: If you do not stabilize and energize mitochondria, no amount of mechanical or pharmacologic sophistication will consistently produce healing.

That is the unifying thesis of this appendix and, in many ways, of the book:

The living chip is only as smart as it is powered.

APPENDIX A: The UCOS Clinical Framework

UCOS Clinical Framework and 12-Week Program

What UCOS is (and is not)

UCOS (Ultimate Cellular Optimization System) is a structured approach to restoring and optimizing cellular function. It is:

- A framework, not a branded protocol.
- Built around the core "chips" from the book: magnesium, B12/folate, zinc, phosphorus/creatine, boron, copper, vitamin C, plus vitamin D and omega-3s.
- Designed as closed-loop practice: test → intervene → retest → refine.

UCOS always starts with terrain (sleep, nutrition, movement, stress), then corrects core deficiencies and imbalances, then only layers advanced tools (NAD^+ support, peptides, senotherapeutics) when foundations are in place.

The AMPK/mTOR seesaw: Balancing growth and cleanup

One of the most critical concepts in longevity medicine is understanding that anabolism (building up) and catabolism (breaking down) are both essential, and neither should dominate continuously.

The drug rapamycin, originally an immunosuppressant, has emerged as a potential longevity intervention by modulating mTOR and enhancing autophagy — though its use in healthy individuals remains investigational and is discussed in detail in Chapter 12.

AMPK (AMP-activated protein kinase) and mTOR (mechanistic target of rapamycin) are the master regulators of this balance. They function as metabolic antagonists, forming a dynamic "seesaw" that determines whether cells prioritize growth, repair, and protein synthesis (mTOR) or cleanup, efficiency, and stress resistance (AMPK).

The ideal state is rhythmic alternation: AMPK dominance during fasting and rest, mTOR dominance during feeding and activity, with neither chronically suppressed or activated.

The AMPK/mTOR balance table

State	AMPK	mTOR	Cellular priority	Outcomes (acute)	Outcomes (chronic)
Fasted / Low energy	↑↑ Active	↓ Inactive	Efficiency, cleanup, stress resistance	- Autophagy ↑	✓ Healthy longevity
				- Mitochondrial biogenesis ↑	- Reduced senescent cells
				- Fat oxidation ↑	- Improved metabolic flexibility
				- Insulin sensitivity ↑	- Lower cancer risk
				- Inflammation ↓	
Fed / High energy	↓ Inactive	↑↑ Active	Growth, protein synthesis, anabolism	- Protein synthesis ↑	✓ Healthy anabolism (if pulsed)
				- Muscle growth ↑	- Muscle mass maintained
				- Glycogen storage ↑	- Tissue repair
				- Autophagy ↓	- Adequate growth hormone signaling
				- Cell proliferation ↑	

Chronic AMPK activation	↑↑↑	↓↓↓	Survival mode,	- Excessive autophagy	✕ DANGER
(prolonged fasting, extreme caloric restriction, chronic metformin without feeding windows)			energy conservation	- Mitochondrial depletion	- Muscle wasting
				- Muscle catabolism	- Mitochondrial dysfunction
				- Fatigue	- Loss of stress resilience
				- Cold intolerance	- Metabolic slowdown
					- Hormonal suppression
Chronic mTOR activation	↓↓↓	↑↑↑	Uncontrolled growth,	- Autophagy suppression	✕ DANGER
(constant feeding, high insulin, sedentary lifestyle, obesity)			no cleanup	- Senescent cell accumulation	- Accelerated aging
				- Insulin resistance ↑	- Cancer risk ↑

				- Inflammation ↑	- Neurodegenerative disease risk ↑
				- Protein aggregation	- Metabolic syndrome
					- Cardiovascular disease

Clinical strategies: How to pulse the seesaw

Morning: AMPK dominant (fasted state)

- Wake up after a 12-16-hour overnight fast (last meal by 7-8 pm, first meal at 10 am-12 pm)
- Morning light exposure (sets circadian clock, supports mitochondrial function)
- Fasted or lightly fueled exercise (aerobic or low-intensity strength)
- Optional: Black coffee (caffeine activates AMPK), green tea (EGCG activates AMPK)
- Metabolic state: Fat oxidation, autophagy, mitochondrial cleanup

Post-workout / Midday: Transition to mTOR

- Breakfast with a protein-rich meal containing 2-3 g leucine (eggs, Greek yogurt, whey protein, chicken)
- Carbohydrates timed to training (sweet potato, rice, fruit) to replenish glycogen
- Metabolic state: Insulin spike, mTOR activation, protein synthesis, muscle repair

Afternoon/Evening: mTOR dominant (fed state)

- Second meal with adequate protein (1.6-2.0 g/kg total daily)
- Resistance training or high-intensity interval training (signals mTOR via mechanical tension and metabolic stress)
- Metabolic state: Anabolism, growth, tissue building

Overnight: Return to AMPK

- Stop eating 2-3 hours before bed (by 7-8 PM)
- Sleep 7-9 hours (growth hormone peaks during deep sleep, facilitates both anabolism and autophagy)
- Overnight fast (12-16 hours total)
- Metabolic state: Autophagy reactivation, mitochondrial repair, cellular cleanup

Pharmacologic and Nutraceutical modulation

AMPK activators (use during fasted/cleanup windows)

Agent	Mechanism	Typical dose	Timing
---	---	---	---
Metformin	Inhibits Complex I, raises AMP/ATP ratio	500-2,000 mg/day (Rx)	Evening, with or after dinner
Berberine	Similar to metformin; AMPK activation	500 mg 2-3×/day	Before meals
EGCG (green tea extract)	Direct AMPK activation	400-600 mg/day	Morning, fasted
Resveratrol	SIRT1 → AMPK axis	250-500 mg/day	Morning or evening
ALA (alpha-lipoic acid)	Enhances AMPK sensitivity	600-1,200 mg/day	Morning, fasted
Exercise	↑ AMP, ↓ ATP → AMPK	30-60 min aerobic or resistance	Morning or early afternoon

mTOR activators (use during fed/growth windows)

Agent	Mechanism	Typical dose	Timing
---	---	---	---

Leucine	Direct mTOR activation via Rag GTPases	2-5 g per meal	Post-workout or with protein meals
Protein (high-quality)	Provides leucine + other EAAs	30-50 g per meal	2-3 meals/day, emphasize post-training
Insulin (endogenous or Rx)	Activates PI3K-AKT-mTOR	N/A (via carbohydrate meals)	Post-workout, afternoon
Resistance training	Mechanical tension → mTOR	3-5 sets, 6-12 reps, progressive overload	Afternoon or early evening
Creatine	Enhances ATP availability for training	3-5 g/day ongoing	Any time; enhances mTOR response to training

mTOR inhibitors (use cautiously, for specific therapeutic goals)

Agent	**Mechanism**	**Typical dose**	**Clinical use**
---	---	---	---
Rapamycin	Direct mTORC1 inhibition	3-10 mg weekly (pulse)	Anti-aging, immune modulation (investigational)
Fasting	↓ insulin, ↓ amino acids → mTOR off	16-24-hour fasts 1-2×/week	Autophagy enhancement, metabolic reset

Warning: The Danger Zones

Chronic AMPK activation (too much catabolism)

- Seen in: Extreme caloric restriction (<1,200 kcal/day), prolonged fasting (>3 days regularly), high-dose metformin without adequate feeding windows, overtraining with inadequate recovery

- Consequences: Muscle wasting, mitochondrial depletion, fatigue, cold intolerance, amenorrhea (women), low testosterone (men), increased cortisol, impaired immune function
- Fix: Add back calories (especially protein and carbs around training), reduce fasting frequency, implement "re-feed" days, reduce metformin dose, or add feeding windows

Chronic mTOR activation (too much anabolism)

- Seen in: Constant snacking, high-carb/high-protein diet without fasting windows, sedentary lifestyle with overfeeding, insulin resistance, obesity
- Consequences: Autophagy suppression, senescent cell accumulation, cancer risk, accelerated aging, metabolic syndrome, neurodegeneration
- Fix: Implement time-restricted eating (16:8 or 14:10), add fasted morning exercise, reduce meal frequency (from 5-6 to 2-3 meals/day), increase physical activity, consider metformin or berberine if insulin-resistant

Patient language: The growth and cleanup cycle

"Your body has two modes: build and clean. You need both, but not at the same time.

Build mode (mTOR) happens when you eat protein and train hard. Your body makes new muscle, repairs tissues, and grows stronger. This is good, you need it.

Clean mode (AMPK) happens when you fast overnight, exercise in the morning, and give your cells a break from constant feeding. Your body removes damaged mitochondria, clears out cellular junk, and fine-tunes everything. This is also good, you need it.

The problem with modern life is we're stuck in build mode 24/7: constant snacking, no real fasting, and sitting all day. Your body never gets a chance to clean up. That's when damaged mitochondria, senescent cells, and metabolic waste pile up, and you age faster.

The solution isn't to fast forever or stop eating protein. It's to pulse both modes:

- Morning: Fasted exercise, fat-burning, cleanup
- Midday/Afternoon: Eat protein, train hard, build

- Overnight: 12-16-hour fast, sleep, cellular repair

This rhythm is how your body is designed to work. We're just restoring the natural cycle."

UCOS flow: From terrain to advanced tools

Use this as the mental "flowchart" for clinical decision-making.

Step 1, Terrain check (Weeks 1-2)

Assess:

- Sleep: <7 hours, irregular timing, non-restorative?
- Nutrition: high in ultra-processed food, low protein, low fresh plants?
- Movement: <5,000 steps/day, no strength training?
- Stress: no daily down-shift practice?

If "yes" to any, begin terrain interventions immediately, alongside labs:

- Sleep hygiene, consistent bed/wake time, dark and cool bedroom.
- Protein anchored meals, more whole foods, fewer added sugars/seed oils.
- Daily walking; 2- 3 resistance sessions per week as tolerated.
- 5-10 minutes/day of breathwork, meditation, prayer, or quiet.

Step 2, Baseline UCOS labs and subjective metrics

Order a core optimization-leaning panel (details in Appendix B):

- RBC magnesium.
- Vitamin B12, folate, homocysteine.
- Zinc, copper, zinc:copper or copper:zinc ratio.
- Vitamin C (plasma, if available).
- 25-OH vitamin D.
- hs-CRP.
- Fasting glucose and insulin.
- Lipid panel (± ApoB if available).
- TSH, free T4, free T3.
- SHBG, total and free testosterone (± estradiol/progesterone as indicated).

Capture subjective baselines (0, 10):

- Energy, mood, sleep quality, pain, cognitive clarity.
- Note weight, waist circumference, resting HR, and HRV if available.

Core Chip repletion (weeks 2-6)

Unless contraindicated and individualized:

- Magnesium, glycinate, malate, or threonate forms, often evening; aim to move RBC Mg into mid, upper reference range.
- Methylated B-complex, includes methylcobalamin, methylfolate (or 5-MTHF), and B6 to support methylation and homocysteine control.
- Vitamin D3 (± K2), titrate toward 40-60 ng/mL where appropriate.
- Zinc, balanced with copper, avoid long-term zinc monotherapy; monitor zinc:copper ratio.
- Vitamin C, typically 500-2000 mg/day, divided, adjusted to bowel tolerance and demand.
- Omega-3 fatty acids, dose per diet and risk profile.
- Creatine monohydrate, commonly ~3-5 g/day if no contraindication, especially in low-meat diets or high-demand states.
- Protein, generally 1.2-1.6 g/kg/day (ideal body weight) unless otherwise indicated.

Aim for ≥80% adherence to this foundation before introducing advanced tools.

System-Directed layers (weeks 4-12)

Use symptoms + labs to identify the primary bottleneck system (Chapter 10).

1. Energy system

Pattern:

- "Can do normal days" but crash with harder weeks, heavy workouts, or intense cognitive loads.
- Prolonged DOMS, reliance on caffeine, "wired-tired" at night.

Typical findings:

- Low/low-normal RBC magnesium.
- Low vitamin D.
- Possible low creatine intake.
- Low-grade inflammatory load (hs-CRP >1, 2).

Core focus:

- Intensify magnesium, vitamin D optimization, creatine.
- Consider NAD^+ precursor (NMN, NR, or niacin-based) when safety and context allow, especially if post-exertional symptoms persist.

2. Structural system (collagen, myelin, vessels)

Pattern:

- Easy bruising, slow wound healing.
- "Tendinous" pain, recurrent sprains.
- Subtle gait or balance changes, proprioceptive drift.
- Gum sensitivity or bleeding.

Typical findings:

- Low or low-normal vitamin C.
- Suboptimal protein intake.
- Copper imbalance (often low copper in the context of zinc use).

Core focus:

- Vitamin C repletion.
- Adequate protein and collagen substrates (glycine, proline, lysine).
- Evaluate copper and zinc:copper balance; address copper deficiency cautiously and avoid excess.

3. Information system (methylation, homocysteine, cognition)

Pattern:

- Brain fog, slowed processing, word-finding issues.
- Mood lability, depression, anxiety.
- Family history of vascular dementia or early strokes.

Typical findings:

- Homocysteine above ≈10-11 μmol/L.
- Borderline or low-normal B12/folate.
- Possible MTHFR/COMT/FUT2 patterns.

Core focus:

- Methylcobalamin, 5-MTHF, B6, and often choline or betaine.
- RBC magnesium for SAMe synthesis and DNA repair.
- Aim homocysteine toward ~6-10 μmol/L where safe, especially in high-risk patients.

4. Security / immune, inflammatory system

Pattern:

- Frequent colds/URIs; prolonged post-viral fatigue.
- Mildly elevated hs-CRP (≈1-3 mg/L).
- "Inflammaging" pattern: vague joint pain, brain fog, low resilience.

Typical findings:

- Low zinc, low vitamin C, low vitamin D.
- Elevated hs-CRP, possibly ferritin or other inflammatory markers.

Core focus:

- Zinc, vitamin C, vitamin D, and magnesium support.
- Consider boron as an inflammatory "voltage" modulator when appropriate.
- Diet: focus on fiber, polyphenols, and omega-3s to support the gut-immune axis.

5. Hormonal voltage system

Pattern:

- "Normal" hormone labs but low libido, PMS/PMDD, perimenopause chaos, flat mood, mid-day crashes.
- Body composition drift despite unchanged inputs.

Typical findings:

- Elevated SHBG with low free testosterone or estradiol.
- Low-normal vitamin D and magnesium.

- Zinc or boron insufficiency, or copper imbalance.

Core focus:

- Address SHBG and free hormone availability (within scope and with appropriate endocrine evaluation).
- Optimize zinc, boron, magnesium, vitamin D.
- Consider genetic sensitivity (COMT/MTHFR) when patients are "high-reactors" to catecholamines or estrogen shifts.

12-Week UCOS Program: Clinical Scaffold

Use this as a template and adapt per patient.

Weeks 1-2: Orientation & baseline

Goals:

- Establish terrain habits.
- Draw labs.
- Capture subjective/objective baselines.

Actions:

- Implement sleep, diet, movement, and stress basics.
- Order UCOS baseline panel.
- Record subjective scores (energy, mood, sleep, pain, clarity) and simple metrics (weight, waist, HR, HRV).

Milestones:

- Labs drawn and reviewed.
- Patient understands five systems and which symptoms map where.

Weeks 3-4: Core chip repletion

Goals:

- Correct universal deficits.
- Watch for early changes in sleep, muscle tension, and energy.

Actions:

- Start magnesium, methylated B-complex, vitamin D3/K2, zinc (with copper balance), vitamin C, omega-3s, creatine as appropriate.
- Anchor sleep and circadian rhythm (consistent timing, morning light).

- Establish resistance training 2-3×/week and daily walking, scaled to capacity.

Metrics:

- Small improvements in sleep onset, muscle relaxation, fewer cramps or palpitations.
- ≥80% adherence to core supplements and terrain habits.

Weeks 5-8: System targeting and energy upgrade

Goals:

- Prioritize one or two systems based on labs and symptoms.
- Add energy/immune layers if indicated.

Actions:

- If homocysteine high → intensify B12/folate/B6, assess protein, consider choline/betaine.
- If hs-CRP >1, 2 → reinforce diet, optimize omega-3s, consider boron, confirm magnesium and vitamin D sufficiency.
- Consider NAD^+ precursor if fatigue/post-exertional symptoms persist despite magnesium and sleep work.
- Maintain manageable, progressive activity: avoid over-zealous training in fragile patients.

Metrics:

- Energy 1-2 points higher on subjective scale.
- Less post-exertional crash.
- Fewer or milder infections and inflammatory flares.

Weeks 9-12: Refinement and advanced tools (if warranted)

Goals:

- Confirm lab movement.
- Decide if patient remains in "foundational rebuild" or is ready for advanced therapies.

Actions:

- Recheck key labs: homocysteine, vitamin D, zinc/copper, hs-CRP, ± vitamin C, hormones.
- Compare lab changes with symptom changes.

- If foundations are robust and a clear need remains (e.g., chronic tendon injury, resistant cognitive issues, persistent sarcopenia), consider:
- NAD^+ precursor as a longer-term mitochondrial support.
- Selected peptides (e.g., BPC-157 for musculoskeletal/gut, TB4 fragments, GHK-Cu for tissue repair) under medical supervision and with quality sourcing.
- Periodic senotherapeutic cycles (e.g., fisetin) as evidence and patient profile allow.

Metrics:

- Homocysteine trending toward <10 μmol/L where appropriate.
- hs-CRP trending toward <1 mg/L if safely achievable.
- Vitamin D trending into the 40-60 ng/mL range (individualized).
- Subjective: energy ≥7/10 most days, better sleep, faster recovery from stress/illness, clearer thinking, more stable mood.

After 12 weeks, most patients have:

- A clear shift in key biomarkers.
- A felt difference in day-to-day life.
- A defined base protocol.
- A prioritized list of which system still needs the most work.

From there, UCOS becomes maintenance plus intelligent iteration, not guesswork.

Concise UCOS clinician checklist

Use this as a one-page internal reference.

A. Terrain

- Sleep 7-9 h, consistent timing, dark/cool room.
- Protein-anchored, minimally processed diet, low added sugar/seed oils.
- Resistance 2-3×/week, 7-10k steps/day, scaled.
- Daily stress down-shift practice.

B. Baseline

- UCOS lab panel (see Appendix B).
- Subjective scores: energy, mood, sleep, pain, cognition (0, 10).
- HR, HRV, weight, waist.

C. Core chips (4-8 weeks)

- Magnesium.
- Methylated B-complex.
- Vitamin D3/K2.
- Zinc with copper balance.
- Vitamin C.
- Omega-3s.
- Creatine (if no contraindication).
- Protein 1.2-1.6 g/kg/day.

D. System-directed layers

- Elevated homocysteine/cognitive, mood → B12/folate/B6, Mg.
- Frequent infections/hs-CRP >1 → zinc, vitamin C, vitamin D, Mg, consider boron.
- Structural issues → vitamin C, protein, copper balance.
- Hormonal symptoms with "normal" labs → SHBG, free hormones, zinc, boron, Mg, vitamin D.
- Neural bandwidth issues → copper, B12, Mg, vitamin C; evaluate myelopathy red flags.

E. Advanced tools (after D)

- NAD^+ precursor.
- Peptides (BPC-157, TB4 fragments, GHK-Cu, others) with supervision.
- Senotherapeutics (e.g., fisetin cycles) as evidence and patient profile allow.

F. Retesting & iteration

- Recheck key labs at 8-12 weeks.
- Adjust doses and priorities.
- Shift from "repair" to "maintenance + strategic upgrade."

Patient-Facing UCOS Quick Start (for handouts)

90-Day Cellular Optimization: UCOS Quick Start

What UCOS does:

- Helps your cells make and use energy better.
- Supports your brain, immune system, hormones, and repair.

Step 1, Terrain (Days 1-7)

- Sleep: 7-9 hours; regular schedule.
- Food: mostly real food; protein at each meal; cut back on sugar and ultra-processed snacks.
- Movement: daily walking; 2-3 strength workouts per week if possible.
- Stress: 5-10 minutes/day of breathing, prayer, or quiet.

Step 2, Baseline (Weeks 1-2)

Ask your clinician about checking:

- Magnesium, B12, folate, homocysteine.
- Zinc and copper.
- Vitamin C and vitamin D.
- hs-CRP (inflammation).
- Fasting glucose and insulin.
- Lipids.
- Thyroid and sex hormones if symptoms fit.

Rate (0-10): energy, mood, sleep, pain, brain clarity.

Step 3, Foundation (Weeks 2-6)

With your clinician, consider:

- Magnesium, methylated B-complex, vitamin D3, zinc (with copper), vitamin C, omega-3s, creatine.
- Focus on consistency.

Step 4, Target your weakest system (Weeks 4-12)

- Energy crashes → extra focus on magnesium, creatine, NAD^+ support.
- Brain/mood/homocysteine → B12/folate/B6 and magnesium.
- Immunity/inflammation → zinc, vitamin C, vitamin D, magnesium, possibly boron.
- Structural (bruising, tendons, slow healing) → vitamin C, protein, copper balance.

- Hormonal ("labs normal but feel off") → SHBG, free hormones, plus zinc, boron, magnesium, vitamin D.

Step 5, Recheck and refine (around Week 12)

- Repeat key labs.
- Re-score your symptoms.
- Decide, with your clinician, what to keep, adjust, or add.

UCOS is not about perfection; it is about direction, moving step by step from "not sick" toward your best function.

APPENDIX B: Lab Assessment and Interpretation

Laboratory Assessment and Interpretation

Purpose and scope

This appendix translates the mechanistic concepts from the main text into a practical laboratory assessment. It is written for clinicians and advanced readers who want to:

- Decide what to test.
- Understand how optimal differs from normal.
- Interpret patterns, not just single values.
- Link lab results to the clinical stories and protocols in this book.

It is not a substitute for clinical judgment, local lab standards, or individualized care.

Normal vs optimal, why ranges matter

Most reference ranges are population-based:

- "Normal" usually means the central 95% of a sampled population, which includes people with subclinical deficiencies and early disease.
- These ranges are useful for ruling out severe pathology but are not designed to define optimal function.

Optimization aims for:

- Values associated with better performance, lower risk, and improved subjective well-being in the literature and in practice.
- Personalized positioning within those bands based on age, sex, comorbidities, medications, and goals.

Clinical implication: a result inside the "normal" range does not automatically mean "good enough" for energy, mood, cognition, cardiovascular risk, or resilience.

Core UCOS panels and preferred markers

Magnesium

Preferred markers

- RBC magnesium (or other intracellular measures when available).
- Serum magnesium (supportive, interpreted cautiously).

Why RBC magnesium

RBC magnesium reflects intracellular stores over time and is less affected by short-term shifts than serum levels. Low RBC magnesium is associated with neuromuscular irritability, cardiometabolic risk, inflammation, sleep disturbance, and cognitive issues.

Typical patterns

- Normal serum magnesium with low-normal or low RBC magnesium → probable tissue-level deficiency.
- RBC magnesium in the upper half of the lab range often correlates clinically with fewer cramps, better sleep, and improved stress tolerance.

Clinical associations

- Muscle cramps, twitches, tightness.
- Insomnia, restlessness, anxiety.
- Palpitations with otherwise normal cardiac workup.
- Constipation and migraines.

B12, folate, and homocysteine

Preferred markers

- Serum B12.
- Methylmalonic acid (MMA).
- Homocysteine.
- RBC folate (or serum folate interpreted in context).

Patterns

- B12 at the low end of reference with elevated MMA and/or homocysteine suggests tissue-level deficiency even without anemia.
- Elevated homocysteine may reflect B12, folate, and/or B6 issues, renal impairment, hypothyroidism, certain drugs, or lifestyle factors.

- Many functional and cardiovascular sources favor an "optimal" homocysteine band around roughly 6-10 µmol/L, with risk rising progressively above that range.

Clinical associations

- Cognitive decline, "brain fog."
- Neuropathy (numbness, paresthesias).
- Mood changes, irritability, depression.
- Vascular risk (endothelial dysfunction, thrombosis).

Zinc and copper

Preferred markers

- Serum or plasma zinc.
- Serum copper.
- Copper:zinc (Cu:Zn) or zinc:copper ratio.

Patterns

- Low zinc with "normal" or high copper → reduced immune function, impaired wound healing, increased infection frequency.
- Elevated Cu:Zn ratio (or low Zn:Cu) is associated with inflammation, oxidative stress, and worse outcomes in several chronic disease states.
- High zinc supplementation without copper can suppress copper and cause hematologic and neurologic problems.

Clinical associations

- Frequent infections, slow recovery.
- Poor wound healing, skin/hair issues.
- Neurologic changes with copper deficiency or excess.
- Taste/smell disturbances with zinc issues.

Vitamin D

Preferred marker

- 25-hydroxyvitamin D (25-OH D).

Patterns

- Lower-normal levels may be inadequate for immune, musculoskeletal, and cardiometabolic optimization in many people, even if not frankly deficient.

- Magnesium and boron influence vitamin D metabolism and utilization, so these must be considered when vitamin D appears "resistant" to supplementation.

Clinical associations

- Low mood, fatigue.
- Increased infection risk.
- Bone health and sarcopenia concerns.
- Possible associations with cardiometabolic and autoimmune risk.

Inflammation and oxidative stress

Preferred markers

- hs-CRP for systemic inflammatory burden.
- 8-OHdG for oxidative DNA damage, when available.
- F2-isoprostanes for lipid peroxidation, when available.

Patterns

- Elevated hs-CRP indicates chronic inflammatory load and is associated with increased cardiovascular and all-cause risk.
- Elevated 8-OHdG and F2-isoprostanes signal ongoing oxidative damage and insufficient antioxidant/repair capacity.

Clinical associations

- Fatigue, brain fog.
- Slow recovery from stress, illness, or exercise.
- Higher long-term risk for cardiovascular and other chronic diseases.

Summary UCOS lab panel (foundation)

For most patients entering a UCOS-style program, a reasonable starting panel includes:

- CBC, CMP, lipid panel (± ApoB).
- RBC magnesium.
- Vitamin B12, MMA, homocysteine.
- Serum zinc, copper, and Cu:Zn or Zn:Cu ratio.
- 25-OH vitamin D.
- hs-CRP.

- Fasting glucose and insulin.
- Thyroid: TSH, free T4, free T3.
- SHBG, total and free testosterone (± estradiol/progesterone or other sex hormones as indicated by age, sex, and history).

Subsequent layers (oxidative stress markers, iron indices, more advanced hormones, mitochondrial and inflammatory markers) can be added as clinically indicated.

Example interpretation patterns

Pattern 1, "Normal labs" but persistent fatigue

Typical findings

- Conventional basic labs "normal."
- RBC magnesium low-normal.
- B12 low-normal; MMA and homocysteine slightly high.
- Vitamin D low-normal.
- hs-CRP mildly elevated.

Interpretation

- Multiple subclinical deficits in energy and repair.
- High daily demand with inadequate magnesium, methylation support, and vitamin D.
- Chronic low-grade inflammation that is increasing energetic load.

Suggested priorities

- Optimize magnesium (toward upper half of RBC range).
- B12, folate, and B6 support; aim homocysteine toward a healthier band.
- Vitamin D repletion.
- Inflammation reduction: whole-food diet, vitamin C, omega-3s, sleep, and stress interventions.

Pattern 2: Frequent infections and poor healing

Typical findings

- WBC counts in lab range.
- Serum zinc low-normal.
- Serum copper high-normal.

- Elevated Cu:Zn ratio (or low Zn:Cu).
- Vitamin D suboptimal.

Interpretation

- Immune "security" underpowered despite structurally normal counts.
- Zinc insufficiency and skewed Cu:Zn ratio impair barrier integrity and immune control.
- Vitamin D insufficiency adds to immune dysregulation.

Suggested priorities

- Zinc repletion with explicit copper monitoring; avoid driving copper too low.
- Vitamin D optimization with adequate magnesium.
- Vitamin C support; consider gut/mucosal support as indicated.
- Follow-up Cu:Zn ratio and hs-CRP.

Pattern 3, Cognitive decline with vague imaging

Typical findings

- MRI: "age-related changes," no major structural pathology.
- B12 low-normal.
- MMA elevated.
- Homocysteine elevated.
- Vitamin D low-normal.
- 8-OHdG elevated if checked.

Interpretation

- Methylation impairment and probable tissue-level B12 deficiency.
- Oxidative stress affecting DNA and neurons.
- Increased risk for further cognitive and vascular decline if unaddressed.

Suggested priorities

- B12 and folate optimization (consider methylation genetics, renal status, and drug interactions).
- B6, magnesium, and choline/betaine as needed to support homocysteine clearance.

- Antioxidant support (vitamin C, polyphenols, lifestyle hormesis).
- Sleep, exercise, and cognitive engagement programs.

Sequencing tests and follow-up

Initial assessment (foundation)

- CBC, CMP, lipid panel.
- RBC magnesium.
- B12, MMA, homocysteine.
- Serum zinc and copper, Cu:Zn ratio.
- 25-OH vitamin D.
- hs-CRP.
- ± fasting insulin, A1c, thyroid, sex hormones depending on context.

Follow-up (≈8-12 weeks)

- Recheck markers directly targeted by interventions (e.g., RBC magnesium, vitamin D, homocysteine, Zn/Cu, hs-CRP).
- Adjust doses and strategies based on actual movement and symptoms.
- Add specialized tests (oxidative stress markers, advanced lipid and mitochondrial markers, hormones) when the foundation is in place and questions remain.

Long-term monitoring

- Once stable, many markers can be checked every 6-12 months.
- Increase frequency during rapid change (illness, major training, pregnancy, weight-loss drugs, menopausal transition, major stressors).

Labs should serve as feedback, not a fixed identity.

Sidebar: EchoLight vs DEXA—the future of body composition assessment

Traditional DEXA:

- Uses ionizing radiation.
- Provides static, episodic data.
- Is useful but less suited to frequent tracking in optimization settings.

REMS-based EchoLight:

- Uses ultrasound, with no ionizing radiation.
- Produces very rapid scans (often 1-2 minutes).
- Provides real-time information on bone density, muscle quality, and fat distribution, including visceral fat estimates, which are critical for cardiometabolic risk.

Clinical use cases

- Patients on GLP-1 agonists or aggressive weight-loss regimens: frequent REMS scans help distinguish fat loss from lean mass loss and guide protein, resistance training, creatine, and anabolic support decisions.
- Older adults on longevity protocols: early detection of bone and muscle fragility allows timely intervention (resistance training, mineral and vitamin support, bone-active therapies) before fractures or sarcopenia become clinically apparent.

Bottom line: REMS/EchoLight is emerging as a practical, low-risk tool for precision body-composition monitoring in regenerative and longevity medicine.

Practical notes

Context is key

- "Low-normal" may be far from optimal for a specific patient.
- Always interpret labs in the context of history, medications, and current demands.

Avoid over-focusing on single numbers

- Look for patterns and clusters, not isolated values.
- Combine labs with clinical pattern recognition from the five-system model.

Beware overcorrection

- Over-supplementation, especially of minerals like zinc and copper, can create new imbalances and toxicities.
- Use follow-up labs and symptoms; avoid trading one problem for another.

Use labs as guides, not labels

- Labs are snapshots and feedback tools.

- They should inform experiments in lifestyle and therapeutics, not become fixed identities.

APPENDIX C: Advanced Biochemistry

Advanced Mechanistic Biochemistry: Clinician's Deep Dive

Introduction for professional readers

This appendix is intended for clinicians, researchers, and advanced readers who want to understand the biochemical and physiological mechanisms underlying the case stories and protocols in the main text. It connects each "chip" to core pathways in mitochondrial bioenergetics, methylation, immune regulation, hormone signaling, and neural function.

For practical laboratory interpretation of these mechanisms, see Appendix B.

Part 1: Mitochondrial bioenergetics and mineral cofactors

Electron transport chain overview

The mitochondrial respiratory chain consists of protein complexes embedded in the inner mitochondrial membrane that transfer electrons from NADH and $FADH_2$ to oxygen, pumping protons to generate the electrochemical gradient used for ATP synthesis.

- Complex I (NADH dehydrogenase): Accepts electrons from NADH; requires FMN and multiple iron, sulfur clusters.
- Complex II (succinate dehydrogenase): Feeds electrons from succinate into the chain via FAD; links the citric acid cycle directly to the ETC.
- Complex III (cytochrome bc_1): Transfers electrons from reduced CoQ (ubiquinol) to cytochrome c.
- Complex IV (cytochrome c oxidase): Transfers electrons to oxygen, forming water; requires copper and heme iron.
- Complex V (ATP synthase): Uses the proton gradient to synthesize ATP; requires magnesium for ATP binding and catalysis.

Coenzyme Q10 (ubiquinone/ubiquinol) shuttles electrons between Complex I/II and Complex III and is essential for efficient ATP production and limiting ROS generation.

Molecular mechanisms of Mitophagy: Quality control at the organelle level

Mitochondrial autophagy (mitophagy) is the selective removal of damaged or dysfunctional mitochondria through autophagy machinery. Unlike general macroautophagy, mitophagy specifically targets mitochondria via sophisticated recognition systems that distinguish "healthy" from "damaged" organelles.

Two parallel pathways mediate mitophagy: the ubiquitin-dependent pathway (PINK1/Parkin) and the ubiquitin-independent pathway (receptor-mediated, primarily BNIP3/FUNDC1). These pathways are complementary rather than redundant, responding to different stress signals and operating in different cellular contexts.

Pathway 1: PINK1/Parkin (Ubiquitin-Dependent Mitophagy)

The surveillance system

PINK1 (PTEN-induced kinase 1) functions as the primary sensor of mitochondrial health. Under normal conditions, PINK1 is continuously imported into healthy mitochondria via the TOM/TIM translocase complex, where it is rapidly degraded by PARL protease in the inner mitochondrial membrane. This keeps PINK1 levels low in functional mitochondria.

When mitochondrial membrane potential ($\Delta\Psi m$) collapses, due to oxidative damage, respiratory chain dysfunction, or ATP depletion, PINK1 import is blocked. PINK1 then accumulates on the outer mitochondrial membrane (OMM), where it undergoes autophosphorylation and becomes enzymatically active.

The tagging cascade

Once stabilized on damaged mitochondria, PINK1 initiates a multi-step tagging process:

1. PINK1 phosphorylates ubiquitin molecules already attached to OMM proteins at serine-65, creating phospho-ubiquitin (pUb). This serves as both a signal and an amplifier.

2. PINK1 recruits Parkin, an E3 ubiquitin ligase normally residing in the cytosol. Parkin binds to pUb on the mitochondrial surface.
3. PINK1 phosphorylates Parkin, releasing it from autoinhibition. Phosphorylated Parkin undergoes conformational change, exposing its RING2 catalytic domain.
4. Activated Parkin ubiquitinates OMM proteins (including mitofusins MFN1/MFN2, VDAC1, Miro, and others), creating dense polyubiquitin chains in K48- and K63-linkage patterns.
5. PINK1 phosphorylates newly added ubiquitin, creating more pUb and amplifying the signal in a positive feedback loop. This results in the rapid "coating" of damaged mitochondria with phospho-ubiquitin chains.

Autophagosome recruitment

The polyubiquitin coat is recognized by autophagy receptor proteins, which serve as molecular bridges:

- OPTN (Optineurin) and NDP52 bind both polyubiquitin chains and LC3 (the autophagosome marker protein), physically linking damaged mitochondria to forming autophagosomes.
- p62/SQSTM1 and NBR1 also participate, though they appear less critical than OPTN/NDP52 for mitophagy specifically.

The autophagosome then engulfs the ubiquitin-coated mitochondrion, fuses with a lysosome, and degrades the mitochondrial contents via acidic hydrolases.

Clinical significance: Parkinson's disease

Loss-of-function mutations in PINK1 or Parkin cause autosomal recessive early-onset Parkinson's disease (PD). Patients with these mutations accumulate damaged mitochondria in dopaminergic neurons, leading to:

- Excessive ROS production
- ATP depletion and energy crisis
- Mitochondrial DNA damage
- Neuronal cell death in the substantia nigra

This demonstrates that efficient mitophagy is not optional; it is essential for neuronal survival, especially in high-energy-demand cells like dopamine neurons.

Aging and PINK1/Parkin decline

PINK1 and Parkin expression decline with age in multiple tissues, including the brain, heart, and skeletal muscle. This decline is associated with:

- Accumulation of depolarized, ROS-producing mitochondria
- Increased oxidative damage to proteins, lipids, and DNA
- Activation of inflammatory pathways (see Section 2.3 below)
- Loss of cellular resilience and stress tolerance

Restoring PINK1/Parkin function, or bypassing it with alternative mitophagy enhancers, is a major target of anti-aging interventions.

Mitochondrial damage-associated molecular patterns (mtDAMPs) and Inflammaging

One of the most important discoveries in aging biology over the past decade is the recognition that dysfunctional mitochondria drive chronic inflammation not merely through reactive oxygen species, but through the release of specific molecular signals that activate innate immune pathways.

These signals, collectively termed mitochondrial damage-associated molecular patterns (mtDAMPs), include mitochondrial DNA (mtDNA), oxidized cardiolipin, mitochondrial RNA, and N-formyl peptides. When released into the cytosol or extracellular space, mtDAMPs trigger ancient pathogen-recognition systems, causing sterile inflammation that accelerates aging and drives age-related diseases.

Two pathways are particularly important: the cGAS-STING pathway (activated by cytosolic mtDNA) and the NLRP3 inflammasome (activated by multiple mitochondrial stressors, including mtROS, cardiolipin, and ATP/ADP imbalance).

The cGAS-STING pathway: Mistaking self for pathogen

Evolutionary background

The cGAS-STING pathway evolved as a defense against viral and bacterial infections. Cyclic GMP-AMP synthase (cGAS) detects double-stranded DNA in the cytosol, a danger signal indicating viral infection or nuclear DNA damage. Upon binding DNA, cGAS produces the second messenger 2'3'-cGAMP, which activates STING (stimulator of interferon genes) on the endoplasmic reticulum.

STING then triggers transcription of type I interferons (IFN-α/β) and pro-inflammatory cytokines via IRF3 and NF-κB.

This system works perfectly against pathogens. The problem arises when mitochondrial DNA leaks into the cytosol from damaged mitochondria.

mtDNA as an endogenous trigger

Mitochondrial DNA is structurally similar to bacterial DNA (reflecting mitochondria's endosymbiotic origin):

- It is circular and double-stranded
- It lacks histones and is packaged with TFAM instead
- It contains unmethylated CpG motifs, a "bacterial signature"

When mitochondrial outer membrane permeabilization occurs, due to PINK1/Parkin failure, excessive ROS, BAX/BAK pore formation, or mechanical rupture, mtDNA escapes into the cytosol. cGAS cannot distinguish mtDNA from viral DNA, so it activates STING, triggering a full-blown type I interferon response.

Consequences of chronic cGAS-STING activation

In acute settings (infection, injury), type I interferon signaling is protective. In chronic settings (aging, mitochondrial dysfunction), it drives pathology:

- Chronic interferon signature: Sustained IFN-α/β production suppresses normal immune function, increases autoantibody production, and promotes T-cell exhaustion
- SASP amplification: Type I interferons upregulate senescence-associated secretory phenotype (SASP) factors, including IL-6, IL-8, and MMP3, which spread senescence to neighboring cells
- Tissue fibrosis: Chronic interferon signaling promotes fibroblast activation and collagen deposition in the liver, lung, heart, and kidney
- Neurodegenerative disease: cGAS-STING activation has been implicated in Alzheimer's disease, Parkinson's disease, and ALS pathology

Clinical evidence in aging and disease

Age-related macular degeneration (AMD): Mitochondrial dysfunction in retinal pigment epithelium (RPE) cells leads to mtDNA leakage, cGAS-STING activation, complement system activation, and drusen deposition, the hallmark pathology of AMD.

Atherosclerosis: Vascular smooth muscle cells with mtDNA defects undergo necrosis rather than apoptosis due to ATP depletion, releasing mtDNA into the extracellular space. This activates cGAS-STING in neighboring endothelial cells and macrophages, driving plaque inflammation and instability.

STING gain-of-function mutations: Patients with constitutively active STING variants develop STING-associated vasculopathy with onset in infancy (SAVI), characterized by systemic inflammation, vasculitis, and interstitial lung disease, essentially, accelerated "inflammaging" from birth.

How mitophagy blocks cGAS-STING

Functional mitophagy prevents cytosolic mtDNA accumulation through two mechanisms:

1. Direct removal: Damaged mitochondria with compromised membranes are engulfed by autophagosomes before mtDNA can escape into the cytosol.
2. mtDNA-trapping vesicles: Even when mtDNA leaks into the cytosol, autophagy machinery can form specialized double-membrane vesicles around cytosolic mtDNA, sequestering it before cGAS can bind. These vesicles then fuse with lysosomes for degradation.

Loss of autophagy (genetic knockout or age-related decline) leads to cytosolic mtDNA accumulation, cGAS-STING hyperactivation, and type I interferon-driven inflammation.

The NLRP3 Inflammasome: Sensing mitochondrial distress

Inflammasome overview

Inflammasomes are multi-protein complexes that activate caspase-1, which cleaves pro-IL-1β and pro-IL-18 into their mature, bioactive forms. IL-1β and IL-18 are potent pro-inflammatory cytokines that drive fever, acute-phase responses, and chronic inflammatory diseases.

Of the many inflammasomes (NLRP1, NLRP3, NLRC4, AIM2, pyrin), NLRP3 is the most strongly associated with aging and metabolic disease.

NLRP3 is a mitochondrial damage sensor

NLRP3 activation requires two signals:

Signal 1 (Priming): TLR or cytokine receptor activation (e.g., LPS, TNF-α) induces NF-κB, which upregulates NLRP3 and pro-IL-1β expression.

Signal 2 (Activation): A diverse array of cellular stressors triggers NLRP3 oligomerization and inflammasome assembly. Mitochondrial dysfunction provides multiple Signal 2 inputs:

1. Mitochondrial ROS (mtROS): The most potent NLRP3 activator. Complex I and Complex III dysfunction generate superoxide, which activates NLRP3 through oxidation of thioredoxin-interacting protein (TXNIP).
2. Oxidized mitochondrial DNA: mtDNA released from damaged mitochondria, especially when oxidized (8-OHdG), directly binds and activates NLRP3.
3. Cardiolipin externalization: Damaged mitochondria externalize cardiolipin from the inner membrane to the outer membrane and cytosolic face, where it serves as an "eat me" signal for mitophagy. If mitophagy fails, externalized cardiolipin also activates NLRP3.
4. Mitochondrial ATP/ADP imbalance: Excessive ATP release (from necrotic cells) or severe ATP depletion (causing ADP accumulation) both dysregulate purinergic signaling and lower the threshold for NLRP3 activation.
5. Mitochondrial calcium overload: Damaged mitochondria fail to buffer cytosolic Ca^{2+}, leading to calcium-dependent NLRP3 activation.

In essence, NLRP3 functions as a broad mitochondrial stress integrator; almost any form of severe mitochondrial dysfunction can trigger it.

NLRP3 and cellular senescence

NLRP3 is central to the senescence-associated secretory phenotype (SASP):

- Senescent cells exhibit chronic low-level NLRP3 activation due to accumulated mitochondrial dysfunction
- IL-1β secretion from NLRP3 amplifies SASP via autocrine and paracrine signaling, upregulating IL-6, IL-8, and other factors

- Blocking NLRP3 (genetic knockout or pharmacologic inhibition with MCC950) reduces SASP, decreases senescent cell burden, and extends healthspan in mouse models

NLRP3 in age-related diseases

Disease	Role of NLRP3	Evidence
---	---	---
Type 2 diabetes	β-cell dysfunction, insulin resistance	NLRP3 knockout protects against diet-induced obesity and insulin resistance
Atherosclerosis	Promotes plaque inflammation, foam cell formation, and instability	NLRP3 inhibitors reduce plaque size and improve stability in ApoE^{-}/$^{-}$ mice
Alzheimer's disease	Microglial activation, Aβ-induced inflammation	NLRP3 knockout reduces Aβ deposition and cognitive decline in AD models
Gout and pseudogout	MSU and CPPD crystals activate NLRP3 → IL-1β	First disease linked to NLRP3; colchicine works partly by inhibiting NLRP3
Parkinson's disease	α-synuclein aggregates activate NLRP3 in microglia	NLRP3 inhibition reduces dopaminergic neuron loss
Heart failure	Chronic IL-1β drives cardiac remodeling and fibrosis	IL-1 blockade (anakinra) shows benefit in some HF trials

How mitophagy suppresses NLRP3

Functional mitophagy blocks NLRP3 through multiple mechanisms:

1. ROS reduction: Removing ROS-producing mitochondria directly lowers mtROS, the primary NLRP3 trigger.
2. mtDNA clearance: Autophagic degradation of damaged mitochondria prevents mtDNA accumulation in the cytosol.

3. Cardiolipin sequestration: Autophagy engulfs mitochondria with externalized cardiolipin before they can activate NLRP3.
4. Energy homeostasis: Mitophagy coupled with mitochondrial biogenesis maintains ATP synthesis, preventing the ATP/ADP imbalance that primes NLRP3.

Conversely, when PINK1, Parkin, or FUNDC1 is deficient, damaged mitochondria accumulate, and NLRP3 activation becomes chronic. This has been demonstrated in PINK1^{-}/$^{-}$ and Parkin^{-}/$^{-}$ mouse models, which exhibit elevated IL-1β, IL-6, and TNF-α across multiple tissues.

Therapeutic Implications: Targeting mtDAMP-Driven Inflammation

Why standard anti-inflammatory drugs often fail in aging

NSAIDs, corticosteroids, and even biologic TNF or IL-6 inhibitors often provide only partial benefit in age-related diseases because they target downstream mediators without addressing the upstream mitochondrial damage that continuously regenerates inflammatory signals.

A more effective strategy is to restore mitochondrial quality control, thereby turning off the mtDAMP signal at its source.

Intervention hierarchy

Tier 1: Restore mitophagy (foundational)

- UCOS implementation: Magnesium, NAD^{+} precursors, CoQ10, vitamins C and E, restore baseline mitochondrial function
- Autophagy enhancers: Spermidine (1-10 mg/day), urolithin A (500 mg/day), time-restricted eating
- Exercise: Aerobic and resistance training upregulate FUNDC1, PGC-1α, and mitochondrial turnover

Tier 2: Direct NLRP3 inhibition (if inflammatory burden is high)

- MCC950: Highly selective NLRP3 inhibitor; in Phase II trials for inflammatory diseases
- Colchicine: Microtubule disruptor that secondarily inhibits NLRP3 assembly; FDA-approved for gout and pericarditis, used off-label for cardiovascular disease (COLCOT trial showed 23% reduction in MACE)

- Beta-hydroxybutyrate (BHB): Ketone body that directly inhibits NLRP3; achievable via ketogenic diet, exogenous ketones, or fasting

Tier 3: cGAS-STING inhibition (investigational)

- STING inhibitors (e.g., H-151, C-176): In preclinical development for autoimmune diseases and cancer
- Mitochondrial antioxidants: MitoQ, SkQ1, SS-31 reduce mtDNA oxidation and leakage

Tier 4: Senolytic therapy

- Fisetin: Clears senescent cells, which are major sources of SASP and chronic NLRP3 activation (see Appendix F)
- Dasatinib + quercetin: Senolytic combination used in clinical trials for idiopathic pulmonary fibrosis, osteoarthritis, and frailty

Monitoring response

Track inflammatory markers:

- hs-CRP: Should decrease from >2 mg/L to <1 mg/L
- IL-6: Often elevated in chronic inflammaging; reduction correlates with clinical improvement
- Circulating mtDNA: Research assay; reduction indicates improved mitophagy

Patient language: Why damaged mitochondria cause inflammation

"Your mitochondria are ancient bacteria that your ancestors captured billions of years ago. They still have bacterial DNA, which is circular and lacks the protective packaging that your human DNA has.

When mitochondria get damaged, they can rupture and leak that bacterial-looking DNA into the cell. Your immune system sees it and thinks, 'Bacteria! Infection!' It launches a full inflammatory attack, even though there's no actual infection.

This is called 'sterile inflammation,' and it's one of the main reasons you feel achy, tired, and inflamed as you age. It's not because you're 'falling apart', it's because your cleanup systems (mitophagy) have slowed down, so damaged mitochondria pile up and keep triggering false alarms.

When we restore mitophagy with the right nutrients, fasting, and exercise, your cells remove the damaged mitochondria before they can leak. The false alarms stop. The inflammation goes down. And you start feeling like yourself again."

Pathway 2: Receptor-Mediated Mitophagy (Ubiquitin-Independent)

Unlike the PINK1/Parkin pathway, receptor-mediated mitophagy does not require ubiquitin tagging. Instead, mitophagy receptors embedded in the outer mitochondrial membrane directly bind LC3 via short amino acid motifs called LIR (LC3-interacting region) domains.

The major mitophagy receptors include:

BNIP3 (BCL2/adenovirus E1B 19 kDa protein-interacting protein 3)

- Upregulated by hypoxia via HIF-1α transcription
- Directly binds LC3 through its LIR motif
- Plays a major role in hypoxic mitophagy (e.g., during ischemia, high altitude, or tumor hypoxia)
- Also involved in developmental mitophagy (e.g., during erythrocyte maturation, where mitochondria are cleared as reticulocytes mature into red blood cells)

NIX (BNIP3L, NIP3-like protein X)

- Closely related to BNIP3; also binds LC3 via LIR motif
- Essential for mitochondrial clearance during red blood cell development
- Knockout mice exhibit severe anemia due to failure to clear mitochondria from maturing erythrocytes

FUNDC1 (FUN14 domain-containing 1)

- Constitutively present on the OMM but kept inactive by phosphorylation under basal conditions
- During hypoxia or mitochondrial stress, phosphatases dephosphorylate FUNDC1 (especially at Ser13), dramatically increasing its affinity for LC3
- FUNDC1 is particularly important in cardiac and skeletal muscle mitophagy

- Exercise strongly upregulates FUNDC1 expression and dephosphorylation, enhancing mitochondrial turnover in response to training stress

BCL2L13 and FKBP8

- Additional mitophagy receptors with LIR motifs
- Less well-characterized but contribute to mitochondrial quality control in specific tissues and stress contexts

Regulation by phosphorylation: the FUNDC1 example

FUNDC1 activity is tightly controlled by reversible phosphorylation:

- Basal state (normoxia, healthy mitochondria): Kinases (e.g., CK2, SRC) phosphorylate FUNDC1 at Ser13, Tyr18, and Ser17, which inhibits LC3 binding. Mitophagy is OFF.
- Stress state (hypoxia, mitochondrial damage): Phosphatases (e.g., PGAM5) dephosphorylate FUNDC1 at Ser13, dramatically increasing LC3 affinity. Mitophagy is ON.

This phosphorylation switch allows FUNDC1-mediated mitophagy to respond rapidly to acute stressors without requiring new protein synthesis or the multi-step PINK1/Parkin cascade.

Pathway overlap and redundancy

PINK1/Parkin and receptor pathways are not mutually exclusive. In some contexts, they cooperate:

- PINK1 can directly recruit OPTN and NDP52 even in the absence of Parkin, achieving "Parkin-independent" PINK1 mitophagy
- Parkin ubiquitination of OMM proteins can enhance receptor-mediated mitophagy by altering mitochondrial membrane properties
- Cells with intact PINK1/Parkin can still use receptor pathways, and vice versa

This redundancy is protective: even if one pathway is impaired (e.g., Parkin mutation in PD), receptor pathways may partially compensate. However, when both systems fail, as is often the case in advanced aging, mitochondrial quality control collapses.

Clinical and therapeutic implications

Targeting mitophagy for intervention

Understanding these pathways opens multiple therapeutic entry points:

1. Enhance PINK1 stabilization: Compounds that mimic ΔΨm loss or block PINK1 degradation could activate the pathway without damaging mitochondria.
2. Bypass Parkin: Direct OPTN/NDP52 recruitment or PINK1-OPTN activation can achieve mitophagy in Parkin-deficient contexts (e.g., PD patients with Parkin mutations).
3. Activate receptor pathways: Exercise, intermittent hypoxia, or pharmacologic FUNDC1 dephosphorylation (via PGAM5 activators) can enhance receptor-mediated mitophagy.
4. Combination strategies: Urolithin A, spermidine, and NAD^+ precursors appear to enhance mitophagy through multiple entry points simultaneously (see Section 5 below).

Monitoring mitophagy in clinical practice

Direct measurement of mitophagy in humans is not yet clinically available, but surrogate markers include:

- Mitochondrial DNA copy number (whole blood or PBMCs): Should increase with enhanced mitochondrial biogenesis and turnover
- Circulating mtDNA fragments: Elevated levels suggest mitochondrial damage and inadequate clearance
- Cardiolipin oxidation products (research assays): Marker of mitochondrial membrane damage
- Functional assessments: VO_2max, lactate threshold, post-exercise recovery kinetics (indirect but practical)

Patient language: explaining mitophagy

"Your cells have two quality-control systems for damaged mitochondria. The first is like an alarm system: when a mitochondrion loses power, a sensor called PINK1 tags it with a 'remove me' signal, and a protein called Parkin coats it with molecular flags. Your cell's recycling machinery (autophagy) recognizes those flags and breaks down the damaged mitochondrion.

The second system is like direct haulers: proteins called FUNDC1 and BNIP3 sit on the mitochondrial surface and bind the recycling machinery directly when the cell is under stress, such as during exercise or low oxygen.

When you're young, both systems work well, bad mitochondria get removed, and your cells build new ones. As you age, these systems slow down. Damaged mitochondria pile up, leak toxic chemicals, and make you tired and inflamed.

Our goal is to restore these cleanup systems with the right nutrients, exercise, and fasting patterns, so your cells can throw out the junk and rebuild fresh, efficient mitochondria."

Magnesium and ATP

Magnesium is required for ATP to function biologically. In cells, ATP is active primarily as Mg-ATP.

- Mg^{2+} binds to the phosphate groups of ATP, reducing charge repulsion and enabling correct enzyme binding and catalysis.
- Hundreds of enzymes require magnesium as a cofactor, many involved in glycolysis, the TCA cycle, and oxidative phosphorylation.
- Low magnesium can create functional ATP deficiency even when total ATP levels are near normal, because the ATP that is present cannot be properly utilized.

Clinical implication: Magnesium status is foundational for any attempt to improve energy metabolism. See Chapter 2 and Appendix B for assessment and optimization targets.

Copper and complex IV

Complex IV (cytochrome c oxidase) contains copper centers essential for electron transfer to oxygen.

- Copper deficiency reduces Complex IV activity, limiting maximal oxidative phosphorylation.
- Reduced Complex IV function leads to decreased ATP production, increased ROS, and impaired function in high-demand tissues such as the brain, heart, and skeletal muscle.

Clinical implication: Copper balance is critical when addressing unexplained fatigue, neurologic symptoms, or myelopathy, especially in patients with a history of zinc supplementation or gastric surgery. See Chapter 8 and Appendix B.

Part 2, Epigenetics, methylation, and B12/folate

The methylation cycle

The methylation cycle generates S-adenosylmethionine (SAM), the universal methyl donor in mammalian cells.

Key steps:

1. Methionine + ATP → SAM (via methionine adenosyltransferase).
2. SAM donates methyl groups to DNA, RNA, proteins, lipids, and neurotransmitters.
3. After donation, SAM → S-adenosylhomocysteine (SAH) → homocysteine.
4. Homocysteine is remethylated to methionine by:

- Methionine synthase (requires vitamin B12 and 5-methyltetrahydrofolate).
- Betaine-homocysteine methyltransferase (uses betaine; liver-dominant).

If B12 and/or folate are insufficient:

- Homocysteine accumulates.
- SAM levels decrease.
- DNA methylation, neurotransmitter synthesis, and myelin maintenance are impaired.

Epigenetic regulation

DNA methylation at CpG sites and histone modifications regulate gene expression without changing the DNA sequence.

- Hypomethylation at repetitive elements can increase genomic instability.
- Hypermethylation at promoters of DNA repair or tumor-suppressor genes can silence protective pathways.
- Nutrient status (B12, folate, choline, methionine) and oxidative stress influence these patterns over time.

Clinical implication: Mild-to-moderate B12 or folate tissue insufficiency can drive cognitive decline, neuropathy, and vascular risk long before classic macrocytic anemia appears. See Chapter 3 and Appendix B for assessment of B12, MMA, and homocysteine.

Part 3, Zinc, immunity, and barrier function

Zinc as an immune gatekeeper

Zinc is required for the development and function of both innate and adaptive immunity.

Roles include:

- T-cell development in the thymus (zinc-dependent transcription factors and signaling).
- B-cell maturation and antibody production.
- Neutrophil and NK-cell activity, including chemotaxis, phagocytosis, and cytotoxicity.
- Cytokine production and regulation.
- Maintenance of epithelial barriers and tight junctions.

Zinc fingers, protein domains stabilized by zinc, are abundant in transcription factors and DNA-binding proteins, making zinc essential for regulated gene expression across the genome.

Clinical implication: Frequent infections, poor wound healing, and impaired vaccine response warrant evaluation of zinc status and zinc:copper balance. See Chapter 4 and Appendix B.

Part 4, Phosphorus, creatine, and the phosphagen system

ATP and phosphocreatine

The phosphagen system provides rapid ATP regeneration during high-intensity efforts.

- ATP stores in muscle are small and turn over in seconds during maximal activity.
- Phosphocreatine (PCr) serves as an immediate buffer:

PCr + ADP → creatine + ATP (via creatine kinase), providing approximately 8-10 seconds of high-power output.

- Phosphorus is required for ATP, phosphocreatine, phosphorylation signaling cascades, and membrane phospholipids.

Clinical implication: Individuals with low phosphocreatine capacity may fatigue early in high-intensity tasks despite adequate baseline energy; creatine supplementation (typically 3-5 g/day) and phosphorus support are relevant here. See Chapter 6.

Part 5, Boron, hormonal regulation, and inflammation

Boron and sex hormones

Short-term boron supplementation in humans can:

- Decrease sex hormone-binding globulin (SHBG).
- Increase free testosterone.
- Alter inflammatory markers such as hs-CRP.

Boron may influence enzymes involved in steroid metabolism and affect receptor sensitivity or binding dynamics, though the exact mechanisms remain under investigation.

Boron, vitamin D, and minerals

Boron appears to:

- Enhance retention and half-life of active vitamin D.
- Reduce urinary loss of magnesium and calcium.
- Support bone mineralization and reduce markers of bone resorption.

Boron and inflammatory signaling

Boron has been associated with the modulation of inflammatory mediators such as TNF-α, IL-6, and hs-CRP, particularly in inflammatory arthritis models.

Clinical implication: Boron is a small but potentially powerful modulator of hormonal availability, vitamin D status, mineral economy, and inflammatory tone. See Chapter 7 and Appendix B.

Part 6: Copper, myelin, and neural function

Copper and myelin integrity

Copper imbalances have been implicated in demyelinating conditions and neuropathies, including copper-deficiency myelopathy.

Mechanisms include:

- Copper-dependent enzymes in myelin lipid synthesis.
- Copper requirements for Complex IV, affecting energy supply in oligodendrocytes and neurons.
- Copper as part of Cu/Zn superoxide dismutase (SOD1), reducing oxidative damage in neural tissue.

Clinical implication: Suboptimal copper status, especially in the context of excessive zinc intake, gastric bypass, or malabsorption, can contribute to gait disorders, sensory changes, and cognitive slowing. See Chapter 8 and Appendix B.

Part 7: Vitamin C, collagen, and oxidative stress

Vitamin C and collagen

Vitamin C is essential for the hydroxylation of proline and lysine residues in collagen, critical for triple-helix stability and crosslinking.

- Without sufficient vitamin C, collagen is structurally weak.
- Effects appear in blood vessels, skin, bone, cartilage, tendons, and gums.

Vitamin C as antioxidant and antioxidant recycler

Vitamin C:

- Directly scavenges reactive oxygen species (ROS).
- Regenerates other antioxidants, including vitamin E and glutathione.
- Concentrates in immune cells (neutrophils, lymphocytes) and supports their bactericidal and antiviral functions.

Clinical implication: In high-stress, high-demand, or inflammatory states, vitamin C demand increases; marginal intake can lead to structural fragility and increased oxidative damage over time. See Chapter 9 and Appendix B.

Part 8: Systems interactions and synergies

Key synergistic relationships include:

- Magnesium + ATP: Enabling energy use across all systems.
- Zinc + Vitamin C: Immune resilience and wound healing.
- Boron + Vitamin D + Magnesium: Hormonal availability, bone health, and mineral retention.
- Copper + Zinc: Balanced antioxidant defense (Cu/Zn SOD), myelin maintenance, and immune modulation.
- B12/Folate + Vitamin C + B6/B2: Methylation, DNA repair, and neurotransmitter synthesis.

These interactions underscore why isolated, high-dose single-nutrient strategies can fail or backfire, and why comprehensive assessment is often needed. See Chapter 10 (Integration) and Appendix A (UCOS framework) for systems-based clinical protocols.

This appendix provides the mechanistic backbone for the clinical stories in the main chapters. Appendix B translates these mechanisms into practical laboratory assessment and interpretation. Appendix D extends this framework into biophysical and frequency-based models of cellular coherence.

APPENDIX D: Biophysical Models

The Body as a Living Frequency System: A Clinician's Deep Dive

Introduction for professional readers

This appendix presents the biophysical rationale for viewing the human body as a coherent electromagnetic and quantum system, a "living frequency". It connects this framework to the cellular architecture, mineral cofactors, and mitochondrial mechanisms described throughout this book. The goal is to provide clinicians with mechanistic anchors and practical applications for integrating frequency-based thinking into longevity, regenerative, and functional medicine practice.

The material here is emerging and speculative in places, but rooted in peer-reviewed quantum biology, chronobiology, and mitochondrial physiology. It is intended for advanced practitioners interested in systems-level coherence and biophysical optimization.

Section 1: From Einstein to Popp: the physics of biological coherence

1.1 Quantum entanglement and non-local correlations

Einstein's 1935 "EPR paradox" introduced the concept of quantum entanglement: two particles can become correlated such that measuring one instantaneously determines the state of the other, regardless of distance. Einstein famously dismissed this as "spooky action at a distance," but subsequent experiments, including John Clauser's and Alain Aspect's Bell-inequality tests, have confirmed that entanglement is a real feature of the quantum world.

Clinical relevance: Emerging quantum biology suggests that entanglement-like correlations may occur within biological systems, particularly in processes involving radical pairs (e.g., cryptochrome-mediated magnetoreception in birds and possibly humans) and in photosynthetic energy transfer. While direct clinical application remains speculative, the paradigm shift is important: if cells can exploit quantum coherence for energy transfer and signaling, then maintaining the conditions that support coherence, redox balance, membrane potential, and mineral cofactors becomes therapeutically significant.

1.2 Biophotons and cellular coherence

Fritz-Albert Popp's work demonstrated that living cells emit ultra-weak photons (biophotons) in the UV-visible range, with intensities of a few to several hundred photons/s/cm^2.

Crucially, these emissions are coherent, exhibiting laser-like properties including long coherence times and stable phase relationships.

Popp proposed that:

- Biophotons originate from a coherent electromagnetic field stored and regulated by DNA.
- They serve as a non-chemical communication channel for intra- and intercellular coordination.
- Healthy tissues show high coherence and efficient photon storage; malignant and aged tissues show reduced coherence and increased "photon leakage."

Clinical relevance: Coherence loss may be an early, upstream marker of cellular dysfunction. Interventions that restore redox balance, membrane integrity, and mitochondrial efficiency may indirectly restore biophoton coherence. This provides a mechanistic rationale for the mineral and cofactor architecture described in Chapters 2 and 9: each cofactor supports a specific node in the electron-transport and redox-signaling system that underlies cellular coherence.

Section 2: Electromagnetic fields, circadian rhythms, and entrainment

2.1 The Schumann resonance and human physiology

The Earth's electromagnetic cavity, formed between the surface and the ionosphere, resonates at approximately 7.8 Hz, with harmonics near 14, 20, and 26 Hz. These frequencies are known collectively as the Schumann resonance. Human brainwave activity overlaps partly with this range (7-14Hz), particularly in the alpha band, and some studies suggest that biological rhythms may entrain to geomagnetic oscillations.

Experimental evidence includes:

- Isolation studies: Subjects shielded from Earth's electromagnetic fields show circadian rhythm destabilization (period drift to 12-56 hours); re-exposure restores 24-hour periodicity.
- Heart rate variability (HRV): Real-time correlations between Schumann Resonance fluctuations and HRV coherence have been documented.
- Cellular respiration: Diurnal geomagnetic variations correlate with respiration rates in plants, worms, and rodents.

2.2 Cryptochromes and radical-pair magnetoreception

The proposed mechanism involves cryptochromes, flavoproteins in the retina and other tissues that, upon light activation, form radical pairs in a quantum-entangled spin state. These pairs are exquisitely sensitive to weak magnetic fields and can transduce geomagnetic information into circadian clock signaling via interactions with PER3 and other clock proteins.

Clinical relevance: Clinicians should consider electromagnetic hygiene as part of circadian and metabolic optimization:

- Minimize nighttime EMF exposure (Wi-Fi, cell phones, Bluetooth) in the sleep environment.
- Encourage morning sunlight exposure to synchronize cryptochrome-mediated clock resetting.
- Consider grounding practices (barefoot contact with Earth) to restore electron flow and entrainment to natural geomagnetic rhythms.

Section 3: Frequency coherence and mineral cofactors— connecting the chapters

3.1 The architecture of coherence

The following table maps the book's chapters to their roles in maintaining cellular frequency coherence:

Chapter	Cofactor / System	Role in Frequency Coherence
---	---	---

Ch. 1	The Living Cell (mitochondria)	Central oscillator; generates membrane potential, ATP, and ROS signals that set cellular "tempo"
Ch. 2	Magnesium	Required for ATP stability, membrane potential, and >300 enzymatic reactions; deficiency disrupts oscillatory enzyme kinetics
Ch. 3	DNA / Epigenetics	DNA may serve as a coherent biophoton antenna; epigenetic marks regulate gene oscillations (circadian genes, redox genes)
Ch. 4	Zinc	Cofactor for SOD and DNA repair enzymes; maintains redox coherence and protects against oxidative "noise"
Ch. 5	Proprioception	Neural integration of body-position signals depends on mitochondrial ATP in sensory neurons; coherence loss → proprioceptive drift, brain fog
Ch. 6	Phosphorus	ATP backbone; phosphorylation cascades are the "pulse" of signal transduction; maldistribution → energy incoherence
Ch. 7	Boron	Modulates membrane potential and hormone signaling; may influence voltage-gated ion

		channels that set cellular oscillation thresholds
Ch. 8	Copper	Cofactor for cytochrome c oxidase (Complex IV) and ceruloplasmin; essential for terminal electron transfer and neural bandwidth
Ch. 9	Vitamin C	Electron donor; protects against oxidative "surge" damage; supports redox coherence
Ch. 10	Integration	Coherence emerges from coordinated function of all subsystems; no single cofactor is sufficient alone

3.2 Methylene blue: tuning the oscillator

Methylene blue (MB) acts as an alternative electron carrier that can bypass damaged segments of the electron transport chain, maintain the proton gradient, and reduce pathological ROS.

From a frequency perspective, MB helps stabilize the mitochondrial oscillator when it is faltering, preventing the loss of membrane potential and ATP pulsatility that underlies coherence loss.

Clinical application: Consider methylene blue in patients with:

- Persistent fatigue despite adequate sleep and nutrition.
- Brain fog or cognitive decline with evidence of mitochondrial dysfunction.
- Circadian rhythm disruption (shift workers, jet lag, insomnia).
- Skin aging or poor wound healing.

Always screen for contraindications (G6PD deficiency, pregnancy) and use pharmaceutical-grade products with certificates of analysis. Dosing is typically low (0.5-4 mg/kg/day) and should be supervised.

Section 4: Clinical assessment of coherence

4.1 Biomarkers and functional tests

While direct biophoton measurement is not yet clinically available, proxies for coherence include:

Domain	Test / Marker	Interpretation
---	---	---
Mitochondrial function	Organic acids (lactate, pyruvate, succinate), GDF15	Elevated lactate:pyruvate ratio or GDF15 suggests mitochondrial stress
Redox status	Glutathione (GSH:GSSG ratio), 8-OHdG, MDA	Oxidative imbalance indicates coherence loss
Circadian rhythm	Salivary cortisol awakening response, melatonin onset, HRV	Blunted rhythms or low HRV coherence suggest desynchronization
Mineral status	RBC magnesium, serum zinc, copper:zinc ratio, phosphorus	Deficiencies or imbalances disrupt cofactor-dependent oscillations
Neurological	Quantitative EEG (alpha power, coherence metrics)	Reduced alpha coherence may reflect impaired brain-frequency regulation

See Appendix B for detailed interpretation of mineral and inflammatory markers.

4.2 Interventions to restore coherence

Intervention	Mechanism	Notes
---	---	---
Morning sunlight (10-30 min)	Synchronizes cryptochrome-mediated circadian clock; stimulates	First-line for all patients with circadian disruption

	mitochondrial biogenesis	
Sleep in darkness; EMF reduction	Allows melatonin secretion; reduces exogenous frequency interference	Remove devices from bedroom; consider EMF shielding if severe
Grounding (barefoot on Earth)	Electron transfer; entrainment to Schumann Resonance	20-40 min/day outdoors
Mineral repletion (Mg, Zn, P, Cu)	Restores cofactor-dependent enzymatic oscillations	Guided by labs; avoid excess copper without monitoring
Methylene blue	Stabilizes mitochondrial oscillator; reduces ROS	Off-label; screen for contraindications; use pharmaceutical-grade
Pulsed electromagnetic field (PEMF)	Externally applied frequency to entrain cellular rhythms	Emerging modality; device quality and evidence vary

Section 5: Integrating frequency medicine into practice

5.1 A layered protocol

1. Foundation: Optimize sleep, light exposure, movement, and nutrition using the cofactors from Chapters 2 and 9. See Appendix A for the UCOS framework.
2. Assessment: Measure mitochondrial, redox, circadian, and mineral biomarkers. See Appendix B.
3. Targeted support: Address deficiencies; consider methylene blue for refractory mitochondrial symptoms.
4. Environmental optimization: Reduce EMF; encourage grounding; consider PEMF where appropriate and evidence-supported.
5. Reassess: Track HRV coherence, subjective energy, cognition, and biomarkers over 8-12 weeks.

5.2 Cautions and contraindications

- Methylene blue: Avoid in G6PD deficiency, pregnancy, and lactation. At oral supplement doses (5-10 mg/day), no published cases of serotonin syndrome have been reported, including in patients on SSRIs, SNRIs, or MAO inhibitors. All documented cases involved intravenous administration at surgical doses (0.74-8 mg/kg). Inform prescribing physician of all concurrent medications. Use pharmaceutical-grade only; avoid industrial dyes.

- PEMF / frequency devices: Evidence is mixed; use only well-characterized devices with peer-reviewed support.
- Grounding: Generally safe; use caution in immunocompromised patients or those with open wounds.

Conclusion: toward a coherent medicine

The paradigm presented here, the body as a living frequency system, does not replace biochemistry; it extends it. Electrons, photons, and electromagnetic fields are not mystical add-ons but measurable, manipulable aspects of cellular physiology.

For clinicians, this means:

- Thinking beyond isolated biomarkers to systemic coherence.
- Recognizing that cofactors like magnesium, zinc, and copper are not just "nutrients" but frequency regulators.
- Understanding that interventions like light, grounding, and methylene blue work, in part, by restoring oscillatory and coherent function at the cellular and whole-body level.

APPENDIX E: Peptide Protocols

Peptide Protocols & Cellular Optimization

The central principle: signals need a system that can respond

Peptides are instructions, not fuel.

This is the single most important concept for understanding why peptide therapy appears to succeed in some patients and fail in others.

BPC-157 signals tissue repair. Thymosin alpha-1 coordinates immune activity. SS-31 stabilizes mitochondrial membranes. GLP-1 agonists modulate appetite, insulin secretion, and glucose regulation.

However, if the receiving cell lacks sufficient energy, raw materials, cleanup capacity, redox balance, or hormonal voltage, the signal may still arrive, but the system will be unable to respond effectively.

This is why UCOS is used first, or at least in parallel.

Rather than "making peptides stronger," UCOS improves the underlying conditions so that peptide signals can be translated into actual structural and functional change:

- NAD^+, PQQ, CoQ10, methylene blue → mitochondrial ATP support
- Spermidine → autophagy and cellular cleanup
- Boron ± prescription SERMs (e.g., enclomiphene) → hormonal voltage (specialist use)
- Zinc, vitamin C, magnesium → essential cofactors for enzymatic and structural processes
- Thoughtful redox modulation → clearer signaling and less oxidative "noise"

When the "living chips" are optimized, clinicians often observe that peptides move from marginal to meaningfully therapeutic. This experience is compelling but still under formal study.

Part 1: Tissue repair & regeneration peptides

BPC-157 (Body protection Compound-157)

Mechanism

Preclinical studies suggest that BPC-157:

- Promotes angiogenesis (upregulation of VEGF and related pathways)
- Enhances fibroblast migration and collagen deposition
- Modulates nitric oxide pathways and may protect vasculature
- Helps stabilize gut barrier function (tight junction proteins)
- Exerts neuroprotective effects in animal models via monoamine modulation

Evidence status: Robust animal data with promising signals in musculoskeletal, gastrointestinal, and neurologic models; human evidence is limited to case reports, small series, and early clinical use, and regulatory status remains unsettled in many countries.

Potential clinical applications (investigational/off-label):

- Tendon, ligament, and muscle injuries (tears, strains, sprains)
- Post-surgical recovery (orthopedic, abdominal)
- Gut healing (ulcers, increased permeability, IBS-like syndromes)
- Neuroprotection (TBI, stroke recovery, peripheral neuropathy)
- Systemic anti-inflammatory support in selected cases

These applications are largely based on preclinical data and early clinical experience rather than on large randomized trials.

Example dosing frameworks

(Investigational; must be individualized and compliant with local regulations.)

- SubQ injection: 250-500 mcg 1- 2×/day, 4-6 weeks (local tissue repair)
- IM injection: 250-500 mcg 1×/day, 4-6 weeks (deeper muscle/tendon)
- Oral/sublingual: 250-500 mcg 1- 2×/day, 6-8 weeks (gut/potential systemic effects)

Injection near the injury is often used for a localized effect; abdominal SubQ for systemic.

UCOS synergy

- Vitamin C (1000-2000 mg/day): Cofactor for collagen hydroxylation. BPC-157 may signal collagen synthesis; vitamin C supports structural quality.
- Zinc (15-30 mg/day, short-term with copper monitoring): Supports wound healing and MMP regulation.
- Mitochondrial support (NAD^+ precursors, CoQ10, Mg): Tissue repair is ATP-intensive.
- Adequate protein (1.6-2.0 g/kg/day in active repair phases): Provides substrate for rebuilding.

Patient language: Explaining BPC-157

"BPC-157 is a peptide signal that tells your body to repair damaged tissue, tendons, ligaments, gut lining, even nerves. It doesn't build tissue by itself; it just gives the command. We pair it with vitamin C, zinc, and enough protein so that when the command is given, your body has the materials and energy to respond."

TB-500 (Thymosin Beta-4)

Mechanism

- Upregulates actin polymerization, promoting cell migration and tissue remodeling
- Supports angiogenesis and vascular endothelial growth
- Appears anti-inflammatory via down-regulation of pro-inflammatory cytokines
- Enhances stem-cell migration in preclinical models

Evidence status: Substantial preclinical literature and some human experience in wound and cardiac models; formal randomized human data are limited, and products/sourcing vary.

Potential clinical applications (investigational/off-label):

- Tendon and ligament injuries (especially chronic or recalcitrant)
- Muscle tears and strains
- Post-surgical healing support
- Systemic inflammation and athletic recovery (theoretical/experiential)
- Hair growth stimulation (largely anecdotal)

Example dosing frameworks

- Loading: 2-5 mg SubQ 2×/week for ~4 weeks
- Maintenance: 2-5 mg SubQ 1×/week for 4-8 weeks

Route is typically systemic (SubQ or IM), not as site-specific as BPC-157.

UCOS synergy

- Collagen support: vitamin C, glycine, proline for structural integrity.
- Omega-3s (2-4 g EPA+DHA/day, if tolerated): Anti-inflammatory synergy and membrane fluidity.

Stacking

A commonly used musculoskeletal stack in regenerative settings:

- BPC-157: 250-500 mcg/day SubQ near injury
- TB-500: 2-5 mg SubQ twice weekly (systemic), 4-6 weeks

Evidence note: This combination is frequently used clinically but has not been tested in large randomized trials.

GHK-Cu (copper peptide)

Mechanism

- Modulates large gene networks related to repair, inflammation, and oxidative stress
- Stimulates collagen and glycosaminoglycan synthesis
- Regulates MMPs and matrix remodeling
- Increases antioxidant enzymes (SOD, catalase)
- May support stem-cell activation and migration in preclinical work

Evidence status: Topical GHK-Cu is well supported in cosmetic/dermatologic literature for skin and wound effects; systemic injectable use is more experimental, with limited formal human outcome data.

Clinical applications

- Topical: skin aging, wound healing, post-procedure repair, scalp/hair support

- Injectable (off-label): musculoskeletal repair, systemic regenerative support in select practices

Example dosing frameworks

- Injectable: 1-5 mg SubQ/IM 3-5×/week for 4-8 weeks (investigational; monitor copper status)
- Topical: 0.1-2% in cream/serum, applied daily, ongoing

Safety notes

Monitor copper and Zn:Cu ratio; avoid use in copper overload disorders (e.g., Wilson disease) or unexplained high copper/low ceruloplasmin.

UCOS synergy

- Vitamin C and protein: support collagen synthesis pathways that GHK-Cu activates.
- Balanced zinc and copper: maintain redox and myelin integrity.

Part 2: Mitochondrial & metabolic peptides

SS-31 (Elamipretide)

Mechanism

- Binds cardiolipin in inner mitochondrial membranes
- Stabilizes ETC architecture and reduces pathological ROS production
- Improves ATP synthesis efficiency
- Protects against mitochondrial permeability transition (apoptosis trigger)

Evidence status: SS-31/Elamipretide has undergone phase II, III trials (e.g., Barth syndrome cardiomyopathy, mitochondrial myopathies) with mixed results; it remains investigational for most indications and is not broadly approved for general fatigue or performance.

Clinical contexts (investigational):

- Mitochondrial myopathies and cardiomyopathies
- Heart failure subsets
- Chronic fatigue with documented mitochondrial dysfunction
- Neurodegenerative diseases (Parkinson's, ALS), early/experimental

- Athletic performance and recovery, theoretical/off-label

Example dosing framework

5-20 mg SubQ daily for 4-12 weeks, sometimes with intermittent schedules (e.g., 5 days on / 2 days off). Use is typically in research settings or specialized centers.

UCOS synergy

- NAD^+ support (e.g., NMN/NR or parenteral NAD): provides NADH for Complex I.
- CoQ10 (100-200 mg/day): ETC carrier; may complement SS-31's structural stabilization.
- Methylene blue (low-dose, e.g., 5-10 mg/day) and PQQ (10-20 mg/day): redox tuning and mitochondrial biogenesis in selected patients, with screening for G6PD deficiency. At oral supplement doses, the serotonin syndrome risk documented with IV surgical doses does not apply.

MOTS-c

Mechanism

- Mitochondrial-derived peptide encoded by mtDNA
- Activates AMPK; improves insulin sensitivity
- Enhances glucose and fatty-acid metabolism
- Protects against metabolic stress and diet-induced insulin resistance in models
- May improve exercise capacity and mitochondrial function in early work

Evidence status: Mostly preclinical with a small number of early human studies; long-term safety and efficacy data in general populations are limited.

Potential clinical applications (investigational/off-label):

- Metabolic syndrome, insulin resistance, prediabetes
- Weight and body-composition support
- Athletic performance and endurance
- Age-related metabolic decline

Example dosing framework

5-15 mg SubQ 2-3×/week for 4-12 weeks, in cycles

UCOS synergy

- L-Carnitine (1000-2000 mg/day): Supports fatty-acid transport into mitochondria.
- Alpha-lipoic acid (300-600 mg/day): Insulin sensitizer; mitochondrial cofactor.
- Omega-3s and vitamin D: anti-inflammatory and metabolic support.

Humanin Mechanism:

- Mitochondrial-derived peptide with anti-apoptotic properties
- Protects neurons from Alzheimer's-related amyloid-beta toxicity
- Improves insulin sensitivity and glucose metabolism
- Neuroprotective and cardioprotective

Clinical uses:

- Alzheimer's disease and cognitive decline (investigational)
- Metabolic dysfunction
- Neuroprotection in aging

Dosing:

- **Investigational:** Varies widely; typically administered in research settings
- **Off-label clinical use:** Limited data; some practitioners use 1-5 mg SubQ 2, 3×/week

UCOS synergy:

- **NAD+, methylene blue, ALCAR**: Comprehensive mitochondrial and neuroprotective support.

Part 3: Immune modulation peptides

Thymosin Alpha-1 , Mechanism:

- Modulates T-cell maturation and differentiation
- Enhances cytotoxic T-cell and NK cell activity
- Upregulates IL-2, IL-3, IFN-gamma production
- Improves immune coordination and reduces chronic viral load
- Proposed anti-aging effects via immune rejuvenation

Clinical uses:

- Chronic viral infections (hepatitis B/C, EBV, Lyme, long COVID)
- Cancer support (adjunct immunotherapy; off-label)
- Immune senescence in aging
- Vaccine response enhancement
- Autoimmune modulation (case-by-case; requires careful monitoring)

Dosing:

Protocol	Dose	Frequency	Duration
---	---	---	---
Standard	1.6 mg	2-3×/week SubQ	3-6 months
Intensive (acute infection)	1.6 mg	Daily	2-4 weeks, then taper

UCOS synergy:

- **Zinc** (15-30 mg/day): Critical for T-cell function and thymic health.
- **Vitamin D** (optimize to 50-80 ng/mL): Supports immune cell differentiation and function.
- **Spermidine** (10 mg/day in Activate365): Autophagy improves T-cell quality and effector function.
- **NAD+**: Immune activation is energy-intensive; NAD+ supports ATP for immune responses.

The Autophagy Goldilocks zone: Why more isn't always better

Mitochondrial autophagy (mitophagy) is essential for cellular health, but it operates within a narrow therapeutic window. Too little allows damaged mitochondria to accumulate and poison the cell with reactive oxygen species; too much removes functional mitochondria and triggers energy collapse.

The danger of over-activation

Similarly, sustained AMPK activation in mammalian cells initially improves mitochondrial function but eventually leads to:

- Excessive mitochondrial clearance and energy deficit
- Dysregulated mitochondrial quality control
- Aberrant decreases in mtDNA copy number
- Loss of mitochondrial stress adaptation capacity

Clinical implications

When designing autophagy-enhancing protocols, avoid stacking too many activators simultaneously without monitoring. The combination of:

- Spermidine (10 mg/day)
- Rapamycin (pulse dosing)
- Prolonged fasting (>3 days)
- High-dose metformin (if prescribed)
- Aggressive caloric restriction (<1,200 kcal/day)

may push beyond the therapeutic window, especially in older adults or those with pre-existing mitochondrial dysfunction.

Warning signs of excessive mitophagy:

- Paradoxical worsening of fatigue despite "clean eating" and fasting
- Unexplained muscle weakness or loss (beyond expected caloric deficit)
- Exercise intolerance (inability to recover, worsening performance)
- Cold intolerance and metabolic slowdown
- Brain fog worsening rather than improving

If these emerge during aggressive autophagy protocols, pull back: reduce fasting frequency, add back calories (especially protein and carbohydrates around training), and consider pulsing autophagy enhancers (e.g., spermidine 5 days on/2 days off) rather than continuous dosing.

The safe approach: Pulsed activation

- Autophagy pulse: Overnight fast (12-16 hours) + morning exercise + spermidine or urolithin A
- mTOR pulse: Post-workout nutrition with leucine-rich protein
- Daily rhythm: AMPK dominant (fasted morning) → mTOR dominant (fed afternoon) → AMPK dominant (overnight)

Bottom line

Patient language:

"Thymosin alpha-1 is like a training sergeant for your immune system. It teaches your T cells to recognize threats, coordinate attacks, and clear infections. But immune cells need energy and nutrients to respond. That's why we pair it with zinc, vitamin D, and NAD+ from UCOS."

LL-37 (Antimicrobial Peptide)Mechanism:

- Broad-spectrum antimicrobial activity (bacteria, viruses, fungi)
- Disrupts microbial membranes
- Modulates immune responses and inflammation
- Enhances wound healing and mucosal barrier function

Clinical uses:

- Chronic infections (sinus, skin, gut, urinary)
- Biofilm disruption (Lyme, SIBO)
- Immune support in immunocompromised patients
- Wound healing (topical or injectable)

Dosing:

- **Injectable:** 100-200 mcg SubQ, 3-5×/week for 4-8 weeks
- **Intranasal:** Compounded nasal sprays for sinus infections
- **Topical:** Creams for skin infections

UCOS synergy:

- **Zinc, vitamin C, vitamin D**: Barrier and immune support.

Part 4: Glp-1 & related metabolic Agonists (6 formulations)

Overview: The GLP-1 revolution and the muscle loss problem

GLP-1 receptor agonists have transformed medical weight management. However, rapid weight loss without proper support leads to:

- 20-30% lean mass loss (muscle, bone, organ tissue) alongside fat loss
- Metabolic slowdown → increased weight regain risk
- Reduced strength, function, and quality of life

The solution: UCOS + resistance training + adequate protein BEFORE and DURING therapy.

The 6 metabolic Agonist formulations you use

1. Semaglutide (Ozempic, Wegovy, Rybelsus)

- Mechanism: Pure GLP-1 receptor agonist → insulin secretion ↑, glucagon ↓, gastric emptying ↓, appetite ↓
- Dosing:
- Subcutaneous (Ozempic/Wegovy): Start 0.25 mg weekly; titrate to 0.5 → 1.0 → 1.7 → 2.4 mg weekly
- Oral (Rybelsus): 7 mg or 14 mg daily on an empty stomach
- Weight loss: 12-15% body weight over 68 weeks (average)
- Lean mass loss: ~25% of total weight lost is lean mass without UCOS intervention

2. Tirzepatide (Mounjaro, Zepbound)

- Mechanism: Dual GIP/GLP-1 receptor agonist → enhanced insulin secretion, improved lipid metabolism, greater weight loss vs semaglutide alone
- Pharmacology: Activates both GLP-1R and GIP receptors; provides complementary metabolic effects
- GLP-1: appetite ↓, glucose control
- GIP: additional glucose-dependent insulin secretion, lipid metabolism
- Dosing: Start 2.5 mg weekly SubQ; titrate to 5 → 7.5 → 10 → 12.5 → 15 mg weekly
- Weight loss: 15-22% body weight (dose-dependent; superior to semaglutide monotherapy)
- Lean mass preservation: Emerging data suggest improved muscle quality (reduced intramuscular fat) even as total lean mass decreases
- Cardiovascular benefit: Superior metabolic outcomes in diabetes and obesity trials

3. Cagrilintide (Amylin Analog)

- Mechanism: Long-acting amylin receptor agonist; complements GLP-1

- Amylin receptors are distinct from GLP-1; they modulate different aspects of appetite, satiety, and glucose regulation
- Acts on hypothalamic amylin receptors 1 and 3 for appetite suppression
- Synergy with GLP-1: Dual mechanism enhances weight loss beyond single-agent therapy
- Dosing: 0.5- 2.4 mg weekly SubQ (typically combined with GLP-1 or tirzepatide)
- Weight loss: When added to GLP-1 or tirzepatide, an additional 5-10% body weight loss
- Use case: Patients who have plateaued on GLP-1 alone; synergistic combination protocols
- UCOS synergy: Same as other GLP-1 agents; cagrilintide adds orthogonal appetite pathway

Clinical note: Often used as "dual therapy" + GLP-1 (e.g., tirzepatide + cagrilintide) for enhanced results

4. Mazdutide (Dual GLP-1/Glucagon Agonist)

- Mechanism: Activates both GLP-1R and glucagon receptor; balanced dual agonism
- GLP-1: Appetite ↓, glucose control
- Glucagon: Lipolysis ↑, energy expenditure ↑, hepatic glucose production are controlled
- Net effect: Greater fat oxidation vs standard GLP-1
- Dosing: Investigational; typical trials use 1.25-5 mg weekly SubQ
- Weight loss: Emerging data show superior lean mass preservation compared to GLP-1 monotherapy (glucagon signals fat preferential oxidation)
- Status: Phase III trials; not yet FDA-approved but available in select longevity clinics via clinical trial access or international sourcing
- Use case: Patients optimizing body composition (maximum fat loss + maximum muscle preservation)

5. Retatrutide (Triple Agonist: GLP-1/GIP/Glucagon)

- Mechanism: First-in-class triple receptor agonist

- GLP-1R: Appetite ↓, glucose control, gastric emptying ↓
- GIP R: Additional glucose-dependent insulin secretion, lipid metabolism
- Glucagon R: Lipolysis ↑, energy expenditure ↑, brown adipose tissue activation
- Synergistic triple effect: Maximal metabolic optimization with balanced lean mass preservation
- Dosing: Start 0.5 mg weekly SubQ; titrate to 1.0 → 1.5 → 2.0 → 2.5 → 3.0 mg weekly
- Weight loss: 18-24% body weight in phase II/III trials (highest of all agents); superior lean mass preservation due to glucagon's anti-catabolic effects
- Metabolic benefits:
- Lowers HbA1c, fasting glucose, lipids
- Improves cardiovascular function
- Enhanced energy expenditure (unlike standard GLP-1)
- Status: FDA breakthrough therapy designation; Phase III trials ongoing; likely approval 2025, 2026
- Use case: Gold standard for advanced weight loss + muscle preservation in patients optimizing for longevity; best used with UCOS

6. Orforglipron (First Oral Non-Peptide GLP-1 Agonist)

- Mechanism: Small-molecule (non-peptide) GLP-1 receptor agonist; oral bioavailability
- Advantage of MODS Max: Orforglipron's weak bioavailability is dramatically enhanced by MODS Max micro-ROS + mucosal opening, making it highly effective despite its small size
- Activates GLP-1R; same downstream effects as peptide semaglutide but taken by mouth
- First daily oral GLP-1 option (vs. weekly SubQ injections)
- Dosing: Oral tablet; typical studies 37.5 → 75 → 150 mg daily (dose-dependent)
- Weight loss: 10-13% body weight; comparable to mid-range semaglutide doses
- Status: FDA approval expected 2025; marketed by Eli Lilly

- Advantage with MODS Max: Combined with MODS Max delivery, orforglipron achieves higher effective bioavailability → better tolerability, and potentially better efficacy than standard oral formulation
- Use case: Patients who prefer oral administration; easier compliance than weekly injections; synergizes with MODS Max products

Clinical pearl: Orforglipron + MODS Max represents a frontier combination; you may be among the first to use this synergy clinically.

The UCOS protocol for metabolic Agonist success (GLP-1, Tirzepatide, Cagrilintide, Retatrutide)

Phase 1: Pre-Agonist optimization (4-8 weeks BEFORE starting)

Goal: Build metabolic and hormonal resilience so weight loss is primarily fat, not muscle.

Interventions:

- Start full UCOS stack (Activate365, Mito365, Renew365, Restore365)
- Testosterone optimization (enclomiphene + boron for men; monitor women case-by-case)
- Baseline body composition (DEXA scan)
- Resistance training 3×/week minimum (focus: compound lifts, progressive overload)
- Protein target: 1.6-2.0 g/kg/day
- Baseline labs: Fasting glucose, HbA1c, insulin, lipids, CMP, CBC, 25-OH D, RBC Mg, total/free testosterone

Rationale: Muscle preservation during caloric deficit requires:

- Anabolic signaling (testosterone, GH via GABA, insulin sensitivity via NAD+/MOTS-c)
- Mechanical load (resistance training)
- Substrate availability (protein, BCAAs, essential amino acids)
- Energy (mitochondrial ATP to support protein synthesis even in deficit)

UCOS provides all of these. Metabolic agonists without UCOS = muscle catabolism.

Body composition tracking with EchoLight (REMS)

During GLP-1 agonist therapy (semaglutide, tirzepatide, retatrutide), precise, frequent body composition monitoring is critical to ensure muscle preservation.

Standard DEXA Limitations:

- Limited to every 8-12 weeks (radiation safety)
- Static snapshot; no real-time feedback
- Cannot distinguish water weight from true muscle loss
- Slower results turnaround

EchoLight (REMS) Advantages:

- Unlimited scan frequency, weekly, biweekly, or monthly, without radiation concerns
- Real-time results, immediate feedback for protocol adjustment
- Precise muscle vs. fat tracking, distinguishes lean mass quality, not just quantity
- Visceral fat measurement, a critical metric for metabolic agonist efficacy
- Faster scans, 1-2 minutes vs. 10-15 minutes
- Lower per-scan cost, can afford more frequent monitoring

Recommended Protocol During GLP-1 Therapy:

Phase	Frequency	Metric Focus
---	---	---
Week 0 (Baseline)	Single EchoLight	Establish body composition, fragility baseline
Weeks 1-12 (Active titration)	Biweekly EchoLight	Track fat loss vs. lean mass; adjust protein/peptides real-time
Weeks 12-24 (Maintenance)	Monthly EchoLight	Monitor stability; prevent rebound
Post-GLP-1 (months 3-12)	Quarterly EchoLight	Long-term composition preservation

Intervention Triggers (Based on EchoLight Data):

- If lean mass loss >10% at any point: Increase protein to 2.0-2.2 g/kg, add creatine, consider CJC-1295 + ipamorelin peptide
- If visceral fat plateaus: Add MOTS-c (5-15 mg 2, 3×/week), increase training intensity
- If bone density declines: Add Sigumir Khavinson peptide, boron 6-10 mg/day, resistance training emphasis

Expected Outcomes with EchoLight Monitoring:

- Fat loss: 15-24% body weight (>90% of total)
- Lean mass preservation: <10% of total weight loss
- Muscle quality improvement: Increased density/strength despite slight mass reduction
- Visceral fat reduction: 30-50% in 24 weeks (major metabolic benefit)

Phase 2: Agonist Initiation + Muscle Defense (Weeks 1-24)

Continue UCOS stack.

Add metabolic agonist:

- Titrate per standard protocols (see above).
- Monitor appetite suppression; ensure protein intake remains >1.2 g/kg/day minimum (ideally 1.6-2.0 g/kg).

Agonist selection:

- Single agent (starting): Semaglutide or tirzepatide
- Advanced (if plateau): Add cagrilintide to tirzepatide; or switch to retatrutide
- Oral option: Orforglipron + MODS Max for daily dosing

Protein strategies when appetite is suppressed:

- High-protein shakes (whey isolate, collagen peptides)
- Front-load protein early in the day
- Small, frequent protein feedings
- Prioritize lean, easily digestible sources (chicken, fish, eggs, Greek yogurt)

Resistance training:

- Maintain 3×/week minimum
- Focus on compound movements: squats, deadlifts, presses, rows
- Progressive overload (add weight or reps weekly)

Body composition tracking:

- DEXA every 8-12 weeks
- Goal: >90% fat loss, <10% lean mass loss
- If lean mass loss >15%, increase protein, add creatine (5 g/day), consider anabolic peptide (e.g., CJC-1295 + ipamorelin)

Labs at 12 weeks:

- Repeat fasting glucose, HbA1c, lipids
- Check total/free testosterone (ensure hormonal support is maintained)
- Adjust UCOS components as needed

Phase 3: Weight Stabilization & Metabolic Reset (Weeks 24-52+)

Goal: Prevent rebound weight gain; lock in new body composition.

Continue:

- UCOS (can reduce to maintenance doses if stable)
- Resistance training (now part of lifestyle)
- Protein 1.2-1.6 g/kg/day
- Metabolic agonist (many patients stay on lower maintenance doses indefinitely)

Metabolic monitoring:

- Resting metabolic rate (RMR) via indirect calorimetry
- If RMR drops >10% beyond what's expected for weight loss → increase reverse dieting, add MOTS-c or other metabolic peptides

Preventing rebound:

- Do not stop agonist abruptly without a transition plan
- Taper dose slowly while reinforcing dietary habits
- Continue UCOS hormonal voltage (testosterone, GABA/GH axis)

- Track weight weekly; intervene early if regain >2-3% body weight

Advanced stacking: Combining metabolic Agonists

The cutting edge of weight loss optimization combines multiple agents for synergistic effects:

Stack	Components	Expected Weight Loss	Lean Mass Preservation	Use Case
---	---	---	---	---
Dual	Tirzepatide + cagrilintide	20-25%	Good (dual mechanism)	Plateau patients; maximum efficacy without triple agonist
Triple	Retatrutide alone	20-24%	Excellent (glucagon preserves muscle)	Gold standard; optimal fat loss + muscle preservation
Oral combo	Orforglipron + MODS Max	12-16%	Moderate (but enhanced by MODS Max)	Patients preferring oral; frontier delivery approach
Peptide + agonist	Tirzepatide + MOTS-c	18-22% + metabolic optimization	Excellent	Refractory cases; orthogonal metabolic signaling

Patient Language: Metabolic Agonist + UCOS Explained

"These newer medications, tirzepatide, retatrutide, or forglipron with MODS Max, are game-changers for weight loss. But they come with a risk: losing muscle along with fat. Muscle is your metabolic engine; lose too much and your metabolism crashes, making weight regain almost inevitable.

That's why we don't just give you the medication and send you home. We start with UCOS 4-8 weeks before the medication to optimize your testosterone levels, mitochondrial function, and muscle-building capacity. We make sure you're eating enough protein and lifting weights. We track your body composition every 8-12 weeks with EchoLight (REMS technology ultrasound for bone density and fragility)

The result? You lose 15-24% of your body weight (depending on which medication), but 95% of that is fat. Your muscles stay strong. Your metabolism stays high. And when you reach your goal weight, you keep it off.

The newest agents like retatrutide actually work WITH your body's fat-burning mechanisms; they don't just kill your appetite, they reprogram your metabolism toward fat oxidation. Combined with UCOS, that's the most powerful weight loss + health preservation platform available today."

The UCOS Protocol for GLP-1 Success

Phase 1: Pre-GLP-1 Optimization (4-8 Weeks BEFORE Starting GLP-1)

Goal: Build metabolic and hormonal resilience so weight loss is primarily fat, not muscle.

Interventions:

- **Start full UCOS stack** (Activate365, Mito365, Renew365, Restore365)
- **Testosterone optimization** (enclomiphene + boron for men; monitor women case-by-case)
- **Baseline body composition** (DEXA scan)
- **Resistance training** 3×/week minimum (focus: compound lifts, progressive overload)
- **Protein target:** 1.6-2.0 g/kg/day
- **Baseline labs:** Fasting glucose, HbA1c, insulin, lipids, CMP, CBC, 25-OH D, RBC Mg, total/free testosterone

Rationale: Muscle preservation during caloric deficit requires:

- **Anabolic signaling** (testosterone, GH via GABA, insulin sensitivity via NAD+/MOTS-c)
- **Mechanical load** (resistance training)

- **Substrate availability** (protein, BCAAs, essential amino acids)
- **Energy** (mitochondrial ATP to support protein synthesis even in deficit)

UCOS provides all of these. GLP-1 without UCOS = muscle catabolism.

Phase 2: GLP-1 Initiation + Muscle Defense (Weeks 1-24)

Continue UCOS stack. Add GLP-1:

- Titrate per standard protocols (see above).
- Monitor appetite suppression; ensure protein intake remains >1.2 g/kg/day minimum (ideally 1.6-2.0 g/kg).

Protein strategies when appetite is suppressed:

- High-protein shakes (whey isolate, collagen peptides)
- Front-load protein early in the day
- Small, frequent protein feedings
- Prioritize lean, easily digestible sources (chicken, fish, eggs, Greek yogurt)

Resistance training:

- Maintain 3×/week minimum
- Focus on compound movements: squats, deadlifts, presses, rows
- Progressive overload (add weight or reps weekly)

Body composition tracking:

- DEXA every 8-12 weeks
- **Goal:** >90% fat loss, <10% lean mass loss
- If lean mass loss >15%, increase protein, add creatine (5 g/day), consider anabolic peptide (e.g., CJC-1295 + ipamorelin)

Labs at 12 weeks:

- Repeat fasting glucose, HbA1c, lipids
- Check total/free testosterone (ensure hormonal support is maintained)
- Adjust UCOS components as needed

Phase 3: Weight Stabilization & Metabolic Reset (Weeks 24-52+)

Goal: Prevent rebound weight gain; lock in new body composition.

Continue:

- UCOS (can reduce to maintenance doses if stable)
- Resistance training (now part of lifestyle)
- Protein 1.2-1.6 g/kg/day
- GLP-1 (many patients stay on lower maintenance doses indefinitely)

Metabolic monitoring:

- Resting metabolic rate (RMR) via indirect calorimetry
- If RMR drops >10% beyond what's expected for weight loss → increase reverse dieting, add MOTS-c or other metabolic peptides

Preventing rebound:

- **Do not stop GLP-1 abruptly** without a transition plan
- Taper dose slowly while reinforcing dietary habits
- Continue UCOS hormonal voltage (testosterone, GABA/GH axis)
- Track weight weekly; intervene early if regain >2-3% body weight

GLP-1 + Peptide Combinations for Advanced Protocols

Goal	GLP-1 Base	Add Peptide	Rationale
---	---	---	---
Maximize muscle preservation	Semaglutide or tirzepatide	CJC-1295 + ipamorelin (GH axis)	GH supports muscle protein synthesis during deficit
Enhance fat oxidation	Tirzepatide	MOTS-c	Dual metabolic optimization
Improve skin during weight loss	Any GLP-1	GHK-Cu (topical + injectable)	Collagen synthesis, skin tightening
Support gut health (nausea)	Any GLP-1	BPC-157 (oral)	Gastric protection, reduced GI side effects

Patient Language: GLP-1 + UCOS Explained

"GLP-1 medications like Ozempic and Mounjaro are incredibly effective for weight loss, but they come with a risk: losing muscle along with fat. Muscle is your metabolic engine; lose too much and your metabolism crashes, making weight regain almost inevitable.

That's why we don't just give you the GLP-1 and send you home. We start with UCOS 4-8 weeks before the medication to optimize your testosterone levels, mitochondrial function, and muscle-building capacity. We make sure you're eating enough protein and lifting weights. We track your body composition every 8-12 weeks with DEXA scans.

The result? You lose 15-20% of your body weight, but 95% of that is fat. Your muscles stay strong. Your metabolism stays high. And when you reach your goal weight, you keep it off."

Patient Language: Metabolic Agonist + UCOS (Tightened)

"Medications like semaglutide, tirzepatide, and the newer multi-agonists are extremely effective for weight loss. Clinical trials show that many people lose significant weight on them. The catch is that a meaningful portion of that loss can be muscle, not just fat, if we do nothing to protect your lean tissue.

Muscle is your metabolic engine. Lose too much of it and your resting metabolism drops, you feel weaker, and it becomes easier to regain weight once the medication is reduced or stopped.

That is why these medications are never a stand-alone plan in this clinic.

Before you start, we spend 4-8 weeks getting your system ready: we optimize your protein intake, support your mitochondria and hormones with a UCOS-style foundation, and get you into a simple, sustainable resistance-training routine. Then, when we add the medication, your body is set up to pull more of the weight loss from fat and to hold on to as much muscle as possible.

We track not just the number on the scale, but also your body composition over time. If we see muscle dropping faster than we like, we adjust quickly, more protein, creatine, training tweaks, or reconsidering the dose and strategy.

The goal is not just to make you lighter. The goal is to make you leaner, stronger, and more resilient, and to give you a way to keep those gains long after the prescription ends."

Part 5: Growth hormone axis peptides

Ipamorelin Mechanism:

- Growth hormone secretagogue (ghrelin mimetic)
- Selective for GH release; minimal effect on cortisol or prolactin
- Short half-life; mimics natural pulsatile GH secretion

Clinical uses:

- Anti-aging, body composition optimization
- Muscle growth and fat loss
- Recovery from injury or surgery
- Improved sleep quality

Dosing:

- **Typical:** 200-300 mcg SubQ, 1-2×/day (morning, pre-bed)
- **Cycle:** 3-6 months on, 1-2 months off

UCOS synergy:

- **GABA** (50 mg in Restore365): may support growth hormone secretion; additive with ipamorelin

CJC-1295 (with or without DAC)Mechanism:

- GHRH (growth hormone-releasing hormone) analog
- **With DAC (Drug Affinity Complex):** Long-acting (half-life 6-8 days); sustained GH elevation
- **Without DAC (Modified GRF 1-29):** Short-acting; used for pulsatile dosing

Clinical uses:

- Body composition, muscle growth, fat loss
- Anti-aging
- Often stacked with ipamorelin for synergistic GH release

Dosing:

- **CJC-1295 DAC:** 1-2 mg SubQ weekly
- **CJC-1295 no DAC (Mod GRF):** 100-200 mcg SubQ, 1-3×/day (often paired with ipamorelin)

Stack example:

- Ipamorelin 200 mcg + CJC-1295 no DAC 100 mcg, both SubQ before bed, 5 days/week

Tesamorelin Mechanism:

- GHRH analog; FDA-approved for HIV-associated lipodystrophy
- Reduces visceral adipose tissue (VAT)
- Improves body composition

Dosing:

- **FDA-approved:** 2 mg SubQ daily
- **Off-label:** Same dosing for non-HIV visceral fat reduction

UCOS synergy:

- Tesamorelin + MOTS-c + UCOS = powerful metabolic remodeling for stubborn visceral fat

Part 6: Cognitive & Neuroprotective peptides

Semax Mechanism:

- Synthetic analog of ACTH (adrenocorticotropic hormone) fragment
- Enhances BDNF (brain-derived neurotrophic factor) expression
- Improves focus, memory, neuroplasticity
- Neuroprotective in stroke and TBI models

Clinical uses:

- Cognitive enhancement, focus, memory
- Neuroprotection (stroke recovery, TBI)
- ADHD (off-label; investigational)
- Anxiety and stress resilience

Dosing:

- **Intranasal:** 300-1,000 mcg (0.3-1.0 mg) per dose, 1-3 times daily" to clarify this is per-dose, not total daily
- **Cycle:** 2-4 weeks on, 1-2 weeks off

UCOS synergy:

- **Methylene blue** (10 mg in Mito365): Crosses BBB; supports mitochondrial function in neurons
- **NAD+** and **ALCAR**: Neuronal ATP and acetylcholine support

Selank Mechanism:

- Synthetic analog of tuftsin (immune peptide)

- Anxiolytic, improves emotional stability
- Enhances learning and memory via modulation of monoamines (serotonin, dopamine)

Clinical uses:

- Anxiety, stress, emotional regulation
- Cognitive enhancement
- Immune modulation (secondary effect)

Dosing:

- **Intranasal:** 0.3, 1.0 mg/day
- **Cycle:** 2-4 weeks

Cerebrolysin Mechanism:

- Peptide mixture derived from porcine brain
- Neurotrophic effects (BDNF, NGF-like activity)
- Neuroprotective in stroke, TBI, Alzheimer's, Parkinson's

Clinical uses:

- Neurodegenerative diseases (investigational in the US; approved in Europe/Asia)
- Stroke recovery
- TBI and concussion

Dosing:

- **IV or IM:** 5-30 mL daily for 10-20 days; repeat courses as needed

UCOS synergy:

- Full mitochondrial and NAD+ support for neuronal energy

Dihexa Mechanism:

- Hepatocyte growth factor (HGF) mimetic
- Promotes synaptogenesis and neuroplasticity
- Proposed cognitive enhancement and neuroprotection

Clinical uses:

- Cognitive decline, Alzheimer's (investigational)
- Cognitive enhancement (off-label; limited human data)
- Critical: NO human clinical trials exist. All human use is experimental and off-label. Dosing extrapolated from animal studies only

Dosing:

- **Highly variable; investigational**
- Oral bioavailability reported; typical experimental doses: 1-5 mg/day

Caution: Limited human safety data; use with extreme care.

P21 (Cerebrolysin-derived)Mechanism:

- LIF inhibition, not direct CNTF agonism
- Neuroprotective, enhances neurogenesis

Clinical uses:

- Cognitive enhancement
- Neuroprotection (TBI, neurodegenerative disease, investigational)

Dosing:

- **Intranasal:** Variable; typically 1-3 mg/day

Part 7: Khavinson Bioregulatory peptides (complete series)

Overview: The Khavinson Peptide System

Developed by Russian gerontologist Vladimir Khavinson, bioregulatory peptides (bioregulators) are short-chain peptides (2-4 amino acids) proposed to restore tissue-specific gene expression and function.

Mechanism hypothesis:

- Bind to specific DNA sequences in target tissues
- Modulate gene transcription and protein synthesis
- "Reset" aging organ function toward youthful patterns

Evidence base:

- **Strong in Russian/European literature:** 40+ years of research, multiple clinical trials
- **Limited Western peer review:** Mechanism plausible (epigenetic modulation), but independent replication needed
- **Clinical use:** Widespread in European/Russian longevity clinics; growing use in US integrative practices

Quality control:

- Source from reputable peptide pharmacies with certificates of analysis

- Watch for contamination and dosing accuracy

General dosing pattern:

- **Cycle:** 10-20 days (daily SubQ or IM)
- **Frequency:** Repeat every 3-6 months or as clinically indicated
- **Stacking:** Can combine 2-3 organ-specific peptides; avoid >3 simultaneously

The Complete Khavinson Series (21 Peptides)

1. Epitalon (Epithalon): Pineal Gland

- **Sequence:** Ala-Glu-Asp-Gly (AEDG)
- **Mechanism:** Proposed telomerase activator; modulates melatonin synthesis; regulates circadian and neuroendocrine function
- **Uses:** Anti-aging, circadian disruption, low melatonin, neuroprotection
- **Dosing:** 5-10 mg total over 10-20 days (e.g., 0.5-1 mg/day SubQ)
- **UCOS synergy:** Melatonin (600 mcg in Restore365) for circadian support

2. Vilon: Thymus (Immunomodulatory)

- **Sequence:** Lys-Glu (dipeptide)
- **Mechanism:** Stimulates T-cell and B-cell function; modulates cytokine expression (IL-1α, IL-1β, IL-8, TNF-α)
- **Uses:** Immune aging, recurrent infections, general immune support
- **Dosing:** 10-20 mg total over 10-20 days
- **UCOS synergy:** Zinc, vitamin D, spermidine (autophagy improves T-cell quality)

3. Thymalin: Thymus (Peptide Complex)

- **Type:** Natural peptide complex from calf thymus (not synthetic like Vilon)
- **Mechanism:** Stronger immune modulation than Vilon; regulates T-cell maturation and differentiation for severe cases
- **Uses:** Severe immune dysfunction, chronic infections, cancer support (adjunct)

- **Dosing:** 10-30 mg over 10 days IM
- **Note:** More potent than Vilon; use for more severe immune issues

4. Thymogen: Thymus

- **Sequence:** Glu-Trp (dipeptide)
- **Mechanism:** Similar to Vilon but with a distinct amino acid sequence; immune modulation
- **Uses:** Immune support, particularly in combination protocols. Synthetic dipeptide (Glu-Trp); similar but distinct from Vilon; use for moderate immune support

5. Cortagen: Brain & Vascular

- **Mechanism:** Neuroprotection, vascular endothelial support
- **Uses:** Cognitive decline, vascular aging, stroke recovery
- **Dosing:** 10-20 mg over 10-20 days
- **UCOS synergy:** Methylene blue, NAD+, ALCAR for neuronal energy

6. Chonluten: Respiratory & Lung

- **Sequence:** Glu-Asp-Gly (tripeptide)
- **Mechanism:** Supports respiratory epithelium and lung function
- **Uses:** COPD, asthma, chronic respiratory conditions, lung aging
- **Dosing:** 10-20 mg over 10-20 days

7. Ventfort: Vascular System

- **Mechanism:** Supports vascular endothelium, improves circulation
- **Uses:** Hypertension, vascular aging, atherosclerosis prevention
- **Dosing:** 10-20 mg over 10-20 days
- **UCOS synergy:** Omega-3s, vitamin C (endothelial support)

8. Cerluten: Brain (Cerebral Cortex)

- **Mechanism:** Neuroprotection, supports neuronal function and plasticity
- **Uses:** Cognitive decline, Alzheimer's, Parkinson's, general brain aging

- **Dosing:** 10-20 mg over 10-20 days
- **UCOS synergy:** Full neuroprotective stack (MB, NAD+, ALCAR, DHA)

9. Pielotax: Kidney

- **Mechanism:** Supports renal function and cellular regeneration in kidney tissue
- **Uses:** Chronic kidney disease, nephropathy, kidney aging
- **Dosing:** 10-20 mg over 10-20 days

10. Chelohart: Heart

- **Mechanism:** Supports cardiomyocyte function, improves cardiac contractility
- **Uses:** Heart failure, post-MI recovery, cardiac aging
- **Dosing:** 10-20 mg over 10-20 days
- **UCOS synergy:** CoQ10, L-carnitine, omega-3s

11. Svetinorm: Liver

- **Mechanism:** Supports hepatocyte function, liver regeneration, detoxification
- **Uses:** Liver disease (NAFLD, hepatitis), detoxification support, liver aging
- **Dosing:** 10-20 mg over 10-20 days
- **UCOS synergy:** ALA, NAC, milk thistle (if using)

12. Stamakort: Gastric Mucosa

- **Mechanism:** Supports gastric epithelium, reduces inflammation, promotes healing
- **Uses:** Gastritis, ulcers, GERD, gastric aging
- **Dosing:** 10-20 mg over 10-20 days
- **UCOS synergy:** BPC-157 (oral) for gut healing

13. Sigumir: Bone & Cartilage

- **Mechanism:** Supports osteoblast and chondrocyte function, bone/cartilage regeneration
- **Uses:** Osteoporosis, arthritis, fracture recovery, musculoskeletal aging
- **Dosing:** 10-20 mg over 10-20 days
- **UCOS synergy:** Boron, vitamin D, magnesium (bone health)

14. Zhenoluten: Female Reproductive System (Ovaries)

- **Mechanism:** Supports ovarian function, hormonal balance
- **Uses:** Menopause symptoms, hormonal imbalance, female reproductive aging
- **Dosing:** 10-20 mg over 10-20 days
- **UCOS synergy:** Boron (estrogen metabolism)

15. Libidon: Male Reproductive System (Prostate/Testes)

- **Mechanism:** Supports testicular and prostate function
- **Uses:** Low testosterone, BPH, male reproductive aging
- **Dosing:** 10-20 mg over 10-20 days
- **UCOS synergy:** Enclomiphene + boron for testosterone optimization

16. Pinealon: Pineal Gland (similar to Epitalon but distinct sequence)

- **Mechanism:** Circadian and neuroendocrine regulation
- **Uses:** Sleep disorders, circadian disruption, pineal aging
- **Dosing:** 10-20 mg over 10-20 days

17. Retinalamin: Retina

- **Mechanism:** Supports retinal cell function, visual health
- **Uses:** Macular degeneration, diabetic retinopathy, age-related vision loss
- **Dosing:** 10-20 mg over 10-20 days IM or parabulbar injection (specialist administration)

18. Cartalax: Muscle Tissue

- **Mechanism:** Supports muscle regeneration and protein synthesis
- **Uses:** Sarcopenia, muscle wasting, athletic recovery
- **Dosing:** 10-20 mg over 10-20 days
- **UCOS synergy:** Creatine, BCAAs, resistance training

19. Bronchogen: Bronchial Tissue

- **Mechanism:** Supports bronchial epithelium
- **Uses:** Chronic bronchitis, asthma, respiratory aging
- **Dosing:** 10-20 mg over 10-20 days

20. Taxorest: Adrenal Glands

- **Mechanism:** Supports adrenal function, stress resilience
- **Uses:** Adrenal fatigue, chronic stress, HPA axis dysfunction
- **Dosing:** 10-20 mg over 10-20 days
- **UCOS synergy:** Adaptogenic support if needed (e.g., rhodiola, ashwagandha)

21. Endoluten: Pineal Gland (Natural Complex)

- **Type:** Natural peptide complex from pineal gland (not synthetic)
- **Mechanism:** Similar to Epitalon; circadian and longevity support
- **Uses:** Anti-aging, circadian disorders
- **Dosing:** Variable; often used in combination with Epitalon

Clinical Use of Khavinson Peptides: A Practical Framework.

When to use:

- Target organ dysfunction identified via labs, imaging, or symptoms
- Anti-aging protocols for patients >50 seeking organ-specific support
- After UCOS foundation is established (3-6 months in)

How to select:

- Match peptide to organ system needing support
- Example clinical scenarios:
- **Cognitive decline** → Cerluten, Cortagen, Epitalon
- **Immune senescence** → Vilon or Thymalin
- **Cardiovascular aging** → Chelohart, Ventfort
- **Kidney disease** → Pielotax
- **Male hypogonadism** → Libidon + enclomiphene/UCOS
- **Female menopause** → Zhenoluten + UCOS

Dosing schedule:

- **Standard cycle:** 10-20 days, daily SubQ or IM (0.5-1 mg/day per peptide)
- **Repeat:** Every 3-6 months

- **Stacking:** Can use 2-3 peptides simultaneously (e.g., Epitalon + Vilon + Cerluten for comprehensive anti-aging)

Monitoring:

- Track organ-specific biomarkers (e.g., creatinine for Pielotax, PSA for Libidon, cognitive testing for Cerluten)
- Patient-reported outcomes (energy, sleep, cognition, pain, etc.)
- Adjust frequency and selection based on response

Part 8: Patient communication templates

Template 1: Patient Language—Why We Start with UCOS Before Peptides

"Peptides are like software updates for your body. BPC-157 is the 'repair tissue' update. Thymosin alpha-1 is the 'boost immune system' update. GLP-1 is the 'reduce appetite and regulate blood sugar' update.

But here's the problem: if your hardware is broken, if your mitochondria are struggling, your cells are full of junk, and your hormones are low, those software updates can't install properly.

That's why we start with UCOS. It's like upgrading your RAM, cleaning your hard drive, and making sure your battery is charged before we run the new software. Once your cells are ready, the peptides work 3-5 times better than they would alone."

Template 2: Explaining GLP-1 + UCOS for Muscle Preservation

"GLP-1 medications like Ozempic and Mounjaro are incredibly effective for weight loss. But they come with a risk: if we don't protect your muscle, you'll lose 20-30% of your weight as muscle rather than fat. When that happens, your metabolism crashes and the weight comes right back.

That's why we don't just hand you the medication and say 'good luck.' We start with UCOS 4-8 weeks before the GLP-1 to optimize your testosterone, energy, and muscle-building capacity. We make sure you're eating enough protein and lifting weights. We track your body composition with DEXA scans every 8-12 weeks.

The result? You lose 15-20% of your body weight, but 95% of it is fat. Your muscles stay strong. Your metabolism stays high. And when you reach your goal, you keep it off."

Template 3: Explaining Khavinson Bioregulators

"Khavinson peptides are like a 'reset button' for specific organs. Each one is designed for a particular tissue, such as the brain, heart, liver, thymus, etc. They're short chains of amino acids that signal your cells to restore youthful gene expression patterns.

They've been used in Europe and Russia for 40+ years with good safety data, but they're still considered investigational in the US. We use them when you have a specific organ that's aging faster than the rest of you, for example, your immune system (Vilon or Thymalin), your brain (Cerluten), or your heart (Chelohart).

We give them in short 10-20-day cycles a few times a year alongside your UCOS foundation. Many patients report feeling like that organ 'woke up' again."

Part 9: Clinician sequencing guide

General Sequencing Principle

Phase 1: UCOS foundation (4-12 weeks)

Phase 2: Add first peptide based on primary clinical goal

Phase 3: Add second peptide or Khavinson bioregulatory if needed (avoid >3 peptides simultaneously)

Clinical Scenario 1: Musculoskeletal Injury

Week 0-4:

- Start UCOS (full stack)
- Adequate protein (1.6-2.0 g/kg/day)
- Can start **BPC-157** immediately (250-500 mcg SubQ near injury, 1-2×/day), exception to "UCOS first" rule for acute injury

Week 4-8:

- Continue BPC-157
- Add **TB-500** (2-5 mg SubQ 2×/week) if injury is severe or chronic
- Track healing progress (pain, range of motion, imaging if indicated)

Week 8+:

- Taper peptides as healing progresses
- Maintain UCOS; add **Sigumir** (bone/cartilage Khavinson peptide) if structural support is needed long-term

Clinical Scenario 2: Chronic Fatigue/Mitochondrial Dysfunction

Week 0-8:

- Start UCOS (emphasize Mito365: MB, PQQ, NAD+, CoQ10 (in Renew365))
- Optimize sleep, circadian rhythm, grounding
- Labs: NAD+ (if available), organic acids, hs-CRP, 25-OH D, RBC Mg

Week 8-16:

- If fatigue persists despite UCOS, add **SS-31** (5-20 mg SubQ daily for 4-12 weeks)
- Consider **MOTS-c** (5-15 mg SubQ 2-3×/week) if metabolic component (insulin resistance, weight issues)

Week 16+:

- Reassess labs and symptoms
- Add **Cortagen or Cerluten** (Khavinson) if neurological/cognitive fatigue is prominent

Clinical Scenario 3: Immune Senescence/Recurrent Infections

Week 0-8:

- UCOS foundation (emphasize zinc, vitamin D, spermidine for autophagy)
- Baseline immune labs: CBC with diff, immunoglobulins, vitamin D, zinc

Week 8-24:

- Add **Thymosin alpha-1** (1.6 mg SubQ 2-3×/week for 3-6 months)
- Consider **Vilon or Thymalin** (Khavinson; 10-20 mg over 10-20 days, repeat every 3-6 months)

Ongoing:

- Monitor infection frequency, severity, duration
- Adjust dosing and frequency based on response

Clinical Scenario 4: Weight Loss with GLP-1

Week -8 to 0 (Pre-GLP-1):

- Full UCOS stack

- Testosterone optimization (enclomiphene + boron for men)
- Resistance training 3×/week
- Protein 1.6-2.0 g/kg/day
- Baseline DEXA

Week 0-24 (GLP-1 Active Phase):

- Start GLP-1 (semaglutide or tirzepatide); titrate per protocol
- Continue UCOS, protein, resistance training
- Add **MOTS-c** (5-15 mg 2-3×/week) if metabolic optimization needed
- DEXA at weeks 12 and 24

Week 24+ (Stabilization):

- Taper GLP-1 to maintenance dose or discontinue slowly
- Continue UCOS long-term
- Monitor for rebound; intervene early if weight trends up

Clinical Scenario 5: Cognitive Decline

Week 0-8:

- UCOS (emphasize Mito365: MB crosses BBB, NAD+ for neuronal ATP)
- Add **omega-3 DHA** (2-4 g/day)
- Cognitive baseline (MoCA, MMSE, or neuropsych testing)

Week 8-16:

- Add **Semax** (intranasal, 0.3-1 mg/day for 2-4 weeks, cycle)
- Or **Cerebrolysin** (5-30 mL IM/IV daily for 10-20 days) if more severe

Week 16+:

- Add **Cerluten or Cortagen** (Khavinson; 10-20 mg over 10-20 days, repeat every 3-6 months)
- Reassess cognition at 6 and 12 months

Part 10: Safety, contraindications, and red flags

General Peptide Safety

- **Source:** Use only pharmaceutical-grade peptides from reputable compounding pharmacies with certificates of analysis (COA)

- **Sterility:** All injectable peptides require sterile technique; use bacteriostatic water for reconstitution
- **Storage:** Most peptides require refrigeration (2, 8°C); some freeze-dried forms are stable at room temperature until reconstituted
- **Expiration:** Reconstituted peptides typically stable 30-60 days refrigerated; check specific peptide guidelines

"Peptide Sourcing and Quality Control:

- Source only from FDA-registered 503B compounding pharmacies or licensed international pharmacies
- Require Certificate of Analysis (COA) showing >98% purity
- Verify sterility testing and endotoxin levels
- Reconstitute with bacteriostatic water using an aseptic technique
- Most peptides require refrigeration (2-8°C); shelf life 30-90 days once reconstituted"

Contraindications

Peptide	Contraindications / Cautions
---	---
BPC-157	Generally well-tolerated; theoretical cancer risk (pro-angiogenic), avoid in active malignancy without oncologist input
TB-500	Same as BPC-157; Angiogenic properties; mixed evidence shows tumor promotion in solid tumors (colon, lung) but tumor suppression in multiple myeloma; avoid in active malignancy; pre-treatment cancer screening recommended
Thymosin alpha-1	Autoimmune disease (case-by-case; may worsen in some patients); pregnancy
GLP-1 agonists	Personal or family history of medullary thyroid cancer or

	MEN2; gastroparesis; pregnancy; pancreatitis history (relative)
Growth peptides (ipamorelin, CJC)	Active cancer; history of cancer (especially hormone-sensitive); uncontrolled diabetes
SS-31	Limited long-term human safety data; monitor carefully
Khavinson peptides	Pregnancy; active cancer (theoretical risk, not well-studied); monitor for allergic reactions

Growth peptides: IGF-1, fasting glucose, HbA1c every 3-6 months

Thymosin alpha-1: CBC with differential, immunoglobulins every 6 months

GLP-1 + UCOS: DEXA every 12 weeks (you have this), add lipase if history of pancreatitis

Red Flags: When to Stop or Adjust

- **Allergic reaction** (rash, swelling, difficulty breathing) → stop immediately; seek emergency care if severe
- **Injection site reactions** (excessive pain, redness, swelling, abscess) → check sterile technique; may indicate contamination or allergy
- **New or worsening symptoms** that don't resolve after stopping peptide → reassess diagnosis; consider alternative causes
- **Cancer diagnosis or progression** → stop angiogenic peptides (BPC-157, TB-500) and growth peptides immediately; consult oncology

Conclusion: The integrated paradigm

Peptide therapy is one of the most powerful tools in regenerative and longevity medicine. But like any tool, its effectiveness depends entirely on the system in which it's used.

A peptide given to a cell with dysfunctional mitochondria, inadequate NAD+ and ATP, poor redox balance, low hormonal voltage, and insufficient raw materials such as protein, vitamins, and minerals is like handing a blueprint to a construction crew with no power tools, no materials, and no foreman. The blueprint is perfect, but nothing gets built.

UCOS solves this.

It restores:

- **Mitochondrial capacity** (NAD+, PQQ, methylene blue, CoQ10)
- **Cleanup and renewal** (spermidine, autophagy)
- **Hormonal voltage** (testosterone via enclomiphene + boron; GH via GABA)
- **Redox signaling** (MODS Max micro-ROS; vitamin C, melatonin)
- **Structural support** (magnesium, zinc, vitamin C for collagen)

When those systems are online, peptides work the way they're supposed to: rapidly, reliably, and transformatively.

This appendix gives you the tools to implement that paradigm in your practice:

- 17+ commonly used peptides with dosing, mechanisms, and clinical use cases
- The complete Khavinson bioregulatory series (21 peptides)
- GLP-1 protocols with muscle preservation strategies
- Patient communication templates
- Clinical sequencing guides for common scenarios

You now have a complete, evidence-based, clinically actionable peptide playbook, integrated with the UCOS foundation that makes it all work.

APPENDIX F: Advanced and Frontier Protocols

Advanced Protocols & Frontier Medicine

Purpose and scope

This appendix is for clinicians and advanced patients who want to integrate cutting-edge modalities into the foundational framework of The Living Cell. It covers:

- Quantum biology and how it connects to daily protocols
- Stem cell banking and expansion for regenerative applications
- Supporting nutrient "chips" (omega-3, leucine & BCAAs, L-carnitine, ALA, fisetin, magnolia)
- Precision redox modulation
- HRV and grounding as coherence tools
- Advanced therapeutics (rapamycin, ozone, DMSO, mistletoe, Rife frequencies, PEMF)
- Biohacking tech stack (Oura, wearables, CGM)
- Patient communication templates and clinician sequencing guides

This is where you practice at the forefront.

Section 1: Quantum biology & the living cell

The four quantum effects in biology

Quantum biology now has several well-supported examples in mainstream literature.

1. Photosynthesis coherence

Light-harvesting complexes in plants and bacteria maintain quantum coherence for hundreds of femtoseconds, enabling extremely high (often >95%) energy-transfer efficiency from antenna complexes to reaction centers.

Mechanism: Excitonic states remain in superposition long enough for energy to effectively "sample" multiple paths simultaneously and select the most efficient route to the reaction center.

Clinical connection: The mitochondrial electron transport chain also depends on tightly coupled electron transfer and minimized energy loss. Ensuring adequate cofactors (NAD^+, CoQ10, cytochrome c) and minimizing redox "noise" with targeted agents (methylene blue, PQQ, vitamin C, melatonin) supports more efficient ATP generation and less heat/entropy loss.

2. Cryptochrome and magnetoreception

Birds and some other animals sense the Earth's magnetic field through radical-pair reactions in cryptochrome proteins in the retina. In mammals, cryptochromes are confirmed core circadian proteins; their role in magnetoreception in humans remains debated but mechanistically plausible.

Mechanism: Blue light activates cryptochrome, creating a spin-correlated radical pair whose reaction yield is exquisitely sensitive to weak magnetic fields (~50 μT). Changes in spin state alter downstream signaling and circadian timing.

Clinical connection:

- Cryptochromes regulate PER/CRY feedback loops in the central clock. Morning light exposure → cryptochrome activation → circadian entrainment.
- Weak electromagnetic fields (e.g., Schumann resonance at ~7.8 Hz) have been proposed to influence biological rhythms via radical-pair sensitivity, but this is still speculative and not clinically proven.

Protocol: Prioritize bright morning light (10-30 minutes outdoors), minimize blue light and EMF load at night, and create a dark, low-noise sleep environment.

3. Enzyme quantum tunneling

Protons and electrons can "tunnel" through energy barriers in enzyme-catalyzed reactions, allowing catalysis at physiological temperatures that classical models struggle to explain.

Examples: Alcohol dehydrogenase, amine oxidases, DNA polymerases, and respiratory chain complexes all show signatures of hydrogen tunneling and coupled protein motions.

Clinical connection: Efficient tunneling depends on precise donor-acceptor distances, protein dynamics, and cofactor status (Mg, Zn,

Cu, NAD^+, FAD, heme). Deficiencies in these cofactors increase effective activation energy, slow reaction rates, and reduce cellular efficiency. Restoring mineral and redox balance is not just "biochemistry"; it optimizes quantum-scale charge transfer.

4. Olfaction and vibrational theory (still debated)

The "vibrational theory" of olfaction proposes that olfactory receptors may discriminate odorants partly by their vibrational spectra, via inelastic electron tunneling, in addition to classical shape/lock-and-key recognition.

Status: Quantum-vibrational models are mathematically and physically plausible and supported by some experimental and theoretical work, but they remain controversial; most experts view smell as primarily shape-based with possible vibrational contributions.

Clinical implication: This is conceptually useful to illustrate how quantum effects can scale to perception, but it should be presented as an evolving hypothesis, not a settled fact.

Biophotons and DNA as antenna (frontier/speculative)

Biophoton emission

Ultra-weak photon emission (UPE) from living cells, on the order of 1-100 photons/s/cm^2 in the UV-visible range, is a reproducible phenomenon.

Key observations:

- Emission patterns correlate with metabolic and oxidative state; higher oxidative stress typically increases photon emission.
- Some work suggests differences in emission between healthy and malignant cells, with cancer cells often showing altered intensity and temporal patterns.
- Mitochondria and chromatin appear to be major sources of UPE.
- Popp and others reported coherence-like properties (narrow-band, laser-like features) in some systems and proposed that biophotons might serve as an intercellular communication channel coordinating growth, differentiation, and repair.

Status:

- The existence of ultra-weak photon emission is well documented.
- Its role as an organized signaling system and its clinical relevance remain unproven hypotheses.

DNA as quantum antenna

Popp and later authors proposed that DNA, with its helical structure and stacked aromatic bases, could act as a broadband electromagnetic antenna or waveguide, storing and regulating coherent fields that orchestrate cellular processes.

Rationale: π-stacked bases and helical geometry support charge-transfer and excitonic interactions that could, in theory, support resonant electromagnetic behavior.

Status: This remains highly speculative. There is no direct experimental proof that DNA functions as a macroscopic "quantum antenna" in vivo. It is a useful conceptual metaphor but should be explicitly labeled as unproven.

Why coherence matters clinically

Quantum coherence can be framed as preservation of information and efficient energy transfer across scales.

Coherent systems:

- Maintain ordered electron and proton flow
- Minimize unnecessary heat and entropy production
- Support stable signaling and adaptability

Decoherence:

- Information loss, mis signaling, and energy dissipation as heat
- Drift toward disorder: inflammation, mitochondrial failure, aging phenotypes

In practice, "supporting coherence" maps onto familiar interventions:

- Redox optimization: Aim for clean, pulsed ROS signaling rather than chronic oxidative noise. Tools: precision redox modulators, methylene blue, vitamin C, melatonin, PQQ, NAC, glutathione support.
- Circadian entrainment: Robust light--dark cycles and timing signals stabilize PER/CRY and clock gene oscillations.

Morning bright light, dim evenings, darkness at night, consistent sleep/wake times.

- Cofactor sufficiency: Mg, Zn, Cu, Se, Fe, B-vitamins, NAD^+, and CoQ10 are required for efficient tunneling, electron transport, and antioxidant enzyme function.
- Mitochondrial support: NAD^+, PQQ, CoQ10, methylene blue, cardiolipin support, and mitophagy/autophagy strategies maintain the quality of the ETC hardware.
- Electromagnetic hygiene: Reducing unnecessary EMF exposure during sleep (especially strong RF sources near the bed) may lower background "noise," though evidence remains limited; this is a low-risk adjunct rather than a primary therapy.

Clinically, "coherence" becomes a design principle: favor interventions that sharpen timing, improve signal-to-noise, and reduce chaotic metabolic drift.

Patient language: explaining quantum biology

"Your cells aren't just chemistry—they're also physics. Your mitochondria use quantum effects to move energy with almost zero waste, your internal clock depends on light-sensitive proteins that respond to tiny signals, and your cells even give off ultra-weak light when they're under stress.

When we fix your nutrients, your light exposure, and your redox balance, we're not just 'adding fuel.' We're tuning a living, quantum-level system so your cells stay organized and efficient instead of drifting into chaos."

Clinician notes: quantum biology in practice

Label levels of evidence clearly:

- Established: photosynthetic coherence, enzyme tunneling, cryptochromes as circadian proteins and magnetoreceptors in birds.
- Debated but serious: vibrational theory of olfaction; magnetoreception in humans.
- Frontier/speculative: biophotons as a communication network; DNA as quantum antenna; Schumann resonance entrainment of biology.

Focus on what is actionable and low-risk:

- Morning light, dark nights, circadian discipline
- Mitochondrial/UCOS optimization
- Redox precision (avoid chronic megadose antioxidants; favor hormetic pulses)

Use coherence as a clinical question:

For any intervention, ask: "Does this restore timing, clarity, and efficiency of signaling or add more noise?"

Section 2: Stem cell banking & regenerative expansion

Overview

This section describes a forward-leaning approach: harvest, bank, and potentially expand a patient's own (autologous) stem or progenitor cells for future regenerative applications. Current or emerging targets include type 1 diabetes, ischemic heart failure, neurodegenerative conditions, and selected neurodevelopmental disorders. Many of these uses remain investigational and, in the US, generally require clinical-trial or IND frameworks.

The process

Harvest:

- Collect autologous cells from bone marrow aspirate, adipose tissue, or mobilized peripheral blood, depending on protocol.
- Ideal timing: when the patient is relatively young and metabolically optimized (after several months of UCOS), so harvested cells represent a "younger, cleaner" biological state.

Banking:

- Cryopreserve cells in liquid nitrogen under GMP conditions.
- Periodic viability and sterility checks are recommended to confirm long-term usability.

Expansion (where permitted):

- Culture and expand cells ex vivo under controlled conditions to increase cell numbers and potentially enrich for specific subtypes (e.g., mesenchymal stromal cells, hematopoietic progenitors).
- In the US, substantial manipulation or expansion typically converts a product into a 351 biologic requiring full FDA biologic licensure or IND oversight.

Application:

- Reinfuse or deliver cells to target tissues for tissue repair and remodeling, immune modulation, or metabolic reset (e.g., β-cell support, myocardial energetics).
- Delivery routes may include IV, intra-arterial, intramyocardial, intrathecal, or targeted organ injections depending on indication and trial design.

STEM CELL SECRETOME AND CELL-FREE REGENERATIVE MEDICINE: THE NEXT FRONTIER

The field of regenerative medicine is undergoing a paradigm shift from whole-cell transplantation to cell-free therapeutic approaches centered on the stem cell secretome—the complete collection of bioactive factors secreted by stem cells, including growth factors, cytokines, chemokines, and extracellular vesicles (particularly exosomes). This transition addresses fundamental limitations of traditional stem cell therapy: poor survival of transplanted cells (often <5% at 24 hours post-injection), rapid systemic clearance, risk of immune rejection, tumorigenicity concerns with pluripotent cells, and ethical constraints on embryonic stem cell sourcing. Mesenchymal stem cells (MSCs) and their secreted exosomes (MSC-Exos) have emerged as the most clinically advanced platform, with 64 registered clinical trials as of January 2025 investigating MSC-derived extracellular vesicles for diseases ranging from graft-versus-host disease to neurodegenerative disorders. The therapeutic potency of these secretory products rivals or exceeds that of parent cells in multiple preclinical models, while offering superior advantages: exosomes are non-immunogenic (lacking MHC surface proteins), exhibit extended shelf stability through lyophilization, can be manufactured at scale from immortalized cell lines, pose zero risk of teratoma formation, and circumvent ethical concerns entirely. Critically, the MSC secretome exerts its effects through paracrine signaling rather than cellular engraftment—growth factors such as VEGF, TGF-β, PDGF, and FGF orchestrate angiogenesis, immunomodulation, and extracellular matrix remodeling, while exosomal cargo (particularly microRNAs like miR-126, miR-146a, and miR-21) reprograms recipient cells toward regenerative phenotypes for days to weeks after delivery. This represents a fundamental reconceptualization: stem cells function primarily as biological factories producing therapeutic molecules, not as replacement tissue themselves.

The most transformative application of secretome-based therapy lies in functional organ replacement and chronic disease management through systemic or targeted delivery systems. In organ regeneration, induced pluripotent stem cell (iPSC)-derived organoids — three-dimensional multicellular structures that recapitulate organ architecture and function — are being developed for transplantation to address the critical shortage of donor organs (over 100,000 patients await transplants annually in the United States alone). These organoids, generated from patient-specific iPSCs to eliminate immune rejection, have successfully produced transplantable liver tissue, generated red blood cells with 200-million-fold expansion from single CD34+ cells (sufficient to produce 500 transfusion units from one umbilical cord blood unit), and created vascularized cardiac, kidney, and intestinal organoids approaching clinical-grade functionality. However, the breakthrough enabling true organ replacement is the integration of organoid technology with secretome enhancement strategies: pre-conditioning organoids with hypoxia or inflammatory cytokines increases their production of pro-angiogenic and immunomodulatory factors by 200-400%, dramatically improving post-transplant vascularization and integration. For chronic diseases, systemically delivered MSC exosomes have demonstrated remarkable efficacy across multiple pathologies. In Type 1 and Type 2 diabetes, exosomes carrying miR-106b-5p and miR-222-3p promote pancreatic β-cell regeneration and restore insulin sensitivity by modulating IRS-1 tyrosine phosphorylation and GLUT4 translocation in muscle and adipose tissue; diabetic wound healing is accelerated 60-80% through exosomal delivery of miR-126-3p and VEGF. In neurodegenerative diseases, MSC exosomes traverse the blood-brain barrier (a feat impossible for parent cells) to deliver neuroprotective miRNAs (miR-124, miR-133b) that reduce amyloid-β plaque load in Alzheimer's disease by 40-55%, promote α-synuclein clearance in Parkinson's disease via MMP-2 upregulation, and restore motor function in stroke and spinal cord injury models through enhanced neurogenesis and angiogenesis. In cardiovascular disease, hypoxia-primed cardiac cell-derived exosomes ("cardiosomes") containing miR-455 and miR-29b reduce post-infarction scar tissue by 50%, increase ejection fraction by 15-25%, and ameliorate diabetic cardiac fibrosis through MMP9 modulation. Phase I/II clinical trials (NCT03384433, NCT04356300) have confirmed the safety and preliminary efficacy of intravenous MSC-exosome infusions, with zero serious adverse events and sustained therapeutic effects lasting 6-24 months after single-dose administration.

Delivery methodologies represent the critical translational bottleneck, with three primary approaches emerging: (1) Combination with platelet-rich plasma (PRP), (2) systemic intravenous administration, and (3) intramuscular depot injection. The PRP-exosome combination leverages synergistic mechanisms: PRP provides supra-physiological concentrations of endogenous growth factors (PDGF, TGF-β, IGF-1) that exhibit burst release kinetics within 48 hours, creating an immediate pro-regenerative microenvironment, while co-delivered exosomes fuse with target cells to deliver sustained genetic reprogramming through miRNA cargo lasting 2-4 weeks. Clinical studies demonstrate that co-injection of PRP with ozone-activated growth factors significantly upregulates cartilage synthesis genes (IGF-1, HIF-1α, BMP2) in osteoarthritis patients, reducing pain scores by 60-75% and improving joint function for at least 8 weeks post-treatment. The addition of MSC exosomes to PRP formulations increases follicular stem cell activation in hair restoration by 3-fold compared to PRP alone, with exosomal miR-218-5p activating the Wnt/β-catenin pathway—the master regulator of hair follicle regeneration—for sustained growth stimulation. For systemic delivery, intravenous infusion of MSC-derived cells or exosomes has proven safe and well-tolerated in completed Phase I/II trials: the landmark CYP-001 trial (NCT02923375) using iPSC-derived mesenchymal stromal cells for steroid-resistant graft-versus-host disease achieved 60% two-year survival with zero treatment-related deaths, tumors, or serious adverse events. Systemic IV delivery enables widespread biodistribution and "homing" to sites of inflammation or injury through chemokine gradients, though 40-60% of cells/exosomes are initially trapped in pulmonary capillary beds before redistribution. To overcome this, intramuscular (IM) injection has emerged as superior for sustained secretome delivery: MSCs injected into skeletal muscle exhibit a 5-month dwell time (versus 3 days for IV delivery), continuously secreting therapeutic factors into the circulation while protected within dense muscle fibers. The high vascular density of muscle tissue provides a conduit for systemic factor release, enabling treatment of distant organs–IM-delivered MSCs successfully treated peripheral arterial disease and colitis through sustained circulating IGF-1 and IL-10 elevation. Most promisingly, small pluripotent stem cells (SPSCs) isolated from peripheral blood represent an autologous, ethically uncontroversial source requiring only 50-100 μL of venous blood. These cells, smaller than 8 μm in diameter, evade pulmonary entrapment when delivered systemically and exhibit multipotent differentiation capacity comparable to bone marrow MSCs. A robust chemical reprogramming protocol now generates hundreds of clinically-compliant human chemically-induced pluripotent stem (hCiPS) cells from small blood samples within 22-24 days using serum-free, pathogen-free conditions suitable for clinical translation. These blood-derived cells can be expanded, loaded into PRP formulations, or differentiated into secretome-producing MSCs for personalized regenerative therapy without invasive bone marrow or adipose tissue harvest.

The convergence of these technologies–standardized exosome production, PRP-based delivery vehicles, systemic biodistribution strategies, and autologous blood-derived pluripotent cells—positions cell-free regenerative medicine as the dominant therapeutic modality for the coming decade. Unlike whole-cell transplantation, which faces regulatory hurdles regarding cell viability, genetic stability, and manufacturing consistency, exosome therapies can be lyophilized, stored at room temperature, dosed precisely, and manufactured under Good Manufacturing Practice (GMP) guidelines with batch-to-batch reproducibility. The field is rapidly advancing toward "off-the-shelf" regenerative biologics: allogeneic MSC exosomes (derived from screened, healthy donors) are non-immunogenic and can be stockpiled for immediate use, while personalized formulations using patient-derived blood SPSCs offer the ultimate precision medicine approach. As multi-omics integration (genomics, proteomics, metabolomics) enables prediction of treatment responders and optimization of exosome cargo composition, the era of rationally designed, cell-free regenerative therapeutics targeting organ failure and chronic disease has definitively arrived. The appendix image visually represents this paradigm: mitochondrial factors, growth factors, and pluripotent stem cell-derived exosomes function synergistically as modular therapeutic units, deliverable through PRP matrices or systemic circulation, to restore tissue function without the complexities of living cell transplantation.

Mechanism: "living chip" upgrade

Stem cells as "template chips":

Multipotent or pluripotent cells can differentiate into specialized lineages (neurons, cardiomyocytes, pancreatic β-cells, immune cells) or exert potent paracrine effects via growth factors, cytokines, and exosomes.

Expansion as chip multiplication:

Banking cells when the patient is biologically younger preserves that "source code." Later expansion under controlled conditions increases the number of high-quality "chips" available when disease or injury emerges.

Reinfusion as system reset:

Fresh, functional cells or their secretome can displace or outcompete senescent cells, modulate immune tone, promote angiogenesis, and remodel fibrotic or damaged tissue, moving the system toward a younger functional state.

This fits the Living Cell model: you are not just upgrading software (signals) but replacing or augmenting hardware (cells) with earlier, healthier versions.

Clinical applications (current evidence)

Condition Proposed mechanism Evidence level (as of mid-2020s)

Type 1 diabetes: Autologous or allogeneic stem/progenitor cells to support β-cell mass, modulate autoimmunity, and improve glycemic control. Early-phase trials and pilot studies; promising but clearly investigational; durability and long-term safety still under study

Congestive/ischemic heart failure: Intramyocardial or intracoronary delivery of autologous bone-marrow-derived cells to improve perfusion, reduce fibrosis, and support cardiomyocyte survival via paracrine signaling (VEGF, IGF-1, HGF). Multiple phase II/III trials; some autologous programs have FDA Breakthrough Therapy designation and ongoing phase III work, but no broad FDA marketing approval yet

Dementia/neurodegeneration: Neural or mesenchymal stem cells to provide trophic support (BDNF, NGF), reduce neuroinflammation, and support synaptic and glial repair Early-phase and small open-label trials; mechanistically plausible, but still highly investigational; long-term outcomes unknown

Autism spectrum disorders: Immune modulation, reduction of neuroinflammation, support of synaptic connectivity via IV or intrathecal MSCs or cord blood products. Preliminary case series and early trials; heterogeneous results; mechanism under active investigation and remains experimental

For all of these, emphasize that most uses remain investigational, with variable regulation by jurisdiction.

Patient language: why bank your cells now

"Think of stem cell banking as saving the best version of your biology. Your cells today are younger and healthier than they will be in 10 or 20 years.

We can harvest and freeze those cells now, when they're in better shape. In the future — if your heart, brain, immune system, or pancreas needs help — we may be able to give you back your own cells as a living upgrade. Not just a drug, not someone else's cells, but your own best cells preserved in time."

Clinician implementation

Ideal candidates:

- Age roughly 30-50, before major chronic disease/organ failure manifests
- Motivated, health-literate patients already engaged with UCOS and foundational lifestyle work
- Patients with strong family histories of CHF, neurodegeneration, or autoimmune disease who understand the investigational nature and cost

Timing of harvest:

- After at least 3-6 months of UCOS and lifestyle optimization to improve mitochondrial function, redox status, glycemic control, and inflammatory markers at the time of collection.

- Consider repeating key labs (hs-CRP, HbA1c, lipid panel, NAD^+ surrogate markers, mitochondrial function proxies) prior to harvest.

Banking logistics:

- Use GMP-compliant facilities with documented viability, sterility, and tracking.
- Ensure clear chain-of-custody and access procedures, and educate patients about ongoing storage fees and long-term commitments.

Reinfusion protocols:

- Should be disease-specific and evidence-based, typically under clinical-trial or registry frameworks.
- Often combined with short-term immunomodulation (e.g., peri-procedural steroids, low-dose rapamycin in some protocols) to improve engraftment and reduce maladaptive inflammation; this remains investigational and must align with protocol and regulatory guidance.

Regulatory note

In the US, most autologous stem cell products that are more than minimally manipulated or used for non-homologous indications are regulated as 351 biologics and require an IND and eventual BLA for marketing approval.

A small subset of autologous cell procedures may fall under 361 regulations if minimally manipulated and used homologously, but the FDA has been increasingly strict in enforcement.

Many regenerative protocols marketed direct-to-consumer fall outside formal approvals; clinicians should:

- Work within FDA-sanctioned clinical trials where possible
- Consult regulatory counsel before building or referring to stem cell programs
- Provide explicit informed consent about investigational status, uncertain long-term risk, and realistic outcome expectations

For your practice, stem cell banking fits best as an optional, high-end adjunct for select patients, layered on top of a strong UCOS foundation, not as a replacement for foundational metabolic and mitochondrial work.

OSKM (Oct4, Sox2, Klf4, c-Myc) are the original "Yamanaka factors" that turn a fully differentiated adult cell back into a pluripotent, embryonic-like state, erasing age-related epigenetic marks and resetting cell identity. In standard iPSC protocols, OSKM are delivered into patient cells in a dish using viral (often lentiviral or retroviral) or non-viral vectors, then switched off once the cells reach pluripotency to avoid uncontrolled growth or tumor formation. Mechanistically, each factor binds specific DNA motifs, recruits epigenetic enzymes, and triggers large-scale chromatin remodeling: DNA methylation patterns are reset, heterochromatin marks such as H3K9me3 are partially erased, and youthful gene expression programs re-emerge, including telomere extension and restoration of mitochondrial function. In this sense, OSKM are not "magic genes" but a programmable switchboard that can move a cell along the axis from old/specialized to young/pluripotent, or– if used for shorter, carefully controlled pulses—toward a younger but still tissue-specific state (partial reprogramming).

In vivo work over the last decade has shown that partial, cyclic OSKM expression can rejuvenate cells and tissues without fully erasing their identity. In a classic premature-aging mouse model, short bursts of OSKM expression improved multiple aging hallmarks (DNA damage, senescence, epigenetic drift), reversed pancreatic and muscle injury, and extended lifespan, without the teratomas seen with continuous OSKM activation. More recent studies have delivered OSK/OSKM via AAV vectors to specific tissues: OSK in retinal ganglion cells restored vision in old and glaucomatous mice without tumor formation over 10-18 months, suggesting that targeted, tissue-specific partial reprogramming can safely roll back cellular age in vivo. Newer work using Cdkn2a-linked OSK AAVs in naturally aged mice delayed systemic aging phenotypes, improved wound healing, and extended lifespan without increasing cancer incidence, reinforcing the idea that context-sensitive OSK expression (only in stressed/aged cells) may be the safest route to broad rejuvenation. At the same time, other models show that strong, continuous OSKM expression in organs like the liver and intestine is lethal, producing organ failure within days, highlighting the narrow therapeutic window and the need for tight spatiotemporal control.

Clinically, this points toward two major future applications. The first is ex vivo rejuvenation and replacement: a small skin biopsy or blood draw is taken, somatic cells are reprogrammed to iPSCs with OSKM in the lab, then redifferentiated into youthful, patient-matched tissues—cardiomyocytes for heart failure, insulin-producing β-cells for diabetes, dopaminergic neurons for Parkinson's disease, or even complex organoids for partial organ replacement. iPSC-derived β-like cells have already restored normoglycemia in diabetic animal models, and iPSC-derived cardiomyocytes and cardiac patches improve contractile function and reduce scar burden after myocardial infarction in preclinical work. Separately, robust protocols now generate massive numbers of blood cells from iPSCs, such as red blood cells expanded 200-million-fold from a single progenitor—pointing toward future autologous transfusion products for anemic, oncology, or chronic kidney disease patients. In this paradigm, your "old" cells become a renewable raw material: they are reset to pluripotency, quality-controlled for genomic integrity, and then rebuilt into whatever tissue your disease requires, with minimal rejection risk because they are genetically your own.

The second application is in-body partial reprogramming to rejuvenate existing tissues without replacing them. Here, OSK/OSKM (or safer, next-generation factor cocktails) are delivered directly into the patient via AAV or similar gene therapy vectors, either systemically or to specific organs. The goal is not to create new pluripotent cells in situ — which carries an obvious cancer risk — but to run reprogramming for carefully timed "micro-cycles" that rewind epigenetic age and restore youthful gene expression while preserving the cell's lineage identity. In cardiovascular applications, partial reprogramming of endothelial cells toward a progenitor-like state has been shown to prevent endothelial-to-mesenchymal transition (EndMT), improve vascular repair, and, theoretically, stabilize atherosclerotic plaques or reverse microvascular rarefaction in heart failure and diabetic vasculopathy. In metabolic disease, OSK-based partial reprogramming in pancreatic and muscle tissue has improved glucose tolerance and repaired injury in older mice, suggesting a path to rejuvenating β-cells and insulin-sensitive muscle without full cell replacement. For the brain and retina, OSK-mediated rejuvenation has already restored vision in glaucoma models and improved neuronal survival, making neurodegenerative conditions an early, compelling target.

Where this interfaces with your "Living Chip" and platelet-rich plasma (PRP) framework is at the level of delivery and microenvironment engineering. PRP is essentially a concentrated, autologous growth-factor bath; it delivers PDGF, TGF-β, VEGF, IGF-1, and other signals that promote local repair but do not fundamentally reset cell age. Exosomes and secretomes from stem cells, by contrast, carry microRNAs and transcriptional regulators that can reprogram target cells at the gene-expression level, functioning as a biologic "software update." In the near future, one can envision PRP "super-cocktails" in which:

- Autologous PRP supplies a safe growth-factor scaffold and fibrin matrix for local retention.
- Lab-engineered exosomes derived from partially reprogrammed iPSCs or youthful MSCs deliver rejuvenating signals (miRNAs and proteins that mimic downstream OSK effects but without inserting OSKM genes).
- In some controlled contexts, very short-acting OSK mRNA or protein—rather than integrating DNA—could be incorporated into the injectate to induce transient, local partial reprogramming, then disappear.

Early clinical-style practice is already moving in this direction with PRP plus exosomes, especially for hair, cartilage, and skin: exosome-enhanced PRP increases hair follicle stem cell activity and wound healing beyond PRP alone, and providers are effectively using exosomes as programmable, off-the-shelf "instructions" layered on top of the patient's own platelets. The logical extension for your book is a future in which a small blood sample yields: (1) PRP for structural support and growth factors, (2) circulating small pluripotent stem cells or easily reprogrammable cells, and (3) a library of rejuvenating exosomes—all recombined into targeted injections for joints, myocardium, pancreas, or brain, or delivered systemically via intramuscular depots that secrete factors into the circulation for months. In that world, "taking your old cells and turning them into new cells" is not just metaphor: OSKM and related factor sets provide the reset switch; iPSC and organoid technologies build replacement tissues; and PRP-plus-exosome delivery gives you a minimally invasive way to deploy these tools to repair or rejuvenate almost any tissue or organ damaged by aging, diabetes, cardiovascular disease, or chronic inflammatory conditions.

Mitochondrial Transplantation and Nanoengineered Mitochondria

Most of this book focuses on improving the function of the mitochondria you already have. A complementary frontier is more radical: replacing or augmenting damaged mitochondria with healthy ones.

Conventional mitochondrial transplantation

Mitochondrial transplantation (MT) involves isolating functional mitochondria from healthy donor cells (autologous or allogeneic) and delivering them to damaged tissues (e.g., ischemic myocardium, spinal cord, lung, or brain). Animal and early translational work suggest that transplanted mitochondria can:

- Integrate into host cells and partially restore ATP production
- Reduce ROS and apoptosis
- Improve functional outcomes in models of myocardial infarction, spinal cord injury, and acute lung injury

Clinical development is early and faces challenges: delivery efficiency, immune recognition, durability of benefit, and manufacturing logistics.

Nanoengineered mitochondria: mNP-Mito and beyond

A 2025 mini-review describes nanoengineered mitochondria as a possible next step in mitochondrial therapeutics. These biohybrid constructs combine isolated mitochondria with nanoparticles, RNA cargo, or targeting ligands in order to enhance function, targeting, and delivery.

One example is PARKIN-mRNA-loaded nanoparticle-engineered mitochondria (mNP-Mito). In this approach, healthy mitochondria are functionalized with nanoparticles carrying PARKIN mRNA. When delivered to cells with mtDNA-related complex I defects, such as models of Leber hereditary optic neuropathy, they appear to serve a dual function: supplying functional respiratory capacity while also promoting mitophagy of damaged host mitochondria through PARKIN expression. In preclinical models, this has been associated with improved complex I function and partial restoration of mitochondrial homeostasis.

This approach fits the "living chip" metaphor perfectly: rather than just tuning software (signals), clinicians could one day swap or augment the hardware (mitochondria) with upgraded units.

Current status:

- Preclinical; not ready for routine clinical use
- Key challenges: scalable manufacturing, targeted delivery, immune compatibility, long-term safety

How it fits UCOS:

- UCOS prepares the terrain—reducing oxidative stress, improving autophagy, and optimizing cofactors.
- In the future, mitochondrial transplantation or nanoengineered mitochondria could be layered on top for patients with severe, localized mitochondrial defects (e.g., cardiomyopathy, optic neuropathy), much like stem-cell therapy but at the organelle level.

Mitohormesis: Pushing Mitochondria Just Enough

Mitohormesis is the principle that mild mitochondrial stress can trigger adaptive responses that increase resilience and longevity, upregulating antioxidant defenses, mitophagy, and mitochondrial biogenesis. Exercise, fasting, cold exposure, and certain drugs (for example, metformin and low-dose ETC inhibitors) all act, in part, through mitohormesis.

Recent work suggests a growing class of mitohormetic small molecules, including derivatives such as harmol and certain resveratrol glycosides, that mildly perturb mitochondrial function to induce adaptive stress responses without overt toxicity. These agents transiently alter mitochondrial redox state or ETC efficiency, activate AMPK, NRF2, and mitophagy pathways, and improve metabolic flexibility and stress resistance in preclinical models.

Your framework is already mitohormetic: methylene blue, exercise, alpha-lipoic acid, and intermittent fasting all push mitochondria into short, controlled stress cycles. The key clinical message is unchanged but can be sharpened: hormesis is dose-, tissue-, and timing-dependent. Agents that look similar on paper (for example, methylene blue, metformin, and emerging mitohormetics) can overshoot if stacked aggressively. Pulsed protocols and careful sequencing (UCOS first, then stressors) are safer than chronic, unmodulated activation.

NAD^+, the Microbiome, and Terrain-First Modulation

Why NAD^+ sits at the center of frontier protocols

Nicotinamide adenine dinucleotide (NAD^+) is a central cofactor in redox reactions, glycolysis, the TCA cycle, and the mitochondrial electron transport chain, and it also serves as a substrate for sirtuins, PARPs, and CD38. Age, chronic inflammation, and metabolic stress drive NAD^+ depletion through increased consumption (PARP/CD38 activation) and impaired salvage pathways. Low NAD^+ limits mitochondrial ATP output, autophagy/mitophagy, and DNA repair, and it is one of the most consistent metabolic signatures of biological aging. For clinicians, this framework supports positioning NAD^+ not as a vanity add-on but as core terrain infrastructure that conditions response to peptides, PBM, HBOT, and other high-end signals.

NAD^+ metabolism and the microbiome

NAD^+ is maintained through three main routes: de novo synthesis from tryptophan, the Preiss-Handler pathway from niacin (NA), and the salvage pathway from nicotinamide (NAM) and related precursors such as NR and NMN. The gut microbiome intersects with all three. Many commensal bacteria express nicotinamidase (PncA), which converts NAM into NA and thereby shifts host metabolism toward the Preiss-Handler route, altering NAD^+ pools in the liver and intestine. Microbial metabolism of tryptophan produces indoles and kynurenine-pathway intermediates that modulate host NAD^+ synthesis and inflammation. Dysbiosis, barrier dysfunction, and chronic LPS exposure upregulate CD38 and PARPs, accelerating NAD^+ consumption.

Clinically, this means NAD^+ repletion is not just about a pill or an IV; it is about the terrain—diet, microbiome composition, and inflammatory load—into which NAD^+ precursors and NAD^+ itself are introduced.

Delivery methods: IV, injectable, oral, and sublingual

Multiple delivery routes are now used in practice. IV NAD^+ achieves 100% bioavailability and very high transient plasma levels, but it is invasive, expensive, time-intensive, and best suited to short, intensive protocols. Parenteral precursors (for example, IM or SC NR/NMN) provide high exposure but share similar cost and logistical constraints, with emerging but still limited comparative data. Oral precursors (NR, NMN, NAM) have pharmacokinetic data showing increased tissue NAD^+ in humans, but bioavailability varies by compound, dose, and microbiome context. Sublingual NAD^+ formulations avoid first-pass hepatic metabolism and can deliver intact NAD^+ directly into the circulation and local tissues, with early data suggesting meaningful increases in intracellular NAD^+ and improved symptom scores at home-use doses.

Current evidence does not support a blanket claim that sublingual or oral NAD^+ is "superior" to IV; IV produces the highest peaks, whereas well-designed daily sublingual or other food-grade NAD^+ strategies can provide sufficient, steady NAD^+ support with far better practicality, adherence, and safety for long-term terrain work.

MODS MAX as a terrain-first NAD^+ amplifier

In the Living Cell framework, MODS MAX is positioned as a foundational terrain-first modulator stack centered on boron, NAD^+ support, and spermidine, designed to improve the cellular terrain so other signals—peptides, red light, exosomes, small molecules—are actually usable. It acts on several levels. Boron modulates steroid hormone bioavailability and vitamin D efficacy, influences inflammatory mediators such as TNF-α and IL-6, and supports mineral economy, thereby optimizing hormonal voltage and structural integrity. NAD^+ support via daily sublingual or food-grade NAD^+ plus appropriate precursors increases intracellular NAD^+, supports sirtuin and PARP activity, enhances mitophagy, and improves mitochondrial resilience, particularly when combined with a microbiome-supportive diet and UCOS-aligned lifestyle changes. Spermidine enhances autophagy and mitophagy, improves cardiac structure and function in preclinical and early human studies, and has been associated with increased lifespan and reduced cardiovascular mortality in epidemiologic data.

Together, this stack is designed to deliver higher and more sustained functional NAD^+ availability at the tissue level over time, compared with episodic IV pulses alone, while simultaneously maintaining autophagic cleanup capacity and hormonal/mineral coherence. In other words, MODS MAX aims to raise the floor of cellular capacity so that every additional therapy—BPC-157, GHK-Cu, SS-31, GLP-1 agonists, PBM, HBOT, exosomes—lands in a system that can respond.

NAD^+, autophagy/mitophagy, and senescence

NAD^+ is tightly coupled to autophagy, mitophagy, and cellular senescence. SIRT1 and SIRT3 are NAD^+-dependent deacetylases that regulate autophagy and mitophagy, mitochondrial biogenesis, and antioxidant responses. Low NAD^+ impairs sirtuin activity, contributing to defective mitophagy, accumulation of dysfunctional mitochondria, and increased mitochondrial DNA damage, which in turn drives cGAS-STING and NLRP3 inflammasome activation. NAD^+ repletion—especially in combination with spermidine, urolithin A, and fisetin—forms a cognitive and vascular autophagy stack that targets both damaged organelles and senescent cells, potentially slowing inflammaging and neurodegeneration. From a clinical standpoint, this argues for NAD^+ support as a prerequisite and amplifier for advanced protocols: the more mitochondrial and autophagic capacity you restore, the more likely other interventions are to produce durable gains rather than transient spikes.

For patients, a simple way to think about this is: NAD^+ is like the currency your cells use to run their power plants and repair crews. As we age, that currency runs low. Rather than occasional big "money drops" with IVs, we use a daily, sublingual NAD^+ stack—paired with the right minerals, hormones, and autophagy support—to keep your cell's bank account consistently funded so all the other advanced therapies you do can actually cash in.

Spermidine, Autophagy, and Cellular Cleanup

Why spermidine matters in terrain-first work

Spermidine is an endogenous polyamine that reliably induces autophagy and mitophagy across multiple tissues, including heart and brain, in preclinical models. It enhances lysosomal function, improves organelle turnover, and supports proteostasis, which together reduce the accumulation of damaged proteins and dysfunctional mitochondria that drive inflammaging and tissue decline. Observational human data associate higher spermidine intake with improved cardiometabolic profiles and reduced cardiovascular mortality, suggesting that sustained low-grade autophagy activation has real-world relevance beyond model organisms. For clinicians, spermidine is best framed not as a stimulant or symptomatic agent but as a background "cleanup signal" that improves the quality of the hardware on which all other therapies run.

Autophagy, mitophagy, and their dependence on energy

Autophagy and mitophagy are energy-dependent programs: the cell must spend ATP to tag, sequester, and recycle damaged components. When NAD^+ is depleted and mitochondrial output is low, autophagic flux is blunted, even if you push on upstream signals, which leads to a vicious cycle — dysfunctional mitochondria generate more ROS and mtDNA leakage, activating cGAS-STING and NLRP3, and further degrading terrain. NAD^+-dependent sirtuins, particularly SIRT1 and SIRT3, sit at the center of this loop by coordinating mitophagy, mitochondrial biogenesis, and antioxidant responses; without adequate NAD^+, spermidine's autophagy push cannot fully translate into durable mitochondrial renewal. This is why, in MODS MAX, spermidine is intentionally paired with daily NAD^+ support and micronutrient repair rather than used as a standalone longevity molecule.

Spermidine inside UCOS and MODS MAX

Within the UCOS framework, spermidine primarily supports the Structural and Security systems: it helps maintain matrix integrity, vascular health, and immune tone by keeping cellular "debris" under control. Mechanistically, it induces autophagy and mitophagy in cardiomyocytes and neurons, supports endothelial function, and improves organelle quality control, all of which are critical for cognitive and vascular aging trajectories. In MODS MAX, spermidine is one of three core levers — alongside NAD^+ support and boron — that target the interlocking failure modes of aging cells: NAD depletion, decline in autophagy/mitophagy, and hormonal/mineral dysregulation. The stack is deliberately designed so that spermidine's cleanup effect reduces senescent burden and mtDNA-driven inflammation, lowering CD38/PARP overactivation and thereby conserving NAD$^+$, while restored NAD$^+$, in turn, enhances sirtuin-driven autophagy and mitochondrial resilience.

The cognitive-vascular autophagy stack

Aging brain structures and vasculature share a common pathology: impaired autophagy/mitophagy, accumulation of misfolded proteins, and the persistence of damaged mitochondria, which fuel chronic inflammation and endothelial dysfunction. MODS MAX operationalizes a practical "cognitive-vascular autophagy stack" by combining NAD$^+$ support and spermidine with UCOS cofactors such as magnesium, vitamin D, omega-3s, and B-complex, then layering on movement and sleep optimization. Where appropriate, adjuncts like urolithin A and fisetin can be added to deepen mitophagy and senolytic effects, but the backbone remains daily NAD$^+$ plus spermidine in a repaired terrain rather than intermittent, high-intensity pulses. In this context, peptides, PBM, HBOT, exosomes, and regenerative procedures are not the primary cleanup tools; they are higher-order signals applied to tissue that spermidine-supported autophagy has already made more responsive.

Clinical use: background, daily, long-term

Clinically, spermidine in MODS MAX is positioned as a moderate, daily, long-term autophagy support, not as an aggressive short-term stack. It is introduced after or alongside UCOS foundational work (micronutrients, glucose-insulin, basic hormones) and together with NAD$^+$ support so that patients have the ATP, cofactors, and hormonal voltage to tolerate increased turnover. Monitoring typically focuses on terrain markers — hs-CRP, Cu/Zn ratio, vitamin D, metabolic parameters, and, when available, cardiometabolic imaging or biological-age proxies — rather than any single spermidine-specific lab. Safety at dietary-range doses is generally good; practical cautions mirror those in the main paper: introduce gradually in frail or highly polypharmacy patients, watch GI tolerance, and integrate into an overall plan rather than layering on top of uncontrolled catabolic stress.

For patients, a simple way to picture this is: NAD$^+$ turns the lights back on in the factory and powers the machines, while spermidine hires and pays the night-shift cleaning crew. When both are running every day, your cells are not just working harder — they are constantly clearing out broken parts, so the advanced therapies you invest in have a clean, well-powered workspace to do their job.

Autophagy, Mitophagy, and Cognitive Decline

Neurodegenerative diseases and age-related cognitive decline are increasingly viewed through an autophagy and mitophagy lens. Several 2024 reviews summarize how impaired autophagic flux and defective mitophagy in neurons contribute to Alzheimer's disease (AD), vascular cognitive impairment, and Parkinson's disease.

Key mechanisms:

- Reduced autophagy → accumulation of misfolded proteins (Aβ, tau, α-synuclein)
- Impaired mitophagy → dysfunctional neuronal mitochondria, ROS, and synaptic failure
- Hyperactive mTOR and insufficient AMPK/SIRT1 signaling in the hippocampus and cortex impede autophagosome formation and lysosomal clearance

The existing stack—NAD^+ support, methylene blue, omega-3s, ALCAR, urolithin A, spermidine, fisetin, exercise—forms a rational "cognitive autophagy" program:

- NAD^+ precursors + SIRT1/3 activation → support neuronal mitophagy and mitochondrial biogenesis
- Urolithin A → enhances mitophagy in muscle and likely brain; crosses the BBB and reduces protein aggregation in models
- Spermidine → enhances general autophagy, including in hippocampal neurons
- Fisetin → senolytic in glial and endothelial cells, reducing SASP-driven neuroinflammation
- Exercise → improves hippocampal mitophagy (via FUNDC1) and BDNF signaling
- Methylene blue → supports ETC efficiency and reduces ROS in neurons
- Omega-3s (DHA-rich) → structural membrane support and anti-inflammatory effects

Hyperbaric Oxygen Therapy (HBOT) as a Mitochondrial and Epigenetic Tool

Hyperbaric oxygen therapy (HBOT) exposes patients to 100% oxygen at pressures typically 1.3-2.0 ATA. Originally used for decompression sickness and wound healing, HBOT is being explored as a longevity and cognitive intervention.

Proposed mechanisms:

- Repeated hyperoxia → relative hypoxia post-session → hypoxia-inducible factor (HIF-1α) cycling → angiogenesis and mitochondrial stress adaptation
- Increased oxygen tension → transient ROS bursts → mitohormesis and upregulation of antioxidant defenses
- Small studies suggesting telomere lengthening and reduced senescent T-cells with specific protocols (e.g., 60 sessions over 3 months)

Evidence remains heterogeneous:

- Some trials report improved cognitive function, perfusion, and quality of life in post-stroke, TBI, and "healthy aging" cohorts.
- Others show modest or no benefit, with outcomes heavily dependent on protocol (pressure, session frequency, total number of dives).

Within your framework, HBOT can be presented as:

- A potential adjunct for cognitive decline, vascular compromise, or stubborn fatigue when foundational UCOS work is already done.
- A costly, time-intensive option where risk is low but benefit is uncertain and patient selection is critical.

You can emphasize that HBOT is not a replacement for mitochondrial nutrition, autophagy modulation, or exercise; at best, it may act as a structured mitohormetic stressor in select patients.

Section 3: Supporting nutrient "chips"

A. Leucine & branched-chain amino acids (BCAAs)

Why leucine matters

Leucine is the most potent of the three BCAAs (leucine, isoleucine, valine) for activating the mechanistic target of rapamycin complex 1 (mTORC1), the central regulator of protein synthesis and anabolic signaling.

Mechanisms:

1. mTORC1 activation: Leucine directly stimulates mTOR via the Rag GTPase-Ragulator complex, leading to downstream phosphorylation of S6K1 and 4E-BP1, which drive ribosomal assembly and translation initiation.
2. Mitochondrial biogenesis: Leucine and BCAAs activate PGC-1α signaling, promoting mitochondrial DNA replication and upregulation of oxidative phosphorylation enzymes.
3. Muscle protein synthesis: Leucine ingestion post-resistance exercise amplifies the rise in muscle protein synthesis (MPS) by 50-100% compared to carbohydrate alone, and enhances mTOR translocation to the muscle periphery where growth occurs.
4. Mitochondrial repair after exercise: BCAAs support mitochondrial membrane repair and reduce oxidative damage following high-intensity or eccentric exercise.

Clinical use cases

- Sarcopenia and age-related muscle loss: 2-3 g leucine per meal can help preserve muscle mass in older adults by overcoming anabolic resistance.
- Post-surgical or post-injury recovery: High leucine intake supports both muscle rebuild and mitochondrial recovery.
- Athletic performance and recovery: 5-10 g BCAAs (with ≥2.5 g leucine) pre- or post-workout enhances MPS and reduces delayed-onset muscle soreness.
- Metabolic flexibility: Leucine can improve insulin signaling in muscle and support glucose disposal, especially when paired with resistance training.

Dosing

- General muscle preservation: 2-3 g leucine per meal, ideally from high-quality protein sources (whey, eggs, meat).
- Targeted supplementation (post-exercise or therapeutic): 3-5 g leucine as part of a 10-20 g essential amino acid (EAA) or BCAA blend.

- Timing: Within 30-60 minutes post-resistance exercise for maximal mTOR/MPS response.

Cautions

- Chronic high-dose BCAA supplementation without balancing other amino acids can suppress uptake of aromatic amino acids (tryptophan, tyrosine, phenylalanine) and may theoretically impair neurotransmitter synthesis over time.
- Kidney or liver disease: Monitor closely; excess amino acid load may stress compromised organs.
- mTOR and longevity: Chronic, unregulated mTOR activation may theoretically accelerate aging in some models. The solution: pulse leucine/mTOR around training and recovery windows, not 24/7.

UCOS synergy

- Creatine + leucine: Creatine supports ATP availability for high-intensity work; leucine directs that energy toward protein synthesis. Together, they optimize both the energy supply and the anabolic signal.
- Magnesium: Required for ribosomal function and protein translation; leucine activates mTOR, but Mg allows the ribosome to execute the command.
- NAD^+ and mitochondrial support: Leucine promotes mitochondrial biogenesis; NAD^+, PQQ, and CoQ10 ensure those new mitochondria are functional and energetically efficient.

Mitohormetic agents are mild mitochondrial stressors that trigger adaptive upregulation (better defenses, more mitochondria), not damage, when dosed and timed correctly.

- Exercise: The most powerful mitohormetic; transient hypoxia, ROS, and energy stress → AMPK, PGC-1α, FUNDC1, mitophagy, mitochondrial biogenesis.
- Fasting / time-restricted eating: Lowers insulin and amino acids, activates AMPK and autophagy, improves metabolic flexibility.

- Metformin/berberine: Mild Complex I inhibition → AMPK activation, improved insulin sensitivity, mitophagy; requires careful use to avoid over-catabolism.
- Alpha-lipoic acid (ALA): Redox modulator that improves mitochondrial enzyme activity and can activate AMPK-linked pathways.
- Methylene blue (low-dose): Alternative electron carrier that reduces ETC bottlenecks and modulates ROS signaling, acting as a redox mitohormetic.
- Sulforaphane / NRF2 activators: Mild oxidative stress → NRF2 activation → antioxidant and detox gene upregulation, mitochondrial protection.
- Emerging small molecules (e.g., harmol, resveratrol derivatives): Under study as targeted mitohormetics that tweak mitochondrial redox or ETC flux to induce adaptive responses without overt toxicity.

Key message: dose, timing, and stacking matter. You pulse mitohormesis into a well-nourished, UCOS-supported system, not on top of starvation, overtraining, or polypharmacy.

NAD⁺ and Mitophagy: A Bidirectional Survival Loop

NAD⁺ (nicotinamide adenine dinucleotide) is best known as an electron carrier in cellular respiration, but it also functions as a critical co-substrate for enzymes that regulate autophagy, DNA repair, and longevity pathways. The relationship between NAD⁺ and mitochondrial autophagy is bidirectional: NAD⁺ promotes mitophagy, and functional mitophagy helps preserve NAD⁺ levels.

This creates either a virtuous cycle (high NAD⁺ → efficient mitophagy → mitochondrial health → preserved NAD⁺) or a vicious cycle (low NAD⁺ → impaired mitophagy → mitochondrial damage → NAD⁺ depletion → cell death).

How NAD⁺ Promotes Mitophagy

1. SIRT1 and SIRT3 activation

The sirtuin family of NAD⁺-dependent deacetylases plays a central role in mitophagy regulation:

- SIRT1 (nuclear and cytoplasmic): Deacetylates and activates key autophagy proteins, including:

- ULK1 (unc-51-like kinase 1), the initiator of autophagosome formation
- ATG5, ATG7, and LC3, core components of the autophagy machinery
- FOXO3, a transcription factor that upregulates autophagy gene expression
- SIRT3 (mitochondrial matrix): Deacetylates and activates:
- FOXO3A, which increases expression of PINK1, Parkin, and BNIP3
- SOD2 (MnSOD), the primary mitochondrial antioxidant enzyme, reduces oxidative damage and the need for excessive mitophagy

When NAD^+ levels are sufficient, SIRT1 and SIRT3 maintain a baseline level of autophagy that continuously removes damaged mitochondria before they accumulate.

2. AMPK activation

NAD^+ indirectly activates AMPK (AMP-activated protein kinase) through two mechanisms:

- Energy sensing: When NAD^+ is high, the NAD^+/NADH ratio signals cellular energy sufficiency, but transient drops in ATP (during fasting or exercise) elevate AMP, activating AMPK.
- SIRT1-LKB1 axis: SIRT1 deacetylates and activates LKB1, the upstream kinase that phosphorylates and activates AMPK.

Once activated, AMPK:

- Phosphorylates ULK1, triggering autophagosome formation
- Inhibits mTOR, lifting the brake on autophagy
- Promotes mitochondrial fission via phosphorylation of MFF and DRP1, facilitating mitophagy of fragmented mitochondria

3. PGC-1α and mitochondrial biogenesis coupling

NAD^+-activated SIRT1 deacetylates PGC-1α (peroxisome proliferator-activated receptor gamma coactivator 1-alpha), the master regulator of mitochondrial biogenesis. This creates a coordinated response:

- Mitophagy removes damaged mitochondria (via PINK1/Parkin and FUNDC1)

- Mitochondrial biogenesis replaces them with new, functional mitochondria (via PGC-1α → NRF1 → TFAM → mtDNA replication)

This "replace while you clear" strategy prevents energy crisis during mitophagic pulses and maintains mitochondrial mass at healthy levels.

How Defective Mitophagy Depletes NAD^+

The reverse relationship is equally important: when mitophagy fails, NAD^+ levels collapse through multiple mechanisms.

1. ROS overproduction and DNA damage

Damaged mitochondria with impaired respiratory chains leak electrons, generating excessive superoxide and hydrogen peroxide. This oxidative burst causes:

- Nuclear and mitochondrial DNA damage: Single- and double-strand breaks accumulate
- PARP (poly-ADP-ribose polymerase) hyperactivation: PARPs detect DNA breaks and catalyze the transfer of ADP-ribose units from NAD^+ to target proteins, consuming vast amounts of NAD^+ in the process
- NAD^+ depletion: In severe oxidative stress, PARP activity can deplete >90% of cellular NAD^+ within minutes, triggering energy failure and cell death

2. Chronic SIRT overactivation

Paradoxically, sustained mitochondrial stress can hyperactivate sirtuins in an attempt to restore homeostasis. When this becomes chronic:

- SIRT1/3 continuously consume NAD^+ without achieving repair, since the damaged mitochondria are not being removed
- NAD^+ demand exceeds synthesis capacity, leading to progressive depletion
- Autophagy and DNA repair machinery both fail due to insufficient NAD^+ for sirtuin and PARP activity

3. Mitochondrial NAD^+ transport dysfunction

Damaged mitochondria often exhibit disrupted NAD^+ transport across the inner mitochondrial membrane. Since mitochondria cannot synthesize NAD^+ de novo and must import it from the cytosol via SLC25A51 and SLC25A52 transporters, damage to these systems causes:

- Local mitochondrial NAD^+ deficiency, even when cytosolic levels are normal
- Impaired SIRT3 activity within the mitochondrial matrix
- Further respiratory chain dysfunction due to insufficient NAD^+ for Complex I

Removing these damaged mitochondria via mitophagy restores normal NAD^+ distribution.

Clinical Implications: NAD^+ Supplementation and Autophagy Priming

Why NAD^+ precursors sometimes "don't work"

Patients and clinicians frequently report variable responses to NAD^+ precursors (NMN, NR, or IV NAD^+). One major reason is autophagy capacity:

If mitophagy is severely impaired (due to aging, sedentary lifestyle, chronic overfeeding, or genetic factors), boosting NAD^+ alone may not rescue function. The elevated NAD^+ activates SIRT1/3 and signals mitochondrial biogenesis, but the damaged mitochondria remain in place, continuing to generate ROS and consume NAD^+ via PARP.

Solution: Prime autophagy before or alongside NAD^+ supplementation

To maximize NAD^+ efficacy:

1. Establish autophagy baseline with:

- Time-restricted eating (12-16 hour overnight fast)
- Spermidine (1-10 mg/day) for 2-4 weeks
- Regular exercise (especially aerobic and resistance training)

2. Then add NAD^+ precursors:

- NMN (250-1,000 mg/day) or NR (300-1,000 mg/day) in the morning
- Consider parenteral NAD^+ (IV or SubQ, 250-500 mg) weekly for 4-6 weeks in severe cases

3. Monitor response:

- Energy and exercise tolerance should improve within 2-4 weeks

- If no improvement, consider adding urolithin A (500 mg/day) or pulsed fasting (24-36 hours monthly) to force mitophagic activation

NAD⁺ precursor rescue in autophagy-deficient models

Animal studies demonstrate this principle clearly: in autophagy-deficient models (*ATG5* or *ATG7* knockout), supplementation with NAD⁺ precursors (NR or NMN) partially rescued:

- Cell survival under stress
- Mitochondrial membrane potential
- Lifespan extension (though not to wild-type levels)

This suggests that NAD⁺ can bypass some autophagy defects by enhancing alternative quality control mechanisms (UPRmt, mitochondrial-derived vesicles, apoptosis of severely damaged cells), but it cannot fully replace functional mitophagy.

The prolonged NAD⁺ elevation paradox

While NAD⁺ boosting is generally beneficial, the article raises an important caution: sustained, supra-physiological NAD⁺ elevation may disrupt mitochondrial homeostasis in some contexts.

Potential mechanisms include:

- Chronic SIRT1 activation → excessive autophagy → mitochondrial depletion (the "double-edged sword" again)
- Dysregulated NAD⁺/NADH ratio → altered redox signaling and metabolic flexibility
- Suppression of adaptive stress responses that require transient NAD⁺ dips

Clinical pearl: Pulse NAD⁺ supplementation rather than using continuous high doses indefinitely. For example:

- Pulse protocol: NMN 500-1,000 mg/day × 8-12 weeks, then reduce to 250-500 mg/day maintenance or 5 days on/2 days off
- Cyclical protocol: High-dose NAD⁺ (IV or oral) during periods of high demand (post-surgery, illness recovery, intense training blocks), then return to baseline UCOS support

Patient Language: The NAD⁺-Mitophagy Loop

"NAD^+ is like the 'battery charge' your cells need to run cleanup and repair systems. When NAD^+ is high, your cells activate proteins called sirtuins, which turn on the recycling machinery that removes damaged mitochondria and builds new ones.

But here's the catch: if your recycling system is broken (poor autophagy), the damaged mitochondria stay in place and keep leaking toxic chemicals. Those chemicals damage your DNA, which triggers emergency repair enzymes (PARPs) that burn through NAD^+ like crazy—depleting the very fuel you need for cleanup.

This creates a vicious cycle: low NAD^+ → poor cleanup → more damage → NAD^+ depletion → cell death.

That's why we don't just give you NAD^+ boosters and call it done. We first fix your autophagy with fasting, exercise, and spermidine—so when we add NAD^+, your cells can actually use it to clear out the junk and rebuild. That's when patients feel the dramatic energy shift."

Patient language: Leucine

"Leucine is like the ignition key for muscle growth. When you eat protein with enough leucine, it tells your muscle cells to start building. But building muscle also requires energy — that's where your mitochondria come in. We optimize your mitochondria with UCOS first, then use leucine-rich protein around your workouts to maximize the anabolic signal. That's how you build muscle even as you age."

B. Omega-3 fatty acids (EPA & DHA): advanced mitochondrial perspective

Why omega-3s matter for mitochondria

Beyond cardiovascular and anti-inflammatory benefits, omega-3 fatty acids are structural and functional components of mitochondrial membranes, especially cardiolipin, the signature phospholipid of the inner mitochondrial membrane.

Mechanisms:

1. Cardiolipin composition and ETC efficiency: EPA and DHA incorporate into cardiolipin, improving membrane fluidity and stabilizing respiratory chain complexes (especially Complex IV). This reduces proton leak and improves ATP synthesis efficiency.

2. Reduction of mitochondrial ROS: Omega-3s in mitochondrial membranes reduce lipid peroxidation and oxidative stress, protecting mtDNA and maintaining organelle integrity.
3. Mitochondrial dynamics: Omega-3 supplementation has been shown to shift the balance toward mitochondrial fusion (via upregulation of mitofusin proteins), supporting a more interconnected, stress-resistant mitochondrial network.
4. Inflammation resolution: EPA and DHA are precursors to specialized pro-resolving mediators (SPMs—resolvins, protectins, maresins) that actively turn off inflammation, allowing tissues to exit chronic inflammatory states and return to homeostasis.
5. Neuronal membrane and synaptic function: DHA is the dominant structural omega-3 in neuronal membranes and synapses, supporting fluidity, receptor function, and neuroprotection.

Clinical use cases

- Cardiovascular risk reduction and triglyceride lowering: 2-4 g/day EPA+DHA can reduce triglycerides by 20-30% and modestly improve HDL and LDL particle size.
- Neurodegeneration and cognitive decline prevention: DHA-rich formulations (≥1 g DHA/day) support synaptic density and may slow cognitive decline in early or prodromal stages.
- Chronic inflammatory conditions (arthritis, IBD, metabolic syndrome): 2-3 g/day EPA+DHA reduces systemic inflammation (hs-CRP, IL-6) by 20-50% in many studies.
- Post-exercise recovery and DOMS modulation: Omega-3s reduce muscle soreness and accelerate recovery by resolving exercise-induced inflammation without blunting adaptation.
- Mitochondrial disease and aging: Omega-3 supplementation improves mitochondrial membrane composition, reduces ROS, and may partially restore bioenergetic capacity in aging or mitochondrial dysfunction.

Dosing

- General health: 1-2 g/day combined EPA + DHA

- Cardiometabolic/neuroinflammatory indications: 2-4 g/day EPA + DHA (often in Rx fish oil trials for high triglycerides)
- Mitochondrial optimization: 2-3 g/day with emphasis on DHA for neuronal support and EPA for systemic anti-inflammatory effects
- Form: Triglyceride or phospholipid forms (e.g., krill oil) generally show better absorption than simple ethyl esters; re-esterified triglycerides are also well absorbed.

UCOS synergy

- Vitamin E: Protects omega-3s from oxidation; consider 200-400 IU mixed tocopherols when using high-dose fish oil.
- CoQ10 + omega-3s: Both improve mitochondrial membrane function; combined use may synergistically enhance ETC efficiency and reduce ROS.
- Leucine + omega-3s: Leucine drives mTOR/muscle protein synthesis; omega-3s reduce post-exercise inflammation and support mitochondrial repair. Together, they optimize both anabolic signaling and recovery.

Patient language: Omega-3 fats

"Your brain and mitochondria are built from omega-3 fats. Without enough of them, your cells are like a computer with a scratched hard drive—slower, noisier, and more prone to errors. We're restoring the structural integrity of every cell membrane, especially in your brain and your energy-producing mitochondria."

C. L-carnitine (including acetyl-L-carnitine)

Why it matters

- Fatty acid transport: Carnitine shuttles long-chain fatty acids into mitochondria via the carnitine shuttle (CPT1/2), enabling β-oxidation for ATP production.
- Brain support (ALCAR): Acetyl-L-carnitine crosses the blood-brain barrier, donates acetyl groups for acetylcholine synthesis, and supports neuronal mitochondrial function and neuroprotection.

- Aging: Endogenous carnitine declines with age; supplementation can improve mitochondrial energetics and fatigue in older adults and in high-demand states.

Clinical use cases

- Chronic fatigue and low energy, particularly on higher-fat or ketogenic diets
- Mild cognitive impairment and age-related cognitive decline
- Heart failure and cardiomyopathy (supporting cardiac mitochondrial ATP production)
- Athletic performance, recovery, and delayed-onset muscle soreness

Dosing

- L-carnitine: 500-2,000 mg/day (split doses often better tolerated)
- Acetyl-L-carnitine (ALCAR): 500-1,500 mg/day for cognitive and neuroprotective support
- Timing: With meals; morning dosing preferred when targeting energy and cognition (avoid high evening doses in sensitive patients due to possible stimulation).

Patient language: L-carnitine as transport system

"Carnitine is the shuttle bus that brings fat into your mitochondria to be burned for energy. If you're tired despite eating well, your shuttle system may be broken. We're fixing the transport."

D. Alpha-lipoic acid (R-ALA)

Why it matters

- Universal antioxidant: Both water- and fat-soluble, active in cytosol and membranes, and can cross the blood-brain barrier.
- Antioxidant recycling: Regenerates vitamin C, vitamin E, glutathione, and CoQ10, extending their functional lifespan.
- Mitochondrial cofactor: Essential cofactor for pyruvate dehydrogenase and α-ketoglutarate dehydrogenase, key TCA cycle enzymes.

- Precision redox modulation: At physiologic doses, ALA tends to fine-tune redox signaling and support hormesis rather than blunt ROS across the board.

Clinical use cases

- Diabetic neuropathy (nerve conduction improvement and symptom relief)
- Mitochondrial dysfunction and metabolic inflexibility
- Adjunct in heavy metal chelation protocols (binds mercury, arsenic, lead—must be used thoughtfully)
- Cognitive and neuroprotective support in metabolic or vascular risk states

Dosing

- General support: 300-600 mg/day
- Neuropathy and therapeutic use: 600-1,200 mg/day (often 600 mg BID in studies)
- Form: R-lipoic acid (R-ALA) is the biologically active enantiomer; racemic ALA works but may require higher doses for equivalent effect.

Patient language: ALA explained.

"ALA is the master antioxidant recycler. It doesn't just block damage — it recharges your other antioxidants so they can work again. It's like a battery charger for your cellular defense system."

E. Fisetin: senolytic & selective autophagy enhancer

Why fisetin matters

Fisetin is a flavonoid found in strawberries, apples, and other plants with two key properties:

- Senolytic activity: Selectively clears senescent (aging, dysfunctional) cells in preclinical models.
- Autophagy and mitochondrial support: Enhances autophagy and mitophagy and synergizes with spermidine for broader cellular cleanup.

Mechanisms

1. Senolytic activity: Senescent cells accumulate with age and chronic stress, resist apoptosis, and drive "inflammaging" via SASP (senescence-associated secretory phenotype). Fisetin

modulates pro-survival and stress-response pathways (e.g., BCL-2 family, PI3K/AKT) to preferentially trigger apoptosis in senescent cells while sparing most normal cells in animal models.

2. SIRT1 activation and longevity signaling: Fisetin activates SIRT1, a NAD^+-dependent deacetylase linked to longevity pathways. Downstream effects include increased mitochondrial biogenesis (via PGC-1α/NRF1/TFAM), enhanced antioxidant defenses (SOD2/MnSOD upregulation), improved DNA repair signaling, and promotion of apoptosis in damaged/senescent cells.
3. Autophagy and mitochondrial support: Increases macroautophagy and mitophagy markers, improving the removal of damaged proteins and dysfunctional mitochondria. Reduces ROS accumulation and helps restore mitochondrial membrane potential and ATP production in preclinical models.

Clinical evidence

- Animal studies: In aged mice, intermittent fisetin administration extended remaining lifespan and reduced age-related pathology across multiple tissues. Improvements were seen in metabolic markers, immune function, and physical performance.
- Human data (emerging): Multiple Mayo Clinic and related senolytic trials are underway (frailty, COVID, metabolic indications). Pilot human studies and open-label experiences use 100-500 mg/day for inflammatory and cognitive endpoints, and intermittent high-dose protocols (~20 mg/kg/day for 2 days) for senolytic purposes. Overall tolerability appears good at these doses; long-term safety is still under active investigation.

Dosing protocols

Strategy 1: Daily maintenance (continuous)

- Dose: 100-500 mg/day

- Best for: General antioxidant and anti-inflammatory support; low-grade autophagy and senomorphic effects; patients not ready for high-dose pulses
- Timing: With meals (fisetin is lipophilic; fat improves absorption)
- Duration: Can be used continuously; consider periodic breaks if very high on total polyphenol intake

Strategy 2: Intermittent senolytic pulses ("hit-and-run")

- Dose: ~20 mg/kg/day (70 kg → ~1,400 mg/day; 80 kg → ~1,600 mg/day; 90 kg → ~1,800 mg/day)
- Schedule: Typically 2 consecutive days per pulse
- Frequency: Monthly (more aggressive) or every 1-3 months (common in senolytic protocols and trials). Some research protocols repeat pulses on days 0-1, then again around days 30-31, 60-61, etc., often in conjunction with regenerative interventions (e.g., PRP, stem cell procedures).

Why pulsing? Senescent cells are cleared in discrete events. Continuous high-dose exposure is likely unnecessary, more expensive, and may increase off-target risk without additional senolytic gain. Pulses mimic successful animal protocols and current human senolytic trial designs.

Bioavailability challenges and solutions

Fisetin has poor oral bioavailability (~5-7%) due to low water solubility and rapid first-pass metabolism.

Options to improve exposure:

- Advanced delivery systems: Nanoparticles, micelles, liposomes, and other enhanced formulations can increase bioavailability several-fold. Look for "bioavailable" or "nano-fisetin" products from reputable manufacturers.
- Take with fat-containing meals: At least with a meal that includes fat; it improves absorption.
- High-dose pulses: Intermittent 1,400+ mg dosing can achieve effective tissue levels despite modest absorption.

UCOS synergy: spermidine + fisetin

Component Primary function Mechanism

Spermidine (in UCOS formulations) General autophagy Hypusination of eIF5A, TFEB activation, enhanced lysosomal function

Fisetin (100-500 mg daily or 20 mg/kg pulses) Senolytic + SIRT1 activation Selective apoptosis of senescent cells + NAD^+-dependent longevity signaling

Taken together: comprehensive cellular cleanup. Spermidine removes damaged components within cells; fisetin removes dysfunctional whole cells; combined use supports lifespan and healthspan in preclinical models

When to consider fisetin

Daily low-dose (100-500 mg) is reasonable for:

- Adults >40-50 with inflammatory or metabolic burden
- Cognitive decline or high neurodegenerative risk
- Post-surgical or post-illness recovery (within overall plan)
- General anti-aging support as part of UCOS

Intermittent high-dose pulses are better for:

- Aggressive senescence clearance (every 1-3 months)
- Adjunct to regenerative procedures (PRP, stem cell therapy, major surgery)
- High-burden patients (multiple comorbidities, post-cancer treatment, severe metabolic disease)

Safety and contraindications

- Generally well-tolerated in available human data at 100-500 mg/day and in short high-dose pulses.
- Common minor side effect: Occasional GI upset at high doses (mitigate by taking with food).
- Cautions:
- Anticoagulants: Fisetin has antiplatelet and anticoagulant interactions similar to other polyphenols; monitor closely if on warfarin or DOACs.
- Chemotherapy: Potential interactions with some chemotherapeutic agents; coordinate with oncology before use in active cancer.

- Immunosuppression: As an immunomodulator, high-dose senolytic pulses may not be ideal in heavily immunosuppressed patients without specialist input.
- Pregnancy: Insufficient safety data; avoid.

Patient language: fisetin as "cellular spring cleaning"

"Your body accumulates senescent cells—cells that are old, broken, and won't die. They sit there pumping out inflammatory signals that age everything around them. It's like having broken furniture in your house that keeps growing mold.

Fisetin is like a cellular spring-cleaning service. It specifically targets broken cells and helps clear them. Combined with spermidine (which cleans up the junk inside cells), you get a complete cleanup: remove the debris inside cells and remove the broken cells themselves.

We use it either as a moderate daily dose for ongoing support or as a high-dose 'pulse' every month or quarter for deeper clearing. Either way, it works best as part of your UCOS stack—the full system that optimizes energy, cleanup, hormones, and resilience."

F. Magnolia officinalis (honokiol & magnolol): mitochondrial protection & nervous system recovery

What is Magnolia officinalis?

Magnolia officinalis bark contains the bioactive neolignans honokiol and magnolol, which have been traditionally used for anxiety, insomnia, and GI complaints. Modern data highlight their roles in GABAergic modulation, mitochondrial protection, autophagy/mitophagy, neuroprotection, and longevity pathways.

Unlike benzodiazepines, these compounds support calm and sleep without clear evidence of tolerance, dependence, or cognitive impairment at usual doses.

Mechanisms:

- GABAergic modulation: Positive allosteric modulation of GABA-A receptors, promoting anxiolytic and sedative effects without receptor downregulation seen with benzodiazepines.
- Mitochondrial protection: Reduces mitochondrial ROS, preserves membrane potential, and supports ATP production under stress.

- Autophagy/mitophagy: Enhances clearance of damaged organelles and proteins, supporting cellular housekeeping.
- Anti-inflammatory: Modulates NF-κB and other inflammatory pathways, reducing systemic and neuroinflammation.

Clinical uses (mostly traditional/emerging):

- Anxiety and stress resilience
- Insomnia and sleep quality
- Neuroprotection (adjunct in cognitive decline, TBI recovery)
- Mitochondrial and metabolic support

Dosing:

- Typical extracts standardized to 1-2% honokiol: 200-400 mg before bed for sleep; 100-200 mg 1-2×/day for daytime anxiety support
- Higher-concentration extracts (e.g., 90% honokiol): 50-100 mg doses

UCOS synergy:

- Pairs well with evening GABA and melatonin for enhanced sleep architecture
- Supports mitochondrial recovery when combined with NAD^+, PQQ, and CoQ10

G. Urolithin A: The Clinically Validated Mitophagy Enhancer

What is Urolithin A?

Urolithin A (UA) is a gut microbiome-derived metabolite produced when specific intestinal bacteria metabolize ellagitannins and ellagic acid, polyphenolic compounds found in pomegranates, walnuts, berries, and certain oak-aged beverages.

Unlike its dietary precursors, urolithin A is the bioactive molecule responsible for mitochondrial and cellular benefits. It cannot be obtained directly from food—it must be produced by gut bacteria or supplemented in its final form.

The microbiome problem: Not everyone produces UA

Approximately 40% of the Western population are "non-converters"—they lack the gut bacterial species (primarily

Gordonibacter spp. and certain *Clostridia*) needed to convert ellagitannins into urolithin A.

Even among "converters," UA production declines with age, antibiotic use, poor diet, and dysbiosis. This means that eating pomegranates or drinking pomegranate juice may provide antioxidant benefits but will not reliably deliver mitophagic effects unless the individual has a healthy, UA-producing microbiome.

Solution: Direct supplementation with urolithin A bypasses the microbiome entirely, ensuring consistent bioavailability regardless of gut bacterial composition.

Mechanisms of action

Urolithin A enhances mitochondrial function through multiple complementary pathways:

1. PINK1/Parkin pathway activation

UA increases PINK1 accumulation on depolarized mitochondria and enhances Parkin recruitment, amplifying ubiquitin-dependent mitophagy. This has been demonstrated in muscle, neurons, and endothelial cells.

2. Direct autophagosome-lysosome fusion

UA appears to enhance autophagosome formation and promote fusion with lysosomes independently of PINK1/Parkin, suggesting it may also activate receptor-mediated mitophagy pathways (though the exact receptors involved are still under investigation).

3. Mitochondrial biogenesis coupling

Like NAD^+ and exercise, UA does not merely remove damaged mitochondria—it also signals the production of new, functional mitochondria via PGC-1α upregulation. This creates a net improvement in mitochondrial quality without depleting mitochondrial mass.

4. Anti-inflammatory effects

By reducing dysfunctional mitochondria, UA lowers mtROS, decreases mtDNA leakage, and suppresses NLRP3 inflammasome activation. In preclinical models, UA reduces IL-6, TNF-α, and other pro-inflammatory cytokines.

5. Neuroprotection

UA crosses the blood-brain barrier and has been shown to reduce α-synuclein aggregation (in Parkinson's disease models), Aβ accumulation (in Alzheimer's disease models), and neuroinflammation.

Human clinical evidence

Urolithin A has moved beyond animal models into well-controlled human trials:

Muscle function and mitochondrial gene expression

A randomized, double-blind, placebo-controlled trial in healthy elderly adults (age 65-90) found that:

- 500 mg UA/day × 4 weeks significantly upregulated 13 mitochondrial-related genes in skeletal muscle biopsies, including genes involved in OXPHOS, mitochondrial biogenesis, and mitophagy
- 1,000 mg UA/day × 4 weeks produced similar effects with a trend toward greater magnitude
- Plasma biomarkers of mitochondrial health (acylcarnitines, ceramides) improved dose-dependently
- No serious adverse events; mild GI upset in <5% of participants

Endurance and muscle performance

Additional studies (published 2022-2023) in middle-aged and older adults showed:

- Improved 6-minute walk distance
- Increased VO_2 peak (maximal aerobic capacity)
- Enhanced mitochondrial ATP production capacity in muscle (measured via ^{31}P-MRS)
- Reduced inflammatory biomarkers (hs-CRP, IL-6)

Lifespan extension in model organisms

- C. elegans (nematode): 45.4% lifespan extension with 50 μM UA
- Drosophila (fruit fly): Significant extension of median and maximal lifespan
- Mouse models: Improved healthspan markers (muscle function, glucose tolerance, inflammation) with chronic UA supplementation; lifespan studies ongoing

Dosing protocols

Daily maintenance (anti-aging, general mitochondrial support)

- Dose: 500 mg/day, taken with or without food
- Duration: Ongoing; can be used continuously or cycled (e.g., 12 weeks on, 2-4 weeks off)
- Best for: Adults >40 with metabolic, cognitive, or musculoskeletal concerns; athletes seeking recovery enhancement

High-dose pulse (aggressive mitophagy activation)

- Dose: 1,000 mg/day × 2 consecutive days
- Frequency: Monthly or quarterly
- Rationale: Mimics fisetin pulse protocol; delivers a concentrated mitophagic "cleanse" without requiring continuous high-dose use
- Best for: Post-illness recovery, post-surgical recovery, or as an adjunct to regenerative therapies (PRP, stem cell procedures)

UCOS synergy

Urolithin A works best when layered onto a functional UCOS foundation:

Component Urolithin A Synergy

Spermidine activates general autophagy; UA specifically enhances mitophagy. Together, they provide comprehensive cellular cleanup.

NAD^+ precursors NAD^+ fuels SIRT1/3, which deacetylate autophagy proteins; UA recruits those proteins to mitochondria. The combination accelerates mitochondrial turnover.

CoQ10 + PQQ UA removes damaged mitochondria; CoQ10/PQQ support the function of remaining mitochondria and stimulate biogenesis of new ones.

Leucine + resistance training UA clears old mitochondria; leucine and training signal mTOR to build new muscle and mitochondria. This creates the "remove and replace" cycle.

Omega-3 fatty acids improve mitochondrial membrane composition (cardiolipin); UA removes mitochondria with damaged membranes. Sequential benefits.

Clinical use cases

Sarcopenia and age-related muscle loss

UA is one of the few nutraceuticals with direct human evidence supporting its ability to improve mitochondrial function in muscle in elderly populations. Combine with:

- Adequate protein (1.6-2.0 g/kg/day)
- Leucine-rich meals (2-3 g leucine per meal)
- Resistance training 2-3×/week
- Creatine monohydrate (3-5 g/day)

Neurodegenerative disease risk or early symptoms

UA crosses the blood-brain barrier and shows neuroprotective effects in multiple models. Consider for patients with:

- Family history of Alzheimer's or Parkinson's disease
- Subjective cognitive decline or MCI
- Post-concussion syndrome or TBI recovery
- Chronic neuroinflammation (elevated hs-CRP, history of CNS infections)

Pair with:

- DHA-rich omega-3s (1-2 g/day)
- Methylene blue (5-10 mg/day, if tolerated)
- NAD^+ support
- Cognitive training and aerobic exercise

Post-viral fatigue and long COVID

Mitochondrial dysfunction is increasingly recognized as central to post-acute sequelae of SARS-CoV-2 (PASC). UA may help by:

- Clearing virus-damaged mitochondria
- Reducing chronic NLRP3 activation
- Restoring muscle oxidative capacity

Combine with:

- UCOS foundation (especially magnesium, B vitamins, CoQ10)
- Graded exercise therapy (very gradual progression)
- Anti-inflammatory support (omega-3s, curcumin, low-dose naltrexone if prescribed)

Athletic performance and recovery

UA enhances mitochondrial quality and quantity, leading to:

- Faster post-exercise recovery
- Improved endurance capacity
- Reduced muscle soreness and inflammation

Best used in:

- Off-season or base-building phases (500 mg/day ongoing)
- Post-competition recovery blocks (1,000 mg/day × 1-2 weeks)
- Injury recovery (500-1,000 mg/day until full function restored)

Safety and contraindications

Urolithin A has an excellent safety profile in completed human trials:

- No serious adverse events in doses up to 1,000 mg/day × 4 weeks
- Mild GI upset (nausea, loose stools) in <5% of users at 1,000 mg; typically resolves with continued use or dose reduction
- No drug interactions identified to date (urolithin A is primarily conjugated and excreted via urine and bile)
- No hormonal effects: Unlike some pomegranate extracts (which contain phytoestrogens), purified UA does not exhibit estrogenic activity

Cautions:

- Pregnancy/lactation: Insufficient data; avoid unless under medical supervision
- Severe renal or hepatic impairment: Use caution; no specific data available yet
- Anticoagulants: Theoretical interaction (polyphenols can have mild antiplatelet effects); monitor INR if on warfarin

Product considerations and the patent landscape

Urolithin A is currently available as a dietary supplement, with the most well-studied formulation being Mitopure® (manufactured by Amazentis/Timeline Nutrition), which holds multiple patents on the synthesis, formulation, and therapeutic use of urolithin A.

Patent note: Nestlé Health Science acquired a stake in Amazentis in 2018 and holds exclusive rights to certain formulations and applications of urolithin A. This has created barriers for other manufacturers seeking to produce standalone UA products in some jurisdictions.

Clinical pearl: If cost is prohibitive or product access is limited, consider:

1. Microbiome optimization to enhance endogenous UA production:

- Daily pomegranate consumption (1 cup fruit or 8 oz juice)
- Walnuts (1-2 oz/day)
- Prebiotic fiber to support *Gordonibacter* and UA-producing bacteria
- Avoid unnecessary antibiotics

2. Combination products: Some manufacturers blend ellagitannins with probiotics or with synergistic mitophagy enhancers (spermidine, PQQ, NAD^+ precursors) to create "mitophagy support" formulas. These may provide similar benefits at lower cost, though direct UA supplementation remains the gold standard for non-converters.

Patient language: Why pomegranate isn't enough

"You may have heard that pomegranates are good for you—they are. But the real magic happens in your gut. Special bacteria take compounds from pomegranates and convert them into a molecule called urolithin A, which tells your cells to clean out damaged mitochondria and build fresh ones.

The problem? About 40% of people don't have those bacteria. Even if you do, stress, antibiotics, and aging weaken them. So you could eat pomegranates every day and still not get the benefits.

That's why we use direct urolithin A supplementation—it guarantees you're getting the active molecule, regardless of your gut bacteria. It's one of the only supplements with real human studies showing it improves mitochondrial function in elderly muscle. And when your mitochondria work better, everything works better: energy, recovery, brain function, and resilience."

SECTION 4: Precision Redox & MODS Max Micro-ROS

The redox paradox

Reactive oxygen species (ROS) are not purely "bad"; they are essential signaling molecules.

- Too little ROS: Blunted signaling, poor adaptation to exercise and stress, impaired immune function and mitophagy.

- Too much ROS: Oxidative damage to lipids, proteins, and DNA; accelerated aging and degenerative disease.
- Goal: A "Goldilocks zone" of brief, controlled ROS pulses that activate adaptive pathways (Nrf2, sirtuins, autophagy) without cumulative damage.

MODS Max design rationale

MODS Max (Mitochondrial-Optimized Delivery System) is built around micro-dosed oxidative signaling rather than blanket antioxidant use:

- Transient barrier opening: A small, localized redox pulse at mucosal surfaces can transiently increase permeability and enhance sublingual/GI absorption—conceptually improving effective dose without GI burden.
- Hormetic pulse: A brief ROS signal upregulates endogenous antioxidant and repair systems (Nrf2 → SOD, catalase, glutathione peroxidase) and stress-response pathways.
- Oscillation shaping: Clean, short-lived pulses support rhythmic redox oscillations and better electron flow, rather than a chronic, noisy oxidative background.

Why this matters

Chronic high-dose antioxidant regimens can paradoxically impair exercise adaptation, immune function, and mitohormesis by suppressing beneficial ROS signaling.

MODS Max takes the opposite stance:

- Pulse, don't suppress.
- Train cells to handle oxidative challenges and upregulate their own defenses instead of shielding them continuously.

Best candidates:

- Mitochondrial dysfunction and chronic fatigue
- Poor nutrient absorption or GI sensitivity to higher oral doses
- Patients needing higher functional doses with minimal GI load

Clinician framing

Think of MODS Max as redox training, not antioxidant replacement:

- Use it to deliver a brief, controlled oxidative "exercise" to the system.

- Layer on top of UCOS when foundational antioxidants and cofactors are in place.
- Monitor clinical response (energy, HRV, recovery, inflammatory markers) rather than chasing ROS lab surrogates, which are noisy and context-dependent.

Patient language: MODS Max training

"Most supplements try to block all oxidative stress. MODS Max does the opposite: it gives your cells a tiny, controlled pulse of oxidative signaling—just enough to wake up your internal defense systems and make everything you take work better. It's like a vaccine for your mitochondria: a small, safe stress that makes you stronger."

SECTION 5: HRV & Grounding

Heart rate variability (HRV) as a coherence biomarker

What HRV is:

HRV measures beat-to-beat variability in heart rate and reflects autonomic balance and adaptability.

- High HRV: Greater resilience, recovery capacity, parasympathetic tone; associated with lower cardiovascular and all-cause mortality.
- Low HRV: Chronic stress, inflammation, poor recovery, and higher risk of adverse events.

Key metrics:

- RMSSD: Time-domain measure strongly linked to parasympathetic activity; higher is generally better during sleep.
- LF/HF ratio: Frequency-domain index of sympathetic/parasympathetic balance; often ~1-2 during wake in healthy individuals and <1 during deep sleep.
- Coherence score (e.g., HeartMath): Reflects ordered, sine-wave-like heart rhythms associated with synchronized breathing, emotional regulation, and vagal tone.

Clinical use with UCOS:

- Track response to UCOS: HRV should trend up over 4-12 weeks as mitochondrial function, redox control, and circadian rhythm improve.

- Guide training:
- Low HRV vs. baseline → favor recovery, lighter training, more sleep and parasympathetic work.
- High HRV vs. baseline → window for higher training load.
- Monitor stress/overtraining: Persistent HRV suppression signals need for intervention (sleep, stress management, nutrient/peptide support).

Devices:

- Oura Ring: Strong for nightly HRV, sleep staging, and readiness trends.
- WHOOP: Athlete-oriented HRV and strain metrics.
- HeartMath Inner Balance: Real-time biofeedback for coherence training.

Patient instructions (Oura example):

- Wear nightly and look at trends, not single nights.
- Each morning, check Readiness Score and HRV trend:
- High readiness + higher HRV → push training.
- Low readiness + lower HRV → prioritize recovery, sleep, parasympathetic work.
- When starting UCOS, peptides, grounding, or new protocols, watch HRV over 4-8 weeks as an objective adaptation marker.

Grounding (earthing)

Proposed mechanisms:

- Direct skin contact with the Earth allows free electrons from the ground to enter the body, potentially neutralizing excess positive charge and modulating local electric fields.
- Pilot studies suggest effects on inflammation, autonomic tone, and sleep quality; mechanisms may include electron transfer and interaction with low-frequency electromagnetic fields (e.g., Schumann resonances), but remain incompletely understood.

Evidence (early but promising):

- Small studies report reductions in pain and inflammatory markers (e.g., CRP), improved HRV, and better subjective sleep.

- Data are preliminary; nonetheless, the intervention is low-risk and cost-free.

Clinical use:

- Low-cost, low-risk adjunct for:
- Chronic inflammation and pain
- Poor sleep and high stress
- Patients interested in coherence-oriented practices

Patient protocol:

- 20-30 minutes barefoot on conductive surfaces daily: grass, soil, sand, unsealed concrete (avoid wood, rubber, asphalt).
- Consider properly grounded mats/sheets indoors where outdoor access is limited; ensure they connect to Earth ground, not just house wiring.
- Timing:
- Morning grounding + light → circadian anchor and autonomic reset.
- Evening grounding → parasympathetic shift before sleep.

Patient language: Grounding explained

"Your body runs on electricity. Grounding is like plugging yourself back into Earth's natural electrical system. It can help calm inflammation, stabilize your nervous system, and improve sleep. It's free, simple, and one of the most underused tools in medicine."

Section 5B: EchoLight (REMS) Advanced Body Composition & Bone Fragility Assessment

What EchoLight is

EchoLight uses REMS (Radiofrequency Echographic Multi-Spectrometry), a quantitative ultrasound technology, to assess bone status and body composition without radiation. Compared with DXA:

- Zero ionizing radiation
- Rapid (1--2 minute) scans with immediate 2D/3D visualization
- Simultaneous assessment of bone and soft tissue (muscle, fat, water)
- Portable and suitable for frequent monitoring

EchoLight vs DXA (clinical perspective)

Parameter	EchoLight (REMS)	Standard DXA
Radiation	None	Ionizing X-ray (cumulative)
Scan time	~1–2 minutes	~10–15 minutes
Frequency of use	Safe for weekly/biweekly monitoring	Typically every 3–12 months
Outputs	Bone status, muscle, fat, water	Bone mineral density; limited composition detail
Portability	Compact, room-flexible	Dedicated room/equipment
Obesity/artifacts	Less sensitive to soft-tissue artifacts	Accuracy reduced in obesity/metal implants

Multiple studies show REMS has diagnostic accuracy for osteoporosis comparable to DXA, with advantages in certain populations (e.g., obesity).

Clinical applications in UCOS + peptides

1. GLP-1 agonist monitoring (high priority)

GLP-1/GIP agonists can produce 15-24% weight loss, with potential lean mass loss if not protected.

- EchoLight allows biweekly monitoring of:
- Lean mass vs fat mass
- Muscle density (a proxy for contractile quality and mitochondrial status)
- Protocol:
- Baseline (week 0): DXA (if desired) + EchoLight.
- Weeks 2-4, 6, 8, 12, 16, 20, 24: EchoLight every 2-4 weeks.
- Intervention triggers:

- If lean mass loss >10-15% of total loss → escalate protein, creatine, resistance training, and consider adding MOTS-c or growth-axis peptides.

2. Peptide therapy response tracking

- Regenerative / mitochondrial peptides (SS-31, MOTS-c, BPC-157, TB-500, Khavinson series):
- Track changes in muscle mass and density over weeks to months.
- Immune/metabolic peptides (thymosin alpha-1, GLP-1):
- Follow visceral fat trends and lean preservation in real time.

3. Training and composition optimization

- Monthly EchoLight scans provide precise trends in muscle and fat, distinguishing true muscle gain from fluid shifts.
- Enables fine-tuning of protein targets, training volume, and adjunct peptides.

4. Aging and bone fragility

- Baseline EchoLight at ~40--50 years for bone status and fracture risk analog.
- Quarterly or biannual scans track bone response to UCOS, resistance training, vitamin D/boron/magnesium, and bone-targeted peptides (e.g., Sigumir).

Bone fragility and REMS

REMS generates:

- Ultrasound parameters (e.g., speed of sound, attenuation) reflecting trabecular and cortical structure.
- A fragility index that correlates with fracture risk similarly to DXA T-scores in published studies.

Clinical actions based on fragility:

- High risk → intensify resistance training; add vitamin D, K2, magnesium, boron; consider Sigumir or other bone-supportive peptides.
- Moderate risk → close monitoring and targeted lifestyle + nutrient support.
- Low risk → maintain UCOS and periodic screening.

Workflow integration

- Initial UCOS intake: EchoLight baseline for body composition + bone status.
- Pre-peptide: Repeat EchoLight after 4-8 weeks of UCOS to establish an "optimized baseline."
- Active therapy:
- GLP-1: Every 2-4 weeks.
- Regenerative/mitochondrial peptides: Monthly or every 6-8 weeks.
- Maintenance: Quarterly in the first year, then 1-2×/year for stable patients.

Patient language: Why Echolight

"We use EchoLight instead of relying only on traditional X-ray bone scans because it's fast, has no radiation, and gives us real-time information. We can see exactly how much fat you're losing and how much muscle and bone you're keeping—week by week.

With older methods, we'd only scan every few months and hope things were going well in between. With EchoLight, if we see you starting to lose muscle instead of fat, we can adjust your protein, training, or peptides right away so you come out leaner and stronger, not just lighter."

SECTION 6: Advanced Modalities

Rapamycin (mTOR inhibition for longevity)

Mechanism

- Inhibits mTORC1, a central nutrient and growth sensor.
- Intermittent mTORC1 inhibition:
- Increases autophagy and mitophagy
- Improves proteostasis and mitochondrial quality control
- Reduces chronic inflammation and some forms of cellular senescence
- In multiple species, rapamycin extends lifespan and healthspan, including improved cardiac, immune, and cognitive function.

Human longevity dosing (off-label)

- Not FDA-approved for anti-aging.

- Common practice patterns in longevity clinics:
- 3-7 mg once weekly (starting at lower end).
- Some experienced clinicians titrate up to 10-20 mg weekly in select patients, with careful monitoring.
- Rationale: Intermittent dosing aims to capture autophagy and longevity signaling while avoiding chronic daily immunosuppression seen in transplant regimens (2-10 mg/day).

Monitoring:

- Baseline and q3-6 months: CBC, CMP, fasting glucose/insulin, lipid panel.
- Watch for:
- Mild hyperglycemia or insulin resistance
- Mild dyslipidemia (↑ TG, LDL)
- Aphthous ulcers/mouth sores (dose-dependent)
- Contraindications: Active infection, uncontrolled immunosuppression, pregnancy, poorly controlled diabetes without risk-benefit discussion.

Patient language: Rapamycin

"Rapamycin is the first drug that consistently extends lifespan in multiple mammal studies. It works by putting your cells into 'deep maintenance mode'—they spend more time cleaning up damage and less time over-growing. We use it in low, once-weekly doses to trigger the cleanup benefits while avoiding the heavy immunosuppression seen at transplant doses."

Clinician notes

- Start low (3-5 mg weekly), reassess labs and side effects at 6-8 weeks, and titrate if appropriate.
- Consider cycling (e.g., 6-8 weeks on, 2-4 weeks off) to allow physiologic reset and psychological comfort.
- Rapamycin stacks well with UCOS: UCOS builds metabolic and mitochondrial capacity; rapamycin periodically deepens autophagy and proteostatic cleanup.

Ozone therapy (systemic and local)

Mechanism

- Hormetic oxidative stress: Ozone generates reactive oxygen intermediates that activate Nrf2 and antioxidant enzymes (SOD, catalase, GPx).
- Immune modulation: Modulates cytokine networks (including IFN-γ, IL-2, TNF-α) and enhances some innate and adaptive responses.
- Rheology and oxygenation: Increases 2,3-DPG in RBCs and improves tissue oxygen delivery.
- Anti-inflammatory: Can reduce pro-inflammatory cytokines and NF-κB signaling in some contexts.

Clinical applications (evidence heterogeneous)

- Chronic infections (Lyme co-infections, chronic viral burdens)
- Autoimmune and inflammatory syndromes (adjunctively)
- Chronic fatigue and fibromyalgia
- Ischemic vascular disease and wound healing
- Adjunctive oncology support (symptom relief, quality of life; not disease-modifying monotherapy)

Protocols:

- Major autohemotherapy (MAH): 100-250 mL of blood mixed with a defined ozone/oxygen mixture and re-infused.
- High-dose "10-pass" ozone: Repeats the MAH cycle multiple times in one session for a larger oxidative pulse.
- Local applications: Limb bagging, topical ozone oils, rectal/vaginal insufflation for localized infections or mucosal therapy.

Evidence highlights:

- Small controlled studies in infections, chronic pain, and COVID-19 show promising effects, but large RCTs remain limited.
- Should be presented as an adjunctive, hormetic therapy, not a panacea.

Patient language: Ozone therapy

"Ozone therapy is a controlled oxidative 'workout' for your cells and immune system. We briefly expose your blood to a small, precise amount of ozone so your body turns on its own antioxidant and repair systems. It's not about killing everything directly— it's about training your system to respond better."

DMSO (dimethyl sulfoxide)

Mechanism

- Exceptional penetration enhancer: crosses skin and mucosa easily and can carry other small molecules with it.
- Potent hydroxyl radical scavenger and anti-inflammatory agent.
- May modulate membrane fluidity and mitochondrial respiration (evidence still emerging).

Clinical use:

- Topical:
- Musculoskeletal pain, tendon/ligament injuries, localized inflammation.
- Often combined with other agents (magnesium, NSAIDs, low-dose peptides) for more targeted delivery.
- Systemic (IV, off-label):
- Used in some centers for stroke, TBI, complex regional pain syndrome, and refractory inflammatory states; must follow institutional protocols.

Dosing:

- Topical: Commonly 50-70% DMSO solutions applied 1-3×/day to intact skin (adjust concentration based on tolerance).
- IV: 0.1-1 g/kg in specific protocols; requires experience due to risks (e.g., hemolysis at high concentration).

Safety:

- Garlic-like odor and taste are common and benign.
- Can cause local irritation, erythema, and itching topically.
- Systemic high-dose use requires monitoring for hemolysis and electrolyte shifts.

Patient language: DMSO delivery mechanism

"DMSO is like a molecular delivery truck. It moves quickly through the skin and deeper tissues, carrying anti-inflammatory compounds with it to exactly where you hurt. It also has its own anti-inflammatory properties, so you get a double benefit."

Mistletoe (Viscum album)

Mechanism

- Immunomodulation: Mistletoe lectins and viscotoxins stimulate NK cells, T-cells, and macrophages and modulate cytokine profiles.
- Pro-apoptotic effects: Induce apoptosis in some tumor cell lines and can inhibit angiogenesis in preclinical models.
- Quality of life: Repeatedly shown in European trials to improve fatigue, appetite, mood, and treatment tolerance in cancer patients.

Clinical use:

- Widely used in European integrative oncology as an adjunct to conventional therapy.
- In the US, available primarily through integrative/anthroposophic protocols; considered investigational.

Dosing:

- Subcutaneous injections 2-3×/week, starting with very low doses (e.g., 0.01-0.1 mg) and titrating based on local skin reaction and systemic tolerance; higher doses (up to ~20 mg) in some regimens.
- Preparations: Iscador, Helixor, Abnoba-Viscum, etc.—each with slightly different profiles.

Evidence:

- Numerous European observational and some randomized studies show improved quality of life and reduced chemotherapy side effects.
- Survival benefit data are mixed and cancer-type specific; mistletoe should not be positioned as a stand-alone cancer cure.

Patient language: Mistletoe and the immune system

"Mistletoe has been part of European cancer care for decades. It helps your immune system better recognize abnormal cells and often makes chemotherapy and radiation easier to tolerate—less fatigue, better appetite, and more stable mood. We use it alongside, not instead of, standard treatment."

Rife frequencies (vibrational medicine)

Concept and mechanism (hypothesized)

- Based on the idea that microorganisms and tissues have specific resonant frequencies.
- Applying matching frequencies might disrupt pathogens or modulate cellular and nervous system activity.
- Mechanisms proposed include resonance effects, subtle electromagnetic modulation, and nervous system entrainment, but none are well proven in vivo.

Evidence status:

- There are no robust, high-quality randomized clinical trials demonstrating pathogen eradication or disease reversal in humans.
- Most data are anecdotal, case reports, or uncontrolled series in chronic infections and pain.

Clinical stance:

- If used, it should be as a clearly labeled experimental adjunct, not as a primary therapy.
- Combine only with strong foundational care (UCOS, evidence-based antimicrobials, immune support).
- Reassess after 4-8 weeks; discontinue if no objective or subjective benefit.

Patient language: Rife therapy as additional treatment

"Rife therapy uses specific electromagnetic frequencies that some believe can help with chronic infections and pain. The science is still very early and not yet conclusive, so we treat it as an optional add-on to a solid medical plan—not a replacement. We'll track how you feel and stop if it's not clearly helping."

PEMF (pulsed electromagnetic field therapy)

Mechanism

- Applies low-frequency, low-intensity electromagnetic pulses to tissues.

- Modulates transmembrane potentials and ion flux (Ca^{2+}, Na^{+}, K^{+}), potentially normalizing cellular signaling.
- Can enhance osteoblast activity and bone healing; improves microcirculation and may support mitochondrial function.

Evidence:

- Bone healing: Strongest evidence; FDA-approved for non-union fractures and some orthopedic indications.
- Pain and inflammation: Trials in osteoarthritis and chronic pain show benefit in pain scores and function.
- Neuro and mito support: Early animal data suggest benefits in brain injury and mitochondrial disorders, but human data are still limited.

Clinical use:

- Post-fracture or post-surgical bone healing
- Osteoarthritis and chronic joint pain
- Chronic pain syndromes and fibromyalgia (adjunct)
- Fatigue and recovery in high-demand patients

Dosing patterns:

- Frequencies commonly in the 1-100 Hz range, depending on device and indication.
- Session length: 10-30 minutes, 1-2×/day or several times per week.
- Intensity: Low-moderate; individualized to comfort.

Patient language: How PEMF works

"PEMF uses gentle magnetic pulses to help your cells reset their electrical gradients and communicate better. It's FDA-approved for helping stubborn fractures heal and has good data for arthritis and pain. In our context, we use it to support pain relief, recovery, and mitochondrial function as part of your broader program."

SECTION 7: Biohacking Tech Stack

Oura Ring (HRV, sleep, readiness)

- What it tracks: Nightly HRV, resting HR, sleep stages, temperature trends, respiratory rate, activity/load.

- Why use it: Non-invasive, high adherence, and one of the best validated consumer tools for longitudinal HRV and sleep trend tracking.
- Clinical application:
- Track UCOS response (energy, sleep, HRV trends).
- Guide training load and recovery.
- Monitor circadian alignment and stress resilience.
- Recommendation: Strongly consider for all longevity-focused patients who are comfortable with wearables.

NAD+ / redox biosensors

Current practical tools (2024-2025):

- Jinfiniti NAD test (intracellular NAD^+):
- Finger-prick/home kit; estimates intracellular NAD^+ status.
- Useful for baseline and follow-up when initiating NMN, NR, or NAD^+ IV programs.
- Genova NutrEval (organic acids & cofactors):
- Comprehensive metabolomics; indirect view of NAD^+/redox through lactate/pyruvate, TCA intermediates, oxidative stress markers.
- Guides broader mitochondrial and redox interventions.

Research-grade biosensors (not clinically available):

- Genetically encoded fluorescent NAD(P)H sensors (e.g., NAPs family): Allow subcellular $NADP^+$/NADPH tracking in live cells; research use only.
- CRISPR-based NAD^+ assays (e.g., HOLMES-type): High-sensitivity lab assays under development.
- NMN biosensors: Experimental tools for intracellular NMN monitoring.

Emerging tech:

- Wearable redox and sweat sensors (glutathione, lactate, oxidative markers) and possibly continuous NAD^+ proxies are in development but not yet approved for clinical use.

Clinical use pattern:

- Check NAD^+/metabolomics before starting NAD-targeted protocols.
- Recheck at 4-8 weeks to confirm biochemical response.
- Repeat annually in high-investment longevity patients.

Continuous glucose monitors (CGM)

- Devices: FreeStyle Libre, Dexcom G7, and successors.
- Why: Real-time glucose curves reveal post-prandial spikes, glycemic variability, and nocturnal dysregulation that fasting glucose/HbA1c often miss.
- Clinical applications:
- Optimize diet (timing, carb type, meal composition).
- Track response to metformin, berberine, GLP-1s, rapamycin.
- Monitor fasting, time-restricted eating, and metabolic flexibility.

SECTION 8: Patient Communication Templates

Template 1: Explaining UCOS

"UCOS stands for Ultimate Cellular Optimization System. It's a 24-hour protocol designed to restore the three core jobs your cells have to do: make energy, clean up damage, and send clear signals.

You'll take three formulas:

- Morning (around 6:30 AM): A non-hormonal testosterone optimizer that tells your body to build and maintain muscle, bone, and energy.
- Morning (upon waking): Take 1 mL Activate365 sublingually (hold 30 seconds) — this is your sublingual primer that activates MODS MAX absorption for the tablets that follow — then immediately take 2 tablets Mito365 + 2 tablets Renew365 (swallow, with or without food).
- Evening (30–60 minutes before bed): Take 1 mL Restore365 sublingually (hold 30 sec), then 1 mL TPrime365 sublingually (hold 30 sec) to optimize sleep, growth hormone, and overnight recovery.

Over 4-12 weeks, most patients report better energy, clearer thinking, deeper sleep, faster recovery, and the sense that their body is 'online' again. We'll track your progress with symptoms, labs, and wearables like your Oura Ring so we can adjust as needed."

Template 2: Explaining stem cell banking

"Your stem cells are your body's master templates for repair. Right now, your cells are younger and healthier than they'll ever be again.

We can harvest a small amount, freeze them, and store them. Years from now, if your heart, brain, immune system, or pancreas needs help, we may be able to thaw those cells, expand them, and give them back to you as a living upgrade from your younger self. It's not a guarantee or a magic bullet, but it's the closest thing we have to biological time travel."

MitoTALEN: Gene Editing for Mitochondrial DNA

Background

Unlike nuclear DNA, mitochondrial DNA (mtDNA) has been notoriously difficult to edit. Standard CRISPR-Cas9 systems cannot be reliably targeted to mitochondria because:

- Cas9 requires a nuclear localization signal and functions in the nucleus
- Mitochondria have double membranes that block most macromolecular entry
- Guide RNA delivery into the mitochondrial matrix is inefficient

This has left inherited mitochondrial diseases—caused by pathogenic mtDNA mutations—without direct genetic therapies.

Enter mitoTALEN (Mitochondrially-targeted Transcription Activator-Like Effector Nucleases):

MitoTALENs are engineered nucleases that can:

1. Enter mitochondria via fusion with mitochondrial-targeting sequences (MTS)
2. Bind specific mtDNA sequences using customizable TALE DNA-binding domains
3. Cleave pathogenic mtDNA selectively, allowing wild-type mtDNA to repopulate the mitochondrial network

Proof of concept

In preclinical models (cell culture and mice with heteroplasmic mtDNA mutations), mitoTALEN treatment:

- Reduced mutant mtDNA from 80-90% heteroplasmy to <10% within weeks
- Restored mitochondrial respiratory function (Complex I and IV activity)
- Improved cellular ATP production and reduced ROS
- Prevented disease progression in mouse models of mitochondrial myopathy

Potential applications

- Inherited mitochondrial diseases: MELAS, MERRF, Leber's hereditary optic neuropathy (LHON), Leigh syndrome
- Age-accumulated mtDNA damage: Targeting common age-related deletions (e.g., "common deletion" at 4,977 bp) to rejuvenate aged tissues
- Cancer: Eliminating oncogenic mtDNA mutations that confer metabolic advantages to tumor cells

Current status and limitations

- Preclinical only: No human trials yet; in vivo delivery remains a major challenge
- Delivery barriers: Viral vectors (AAV) can deliver mitoTALEN genes, but systemic mitochondrial transduction is inefficient
- Off-target effects: TALENs are more specific than older zinc-finger nucleases but not perfect; risk of cleaving similar sequences in nuclear or wild-type mtDNA
- Regulatory hurdles: Germline editing of mtDNA (if applied to oocytes or embryos) raises ethical and legal concerns similar to nuclear genome editing

Clinical relevance for longevity medicine

While mitoTALEN is not yet ready for clinical use, it represents a potential future therapy for:

- Patients with confirmed pathogenic mtDNA mutations and progressive disease
- Reversal of age-accumulated mtDNA damage as a rejuvenation strategy
- Targeted elimination of tumor-associated mtDNA mutations in metabolic cancer therapies

Evidence level: Experimental; preclinical only. Not clinically available.

Timeline: Realistically, 5-10+ years before human trials, assuming delivery and safety challenges are solved.

Patient language (if asked):

"Scientists are working on a way to 'edit' the DNA inside your mitochondria—the tiny power plants in your cells. Right now, if you inherit a broken mitochondrial gene, there's no way to fix it. This technology, called mitoTALEN, acts like molecular scissors: it cuts out the bad gene and lets the good copies take over.

It's still in the lab, not available for patients yet. But in 10-20 years, it might be possible to reverse inherited mitochondrial diseases or even undo some of the mitochondrial damage that builds up as we age."

INSERTION CHECKLIST

Template 3: Explaining quantum coherence

"Your cells aren't just chemistry—they're also physics. Your mitochondria use quantum effects to move energy with almost no waste. Light-sensing proteins in your eyes help set your circadian clock. Your DNA likely acts as an information antenna, helping coordinate what happens in the cell.

When we tune your nutrients, light exposure, sleep, and redox balance, we're not just 'adding vitamins.' We're tuning a living quantum system so it stays organized and efficient instead of drifting into chaos. That's why the timing of your light, the form of your magnesium, and even the tiny oxidative pulse in MODS Max matter—we're designing for coherence, not just basic adequacy."

SECTION 9: Clinician Sequencing Guide

Phase 1: Foundations (weeks 0-4)

Lifestyle and environment:

- Sleep: 7-9 hours, dark, cool bedroom; fixed wake time.
- Light: 10-30 minutes of outdoor morning light; minimize blue light after sunset.
- Movement: 3-5 sessions/week (Zone 2 cardio + 2-3 strength sessions).

- Nutrition: Whole-food diet, 1.2-1.6 g/kg protein, low ultra-processed intake, evening eating window compressed as tolerated.

Baseline labs:

- CBC, CMP, lipid panel, hs-CRP
- 25-OH vitamin D, RBC magnesium
- Zinc, copper (± Zn/Cu ratio)
- Total and free testosterone, LH, FSH, SHBG, estradiol

Foundational supplements:

- Magnesium glycinate: 400-600 mg/day
- Vitamin D3: 2,000-5,000 IU/day (titrated to 40-60+ ng/mL)
- Methylated B-complex
- Omega-3: 1-2 g EPA+DHA/day

Phase 2: UCOS + hormonal voltage (weeks 4-12)

- Initiate full UCOS stack (Activate365, Mito365/Mito365 Pro, Restore365).
- Add non-hormonal testosterone optimizer (e.g., enclomiphene + boron + MODS Max) when appropriate.
- Introduce Oura Ring (or equivalent) for HRV/sleep/readiness tracking.
- Start daily grounding (20-30 minutes).

Targets:

- Subjective: better energy, sleep, libido, recovery.
- Objective:
- Rising or normalized total/free testosterone with preserved LH/FSH.
- HRV trending upward versus personal baseline.
- hs-CRP and other inflammatory markers trending down.

Re-lab at 8-12 weeks: hormones, hs-CRP, RBC Mg, Zn/Cu, ± NAD^+ markers.

Phase 3: Advanced optimization (weeks 12+)

Tailor according to the dominant phenotype:

If metabolic/mitochondrial dysfunction persists:

- Add L-carnitine (1,000-2,000 mg/day).
- Add ALA (300-600 mg/day, higher in neuropathy if needed).
- Consider off-label rapamycin (3-7 mg weekly) with structured monitoring.

If chronic infection / immune dysfunction:

- Consider ozone therapy (MAH or high-dose protocols in experienced centers).
- Add thymosin alpha-1, mistletoe (in integrative oncology or severe immune dysfunction), and other immunomodulators as indicated.
- Rife/frequency-based tools only as clearly labeled adjuncts.

If tissue repair is primary:

- BPC-157, TB-500, GHK-Cu, and appropriate Khavinson peptides.
- Add PEMF and targeted rehabilitation.

If cognitive/neurologic issues dominate:

- ALCAR (500-1,500 mg/day).
- Methylene blue-based formulations (with ALA, B6) when appropriate and safe.
- Morning light, grounding, cognitive peptides (Semax, Selank, Cerebrolysin) as indicated.

If stem cell therapy is considered:

- Harvest and bank after 3-6 months of UCOS to maximize cellular quality.
- Reinfuse only within disease-specific, well-designed protocols and regulatory frameworks.

Phase 4: Maintenance & monitoring

- Continue UCOS long-term, or in 12-week on / 4-week off cycles based on patient preference and response.
- Labs: every 6-12 months (more often during major therapeutic changes).
- Continuous: HRV, sleep, readiness (Oura/WHOOP), CGM when needed.

- Adjust stacks for life stress, changes in training, new diagnoses, and aging.

Conclusion: Practicing at the forefront

This appendix is about integrating:

- Biochemistry: Nutrients, hormones, cofactors, and redox.
- Biophysics: Quantum coherence, redox oscillations, electromagnetic environment.
- Regeneration: Stem cells, peptides, autophagy/mitophagy.
- Systems thinking: Circadian biology, HRV, and multi-scale feedback.

The living cell is simultaneously:

- A biochemical factory (substrates, enzymes, hormones).
- A quantum-informed information system (coherence, tunneling, radical pairs).
- A self-repairing architecture (stem cells, autophagy, senolytics).
- A frequency-tuned oscillator (circadian and electromagnetic rhythms).

Patients come not just for more inputs, but for precision tuning of how those inputs interact. This framework gives you a way to design, sequence, and monitor that tuning — from molecules to mitochondria to whole-person function.

SECTION 9: Clinician Sequencing Guide

Purpose

This section provides a staged blueprint for layering UCOS, MODS MAX, NAD^+ support, peptides, advanced therapeutics, and regenerative tools in real patients. It is not a rigid protocol but a decision framework you can adapt to individual risk, resources, and goals.

Phase 1: Foundational Terrain (Weeks 0-8)

Goals

- Stabilize sleep, circadian rhythm, and autonomic tone.
- Normalize glycemic control and basic metabolic markers.
- Begin NAD^+ repletion, autophagy support, and redox coherence before adding "high-voltage" signals.

Core moves

- UCOS foundation: protein, electrolytes, omega-3s, magnesium, B-vitamins, vitamin D/K_2, trace minerals, and mitochondrial cofactors (CoQ10, carnitine, alpha-lipoic acid as indicated).
- MODS MAX: daily boron, NAD^+ support, and spermidine as your terrain-first stack, titrated to tolerance.
- Lifestyle: sleep window, light hygiene (morning light, dark evenings), movement prescription, stress tools (HRV biofeedback, breathing, grounding).

When to stay in Phase 1 longer

- HRV is persistently low or erratic.
- hs-CRP, fasting insulin, or triglycerides remain markedly abnormal.
- Patient is overwhelmed, anxious, or non-adherent. In these cases, delay escalation and simplify.

Phase 2: Peptide Initiation & Hormonal Optimization (Weeks 8-12)

Goals

- Add targeted signaling molecules once the terrain can respond.
- Normalize or optimize sex hormones, thyroid, and adrenal tone without overshooting into hyperstimulation.

Core moves

- Mitochondrial/cognitive peptides: start low-dose, low-frequency options (e.g., SS-31/Elamipretide where available, cerebrovascular peptides, or nootropic peptides) in patients with clear fatigue or cognitive burden.
- Repair peptides: BPC-157, TB-500, GHK-Cu, and related agents for musculoskeletal, GI, and skin/tissue repair as indicated.
- Hormones: normalize estradiol/progesterone, testosterone/DHEA, thyroid, and cortisol curves, aiming for physiologic—not supraphysiologic—ranges.

Monitoring

- Subjective energy, sleep quality, pain, cognition.
- HRV, resting heart rate, and basic labs.

- Watch for early signs of over-activation (insomnia, agitation, palpitations) and back down if needed.

Phase 3: Advanced Optimization & Regenerative Escalation (Weeks 12+)

Goals

- Layer in advanced therapeutics (rapamycin, ozone, HBOT, PBM, GLP-1/GIP, exosomes, stem cell banking) in patients with stable terrain.
- Begin discussing future-facing options (mitochondrial transplantation, partial reprogramming trials) for appropriate candidates, with a clear boundary around what is investigational.

Core moves

- Rapamycin: carefully dosed, intermittent regimens in metabolically suitable patients, with attention to glycemic markers, lipids, wound healing, and infection risk.
- Ozone, mistletoe, and immunomodulators: for chronic infections, cancer-adjacent care (with oncology), and autoimmunity, layered on UCOS and MODS MAX.
- GLP-1/GIP agonists: for obesity/metabolic syndrome, paired with resistance training, protein targets, EchoLight/DEXA monitoring to protect lean mass.
- Regenerative work: PRP, PRP+exosomes, joint/tendon injections, hair and skin protocols, — available and appropriate—stem cell banking and cell-free secretome therapies.

Who qualifies for escalation

- Demonstrated adherence through Phases 1-2.
- Stable or improving HRV, labs, and functional scores.
- Psychological readiness and realistic expectations about risk, cost, and benefit.

Phase 4: Maintenance, Monitoring & Micro-Cycles

Goals

- Convert gains into durable trajectories.

- Use gentle "micro-cycles" of stress (mitohormesis) and repair rather than constant maximal stimulation.

Core moves

- Ongoing UCOS + MODS MAX: keep the daily backbone in place.
- Periodic senolytic/autophagy pulses: fisetin, urolithin A, spermidine intensification, short rapamycin cycles, or fasting blocks as appropriate.
- Intermittent peptide "holidays": cycle off certain peptides to assess whether gains are maintained and reduce receptor desensitization.
- Regenerative re-touch: occasional PRP, exosome, or PBM blocks for joints, brain, or skin as clinically indicated.

Monitoring tools

- HRV and sleep metrics (Oura/WHOOP).
- Body composition and bone status (EchoLight or DEXA).
- Lab panel cadence: at least annually for low-risk patients, more often for high-complexity or on advanced therapeutics (rapamycin, GLP-1, immunomodulators).

Clinician mindset

Think in 12-week blocks. Each quarter, ask:

- What terrain gains are now stable?
- What symptom clusters remain?
- Is the patient asking for escalation, or would they benefit more from consolidation and simplification?

SECTION 10: Clinical Decision Tree & Integration Map

Purpose

This section provides a conceptual "you are here" map so you can decide where to start, how far to escalate, and when to pause or refer. It is meant to guide judgment, not replace it.

10.1 High-Level Decision Flow

Patient presents → Comprehensive intake (history, meds, goals, labs, HRV, body comp)

↓

Is the terrain deconditioned? (poor sleep, high inflammation, dysglycemia, low HRV)

↓

YES → Phase 1: UCOS + MODS MAX (Weeks 0--8), then reassess

NO → Proceed directly to phenotype-driven optimization

↓

Dominant phenotype?

├─ Metabolic/mitochondrial

│ → Prioritize NAD^+ stack, mitochondrial nutrients, GLP-1/GIP (if indicated),

│ ALA, carnitine, urolithin A, structured exercise and mitohormesis.

├─ Immune/infectious/oncology-adjacent

│ → Ozone (where legal), thymosin α-1, LDN, mistletoe (with oncology),

│ gut repair, redox precision.

├─ Tissue repair/pain

│ → BPC-157, TB-500, GHK-Cu, PRP ± exosomes, PBM, mechanical rehab.

├─ Cognitive/psychiatric/neurodegenerative

│ → DHA-rich omega-3, ALCAR, methylene blue (low dose), NAD^+,

│ urolithin A, HRV training, sleep architecture repair, PBM.

└─ Regenerative / longevity-forward

→ Stem cell banking (after terrain work), secretome/exosome programs,

enrollment in partial reprogramming or mitochondrial trials when available.

↓

Monitor response (symptoms, HRV, labs, imaging)

↓

Improve, plateau, or regress?

├─ Improve → Consolidate, then consider targeted escalation.

├─ Plateau → Adjust dose, timing, or stack; address bottlenecks (sleep, trauma, relationships).

└─ Regress → De-escalate, check adherence, review drug--supplement interactions,

screen for new diagnoses, consider referral.

10.2 When to Pause, Simplify, or Refer

Pause or de-escalate when:

- New or unexplained symptoms arise soon after adding multiple interventions.
- HRV and sleep deteriorate despite "more" inputs.
- The patient is overwhelmed by complexity or cost.

Simplify to:

- UCOS basics, MODS MAX, one or two highest-yield agents.
- Clear lifestyle anchors: sleep, steps, resistance training, light.

Refer or co-manage when:

- Active malignancy or high-risk cancer history (coordinate with oncology for rapamycin, mistletoe, exosomes, or stem-cell-adjacent work).
- Significant uncontrolled psychiatric illness or substance use disorder.
- Complex autoimmune, genetic, or mitochondrial disease needing specialty input.

How This Fits with the Living Chip Model

Use this language in the book and in consults:

- UCOS and MODS MAX are the **motherboard and power supply**—they stabilize voltage, timing, and signal-to-noise.
- Peptides, hormones, and small molecules are **firmware updates**—they refine how circuits fire and recover.
- PRP, exosomes, stem cells, and future mitochondrial or OSK-based tools are **hardware upgrades**—they replace or augment damaged components with younger or better-performing units.

When you feel tempted to add "one more thing," ask:

Does this intervention sharpen timing, improve coherence, and support repair—or does it add more noise to an already overloaded system?

Appendix G: Glossary of Terms

This glossary defines key scientific, medical, and technical terms used throughout the book. Terms are listed alphabetically for quick reference.

8-OHdG (8-hydroxy-2'-deoxyguanosine): A biomarker of oxidative DNA damage; elevated levels indicate oxidative stress.

ADP (Adenosine Diphosphate): The low-energy form of ATP; converted back to ATP by mitochondria.

Anabolic: Building up; promoting growth, repair, and protein synthesis. Opposite of catabolic.

Apoptosis: Programmed cell death; a normal process for removing damaged or unnecessary cells.

ATP (Adenosine Triphosphate): The universal energy currency of cells; produced primarily by mitochondria.

Autophagy: Cellular "housekeeping"; the process by which cells break down and recycle damaged proteins and organelles.

BCAA (Branched-Chain Amino Acids): Leucine, isoleucine, and valine; amino acids that activate mTOR and support muscle protein synthesis.

Bioavailability: The proportion of a nutrient or drug that enters circulation and is available for use by the body.

Biophotons: Ultra-weak photon emissions from living cells; proposed as a form of cellular communication.

Cardiolipin: A signature phospholipid of the inner mitochondrial membrane; essential for electron transport chain function.

Catabolic: Breaking down; the opposite of anabolic. Chronic catabolism leads to muscle and tissue loss.

Circadian Rhythm: The body's internal 24-hour clock; regulated by light exposure and critical for hormone release, sleep, and metabolism.

CoQ10 (Coenzyme Q10): An electron carrier in the mitochondrial respiratory chain; also functions as an antioxidant.

Coherence: In biophysics, the preservation of information and efficient energy transfer across scales; loss of coherence leads to metabolic "noise" and dysfunction.

Complex I: II, III, IV, V: Protein complexes in the mitochondrial electron transport chain; Complexes I-IV pump protons, and Complex V (ATP synthase) uses the gradient to make ATP.

Copper:Zinc Ratio (Cu:Zn): The ratio of serum copper to zinc; elevated ratios are associated with inflammation and oxidative stress.

Cryptochrome: A light-sensitive protein in the retina and other tissues; critical for circadian clock regulation and possibly magnetoreception.

DEXA (Dual-Energy X-ray Absorptiometry): A scan used to measure bone density and body composition (fat vs. lean mass).

EchoLight / REMS: Ultrasound-based technology for bone density and body composition assessment; no radiation, allowing frequent monitoring.

Electron Transport Chain (ETC): A series of protein complexes in the inner mitochondrial membrane that generate ATP via oxidative phosphorylation.

Enclomiphene: A selective estrogen receptor modulator (SERM) that raises endogenous testosterone by blocking negative feedback in the hypothalamus and pituitary.

Entanglement: A quantum phenomenon in which particles become correlated and instantaneously affect each other regardless of distance; proposed to occur in biological systems.

Epigenetics: Changes in gene expression that do not involve alterations to the DNA sequence itself; influenced by nutrients, stress, and environment.

F2 Isoprostanes: Biomarkers of lipid peroxidation and oxidative stress.

GLP-1 Agonists: Drugs that mimic glucagon-like peptide-1; used for weight loss and glucose control (e.g., semaglutide, tirzepatide).

Homocysteine: An amino acid byproduct of methionine metabolism; elevated levels are associated with cardiovascular and neurodegenerative risk.

Hormesis: A beneficial biological response to low-dose stressors (e.g., exercise, fasting, cold exposure, controlled ROS).

hs-CRP (High-Sensitivity C-Reactive Protein): A marker of systemic inflammation; levels >1-2 mg/L suggest chronic inflammatory burden.

HRV (Heart Rate Variability): The variation in time between heartbeats; higher HRV generally indicates better autonomic nervous system function and resilience.

Leucine: The most potent branched-chain amino acid for activating mTOR and muscle protein synthesis.

Liposomal: A delivery system that encases nutrients in lipid (fat) spheres to improve absorption.

Methylation: The addition of a methyl group ($-CH_3$) to molecules; critical for DNA regulation, neurotransmitter synthesis, and detoxification.

Mitochondria: The "powerhouses" of the cell; organelles that produce ATP via oxidative phosphorylation.

Mitochondrial DNA (mtDNA): Genetic material inside mitochondria; inherited maternally and vulnerable to oxidative damage.

Mitophagy: Selective autophagy of damaged mitochondria; essential for maintaining a healthy mitochondrial network.

MODS (Mineral Oxide Delivery System): A delivery technology that uses controlled micro-ROS pulses to enhance nutrient absorption and provide hormetic signaling.

mTOR (Mechanistic Target of Rapamycin): A master growth regulator; activated by leucine, insulin, and resistance training; promotes protein synthesis and cell growth.

NAD$^+$ (Nicotinamide Adenine Dinucleotide): A critical coenzyme for cellular energy production, DNA repair, and sirtuin activation; declines with age.

Neuropathy: Damage or dysfunction of nerves; often presents as numbness, tingling, or pain.

Oxidative Phosphorylation (OXPHOS): The mitochondrial process of generating ATP using oxygen and the electron transport chain.

Peptide: A short chain of amino acids; used therapeutically to signal specific cellular responses (e.g., BPC-157, thymosin alpha-1).

PGC-1α: A master regulator of mitochondrial biogenesis; activated by exercise, fasting, and certain nutrients.

Phosphocreatine (PCr): A high-energy phosphate compound in muscle; provides rapid ATP regeneration during high-intensity activity.

Proprioception: The sense of body position and movement in space; it depends on sensory neurons and cerebellar integration.

Redox Balance: The equilibrium between oxidants (ROS) and antioxidants; optimal balance supports signaling; imbalance causes damage.

ROS (Reactive Oxygen Species): Molecules like superoxide and hydrogen peroxide serve as signaling molecules at low levels but cause oxidative damage at high levels.

SAM (S-Adenosylmethionine): The universal methyl donor in cells; required for DNA methylation, neurotransmitter synthesis, and other processes.

SASP (Senescence-Associated Secretory Phenotype): Inflammatory cytokines and factors released by senescent cells drive "inflammaging."

Senescent Cells: "Zombie cells"; old, non-dividing cells that resist apoptosis and secrete inflammatory signals (SASP).

Senolytic: An agent that selectively clears senescent cells (e.g., fisetin, quercetin + dasatinib).

SHBG (Sex Hormone-Binding Globulin): A protein that binds testosterone and estradiol in the blood; high SHBG reduces free (bioavailable) hormone levels.

Sirtuin: A family of NAD^+-dependent enzymes involved in DNA repair, inflammation control, and longevity pathways (e.g., SIRT1, SIRT3).

Spermidine: A polyamine that activates autophagy and promotes longevity in multiple species.

TCA Cycle (Tricarboxylic Acid Cycle): Also called the Krebs cycle, a metabolic pathway in mitochondria that generates electron carriers (NADH, $FADH_2$) for the ETC.

UCOS (Ultimate Cellular Optimization System): A structured framework for restoring and optimizing cellular function through terrain, core chips, system targeting, and advanced tools.

Warburg Effect: The observation that cancer cells preferentially ferment glucose into lactate even in the presence of oxygen; linked to mitochondrial dysfunction.

Zinc Fingers: Protein structures stabilized by zinc; essential for DNA-binding and gene regulation.

Appendix H: 30-Day Living Chip Quick Start

This guide gives you immediate, actionable steps to begin optimizing your cellular function. It's designed for patients who want to start now while they learn the deeper science from the main chapters.

The core principle

Your body is made of trillions of "living chips", cells that need three things to function:

1. Energy (ATP from mitochondria)
2. Cleanup (autophagy to remove damaged components)
3. Signals (hormones, nutrients, and information flow)

This 30-day program builds the foundation for all three.

Week 1-2: Terrain optimization

Before adding any supplements, fix the environment in which your cells live.

Sleep (7-9 hours/night)

- Go to bed and wake up at the same time every day (even weekends)
- Make your bedroom dark, cool (65-68°F), and quiet
- No screens 1 hour before bed

Morning Light (10-30 minutes)

- Get outside within 30 minutes of waking
- No sunglasses (unless medically required)
- This sets your circadian clock and supports mitochondria

Protein at Every Meal

- Target: palm-sized portion of protein 3×/day
- Best sources: eggs, fish, chicken, beef, Greek yogurt, cottage cheese
- Why: Your cells need amino acids to rebuild

Movement (Daily)

- Walk 7,000, 10,000 steps/day

- Add 2-3 resistance training sessions/week if possible (bodyweight squats, push-ups, rows)
- Movement signals your cells to adapt and grow stronger

Stress Down-Shift (5-10 minutes/day)

- Breathing exercises, prayer, meditation, or simply sitting in silence
- Your cells can't repair under constant stress

Track Your Baseline:

- Rate these daily (0-10 scale):
- Energy level
- Sleep quality
- Brain fog
- Pain level
- Mood

Week 3-4: Core cellular chips

Now layer in foundational nutrients. Start one at a time every 2-3 days so you can track how you feel.

Magnesium Glycinate

- Dose: 400-600 mg in the evening
- Why: Required for ATP function, sleep, muscle relaxation
- What to expect: Better sleep, fewer cramps, calmer nervous system

Vitamin D3 (+ K2)

- Dose: 2,000-5,000 IU/day with a meal
- Why: Immune function, bone health, mood, hormone regulation
- What to expect: Gradual improvement in mood, energy, and resilience over 4-8 weeks

Omega-3 Fatty Acids (EPA + DHA)

- Dose: 1-2 g/day combined EPA + DHA
- Why: Brain structure, mitochondrial membranes, inflammation resolution
- What to expect: Less joint stiffness, better focus, improved recovery

Methylated B-Complex

- Includes methylcobalamin (B12), methylfolate (B9), and B6
- Why: Energy production, methylation, homocysteine control, brain function
- What to expect: Clearer thinking, better energy, improved mood

Zinc (balanced with copper)

- Dose: 15-30 mg/day zinc (short-term); monitor copper levels if using long-term
- Why: Immune function, wound healing, DNA repair
- What to expect: Fewer infections, faster healing

Week 4+: Identify Your Weakest System

By now, you've built a solid foundation. Next, target your primary bottleneck. Use the symptoms below to guide you.

Energy System (Fatigue, crashes, poor recovery)

- Add: Creatine monohydrate (3-5 g/day), CoQ10 (100-200 mg/day)
- Consider: NAD^+ precursors (NMN or NR), PQQ for mitochondrial biogenesis

Structural System (Easy bruising, slow healing, joint pain, gum bleeding)

- Add: Vitamin C (1,000-2,000 mg/day), collagen peptides (10-20 g/day)
- Ensure: Adequate protein (1.6-2.0 g/kg/day)

Information System (Brain fog, memory issues, mood swings)

- Labs: Check homocysteine, B12, folate
- Add: Extra methylated B12 and folate, choline, or betaine
- Consider: Acetyl-L-carnitine (ALCAR, 500-1,500 mg/day)

Security System (Frequent infections, slow recovery from illness)

- Add: Extra zinc (30 mg/day short-term), vitamin C (2,000+ mg/day), vitamin D (optimize to 40-60 ng/mL)
- Consider: Probiotic with diverse strains

Hormonal Voltage System (Low libido, "normal" labs but feel off, body composition changes)

- Labs: Check SHBG, total and free testosterone, vitamin D, zinc, boron
- Men: Consider non-hormonal testosterone support (see Appendix K)
- Women: Work with a hormone-literate clinician

Track your progress

At Day 30, re-rate your symptoms (0-10):

- Energy
- Sleep quality
- Brain fog
- Pain
- Mood

Expected Results:

- Energy: +2, 4 points improvement
- Sleep: +1, 3 points improvement
- Brain fog: +1, 3 points improvement
- Mood: More stable, resilient

If you're not seeing improvement, revisit:

1. Sleep and stress (Are you really consistent?)
2. Protein intake (Are you getting enough?)
3. Supplement quality (Are you using high-quality, bioavailable forms?)
4. Underlying conditions (Do you need labs or medical evaluation?)

Next steps

- If feeling significantly better: Continue this foundation for 90 days, then consider advanced optimization (Chapter 12, Appendices A, E, F)
- If plateaued or minimal improvement: Work with a clinician trained in functional or longevity medicine to dig deeper (labs, system analysis, advanced protocols)
- If dramatic improvement: You've identified your primary bottleneck. Maintain the foundation and fine-tune as needed.

Remember: You are not broken. You are a collection of living chips that have been under-resourced and overwhelmed. Give them what they need, and they will reward you with energy, clarity, resilience, and function.

Start today. Track your progress. Trust the process.

Appendix I: Representative UCOS-Aligned Formulations

Purpose and disclosure

The principles in this book are mechanism- and ingredient-based, not brand-specific. The goal is to restore cellular function through terrain optimization, core micronutrient repletion, and system-targeted support, regardless of product source.

That said, patients and clinicians frequently ask, "What products actually implement these principles in clinically relevant doses?"

The table below provides examples of commercially available formulations that align with the UCOS framework. These are not the only options, and this is not a product catalog. Quality sourcing, third-party testing, certificates of analysis, and professional guidance remain essential when selecting any supplement.

Disclosure: The author is affiliated with Best 365 Labs, which produces UCOS-aligned formulations. This relationship does not change the science in this book, which stands independent of any product line. Where Best 365 Labs products are mentioned, they are offered as examples of the principles in action, not as exclusive recommendations.

UCOS-Aligned Formulation Examples

System / Goal	**Representative Product**	**Key Ingredients**	**Dosing Notes**	**Chapter Reference**
---	---	---	---	---
Mitochondrial Energy & NAD^+ Support	Mito365, Mito365 Pro, Triple MB	NAD^+ precursors (NMN or NR), PQQ, CoQ10, methylene blue (10 mg), acetyl-L-carnitine, alpha-lipoic acid	Morning dosing; take immediately after Activate365 sublingual primer (with or without food); screen for G6PD deficiency	Ch. 1, 10, Appendix X

			before using methylene blue	
Cognitive Function & Memory	Memory Pro, ADHD 365, Brain Fog Support	Phosphatidylserine, bacopa monnieri, citicoline, methylated B-complex, acetyl-L-carnitine, alpha-lipoic acid, low-dose methylene blue	AM dosing; avoid evening if stimulating	Ch. 3, 5, 8
Non-Hormonal Testosterone Optimization	Testosterone Optimizer (non-hormonal)	Enclomiphene citrate (12.5-25 mg), boron (6-10 mg), vitamin C, MODS Max (mineral oxide delivery system)	Prescription enclomiphene required in most jurisdictions; monitor LH, FSH, total/free testosterone, estradiol	Ch. 7, 11, Appendix A
Sleep & Recovery	Restore365	GABA (50 mg), melatonin (600 mcg), magnesium glycinate, L-theanine, honokiol/magnolol (magnolia extract)	Evening dosing, 30–60 min before bed; follow with TPrime365 sublingually (hold 30 sec); start with half dose if sensitive to melatonin	Ch. 2, 10, Appendix F
Autophagy & Cellular Cleanup	Activate365	Spermidine (10 mg), resveratrol or pterostilbene, quercetin, NAD^+ support	Upon waking, sublingually (hold 30 sec); sublingual primer that activates MODS	Ch. 10, 11, Appendix F

			MAX absorption for Mito365 and Renew365 tablets taken immediately after	
Foundational Minerals & Vitamins	UCOS Foundation Stack	RBC magnesium-optimizing dose, methylated B-complex (methylcobalamin, 5-MTHF), zinc (15-30 mg), vitamin D3 (2,000-5,000 IU), vitamin C (500-1,000 mg), omega-3s (1-2 g EPA+DHA), boron (3-6 mg)	Core daily support; adjust doses based on labs	Ch. 2, 3, 4, 7, 9, 10
Senolytic & Anti-Aging	Fisetin (standalone or in blends)	Fisetin (100-500 mg daily maintenance, or 20 mg/kg × 2 days pulsed monthly/quarterly)	Use bioavailable or liposomal forms; take with fat-containing meals	Appendix F
Structural Support (Collagen, Joints)	Collagen + Vitamin C formulations	Hydrolyzed collagen peptides (10-20 g), vitamin C (1,000+ mg), glycine, proline, copper (balanced)	Post-workout or with meals; pairs with BPC-157 peptide if used	Ch. 8, 9, Appendix E

Immune & Barrier Support	Zinc + Vitamin C + D blends	Zinc (30 mg short-term), vitamin C (1,000-2,000 mg), vitamin D3 (2,000-5,000 IU), quercetin (500 mg)	Use therapeutic ally during illness or high-demand periods	Ch. 4, 9

Quality standards to look for (any brand)

When selecting UCOS-aligned products, prioritize:

1. Third-party testing: Look for certificates of analysis (CoA) confirming purity, potency, and absence of contaminants (heavy metals, microbes).
2. Bioavailable forms:

- Magnesium: glycinate, malate, or threonate (not oxide)
- B12: methylcobalamin or adenosylcobalamin (not cyanocobalamin)
- Folate: 5-MTHF or methylfolate (not folic acid)
- Zinc: picolinate, citrate, or glycinate
- Vitamin C: ascorbic acid or liposomal for higher doses
- Omega-3s: triglyceride or re-esterified triglyceride forms (better than ethyl esters)

3. Clinically relevant doses: Many multivitamins use "window dressing" doses (e.g., 10 mcg of B12 when 500-1,000 mcg is often needed). Check labels.
4. No unnecessary fillers: Avoid products loaded with artificial colors, flavors, or low-quality excipients.
5. GMP certification: Look for manufacturing facilities certified under Good Manufacturing Practices (FDA-registered, NSF, or equivalent).

A Note on "Proprietary Blends"

Be wary of products that list a "proprietary blend" without disclosing the doses of individual ingredients. You need to know how much of each active ingredient you're getting to assess clinical relevance and safety.

Final thought

The best product is the one that:

- Contains the right ingredients in the right forms and doses
- Has been tested for quality
- Fits your budget and compliance
- Is guided by a clinician who understands your labs and goals

This book gives you the blueprint. The products are tools to implement it. Choose wisely, test regularly, and adjust based on results.

References and Further Reading

APPENDIX H: References and Further Reading

Purpose and scope

This appendix provides a curated set of references and further reading for clinicians, researchers, and advanced readers who want to go deeper into the science underlying the concepts and protocols in this book. The references are organized by chapter/topic rather than a strict citation format to keep them practically usable.

CHAPTER 1: Mitochondria and Cellular Energy

Core mitochondrial biology:

- Genome.gov, "Mitochondria" overview of structure and function
- NCBI Bookshelf, "The Mitochondrion" in Molecular Biology of the Cell
- Nature / Scitable, "Mitochondria, Cell Energy, ATP Synthase" learning module
- Reviews on mitochondrial energy production, ROS, and signaling

ATP and energy turnover:

- General reviews on ATP as the cellular energy currency and its turnover in high-demand tissues

CHAPTER 2: Magnesium

Magnesium in health and disease:

- Narrative and mechanistic reviews on magnesium's role in energy metabolism, neuromuscular function, and cardiovascular health

Clinical aspects:

- Work summarizing magnesium's links to fatigue, sleep, mood, blood pressure, and metabolic health

CHAPTER 3: B12, Folate, and Methylation

Vitamin B12 and neurological function:

- Reviews of neurologic manifestations of B12 deficiency, including cognitive and psychiatric aspects, and the importance of MMA and homocysteine as functional markers

Methylation and epigenetics:

- Articles summarizing methylation pathways, homocysteine metabolism, and implications for brain and vascular health

CHAPTER 4: Zinc and Immune Function

Zinc as an immune "gatekeeper":

- Reviews describing zinc's role in T-cell, B cell, NK cell, and barrier function, and its impact on infection risk and immune aging

Zinc fingers and gene regulation:

- Mechanistic overviews of zinc finger proteins in transcription and gene expression control

CHAPTER 5: Navigation and Proprioception (Seven Planes)

Vestibular and proprioceptive physiology:

- Standard neurophysiology references on vestibular function, proprioceptive pathways, and cerebellar integration

Energy demand of neural systems:

- Reviews highlighting the high metabolic cost of cerebellum, visual cortex, and sensorimotor systems, and their vulnerability to energy deficits

CHAPTER 6: Phosphorus and Creatine

Phosphocreatine and the phosphagen system:

- Overviews of phosphocreatine's role in rapid ATP regeneration, especially in skeletal muscle and brain

Creatine and performance:

- Work summarizing creatine's effects on phosphocreatine stores, exercise performance, and, in some contexts, cognitive support

CHAPTER 7: Boron and Hormonal Regulation

Boron and sex hormones:

- Human trials examining boron's effects on SHBG, free testosterone, inflammatory markers, and vitamin D metabolism

Boron in human health:

- Integrative reviews describing boron's roles in bone health, mineral metabolism, hormone regulation, and inflammation

CHAPTER 8: Copper and Neural Function

Copper and myelin/neurology:

- Studies linking copper deficiency to myelopathy, neuropathy, and demyelinating processes, and exploring copper abnormalities in neurological diseases

Copper in energy metabolism:

- Reviews discussing copper in Complex IV (cytochrome c oxidase) and its impact on neuronal energy

CHAPTER 9: Vitamin C, Collagen, and Oxidative Stress

Vitamin C overview:

- Comprehensive fact sheets on vitamin C's biochemical roles, clinical uses, and safety

Vitamin C and immune function:

- Reviews and FAQs from major medical centers summarizing vitamin C's role in infection prevention, treatment, and recovery

Collagen synthesis and structural roles:

- Clinical and mechanistic work on vitamin C's role in collagen hydroxylation, connective tissue integrity, and wound healing

Vitamin C as antioxidant:

- Reviews on vitamin C's role in antioxidant networks, interaction with vitamin E, and potential in high-dose contexts

CHAPTER 10: Integration

Systems and multi-nutrient interactions:

- Reviews discussing how combinations of vitamins and minerals affect fatigue, cognition, energy, and chronic disease risk

CHAPTER 11: The Electrical Cascade of Cellular Dysfunction

Electrical physiology and grid failure:

- Research on neuronal energy failure, ion gradient collapse, excitotoxicity, and cascade dynamics in acute and chronic neurological conditions

CHAPTER 12: Future Directions and Optimization

Biology, data, and AI:

- Work highlighting the use of multi-omics, machine learning, and advanced analytics to understand complex health patterns, aging trajectories, and personalized interventions

General Preventive and Lifestyle Medicine:

- Overviews from major health organizations and academic centers on sleep, exercise, nutrition, and stress management as foundational pillars of health

How to use this appendix

For clinicians:

- Use chapter/topic sections as a quick launch point when you want to refresh background science or provide patients with high-level references
- Combine these with more detailed, peer-reviewed resources accessible through medical libraries and databases

For advanced readers:

- Start with the more accessible resources, such as health system fact sheets and narrative reviews
- Progress to primary literature and systematic reviews as interest and background allow

This appendix is not a complete bibliography and does not attempt to list every study referenced implicitly in the book. It highlights key nodes in the evidence network so that you can explore further, build your own reference library, and adapt the framework in this book to emerging research over time.

Full References

Full References

2.

3. A 1-page style sheet for you + the editor.

1. Master References (Numbered, Vancouver Style)

Master References

1. Mitchell P. Coupling of phosphorylation to electron and hydrogen transfer by a chemiosmotic type of mechanism. Nature. 1961;191(4784):144, 8.
2. Mitchell P. Compartmentation and communication in living systems. Eur J Biochem. 1979;95(1):1, 20.

3. Hatefi Y. The mitochondrial electron transport and oxidative phosphorylation system. Annu Rev Biochem. 1985;54:1015, 69.
4. Yoshida M, Muneyuki E, Hisabori T. ATP synthase, a marvellous rotary engine of the cell. Nat Rev Mol Cell Biol. 2001;2(9):669, 77.
5. Sazanov LA. A giant molecular extractor. Science. 2015;347(6217):34, 5.
6. Kroemer G, Zamzami N, Susin SA. Mitochondrial control of apoptosis. Immunol Today. 1997;18(1):44, 51.
7. Romani AMP. Magnesium in health and disease. Mol Aspects Med. 2007;26(4, 5):193, 262.
8. de Baaij JHF, Hoenderop JGJ, Bindels RJM. Magnesium in man: implications for health and disease. Physiol Rev. 2015;95(1):1, 46.
9. Gröber U, Schmidt J, Kisters K. Magnesium in prevention and therapy. Nutrients. 2015;7(9):8199, 226.
10. Lindberg JS, Zobitz MM, Poindexter JR, Pak CYC. Magnesium bioavailability from mineral water and synthetic magnesium oxide. J Am Coll Nutr. 1990;9(1):48, 55.
11. Coudray C, Rambeau M, Feingold N, et al. Study of magnesium bioavailability from ten organic and inorganic Mg salts in healthy human subjects. Magnesium Res. 2005;18(4):215, 23.
12. Tardy AL, Pouteau E, Marquez D, et al. Vitamins and minerals for energy, fatigue and cognition: a narrative review. Nutrients. 2020;12(1):228.
13. Stover PJ. Physiology of folate and vitamin B12 in health and disease. Nutr Rev. 2004;62 Suppl 1:S3, 12.
14. Mattson MP, Shea TB. Folate and homocysteine metabolism in neural plasticity and neurodegenerative disorders. Neuromolecular Med. 2003;3(2):79, 94.
15. Selhub J, Miller JW. The pathogenesis of homocysteinemia. Am J Clin Nutr. 1992;55(1):131, 8.
16. Herrmann W, Obeid R. Homocysteine: a biomarker in neurodegenerative diseases. Clin Chem Lab Med. 2011;49(3):435, 41.

17. Refsum H, Ueland PM, Nygård O, Vollset SE. Homocysteine and cardiovascular disease. Annu Rev Med. 1998;49:31, 62.
18. Prasad AS. Zinc in human health: effect of zinc on immune cells. Mol Med. 2008;14(5, 6):353, 7.
19. Shankar AH, Prasad AS. Zinc and immune function: the biological basis of altered resistance to infection. Am J Clin Nutr. 1998;68(2 Suppl):447S, 63S.
20. Eide DJ. Zinc transporters and the cellular trafficking of zinc. Biochim Biophys Acta. 2006;1763(7):711, 22.
21. Vallee BL, Falchuk KH. The biochemical basis of zinc physiology. Physiol Rev. 1993;73(1):79, 118.
22. Stryer L, Berg JM, Tymoczko JL. Biochemistry. 7th ed. New York: W.H. Freeman; 2011.
23. Wyss M, Kaddurah-Daouk R. Creatine and creatinine metabolism. Physiol Rev. 2000;80(3):1107, 1213.
24. Cullen KE, Brooks JX. Proprioception and the predictive sensing of active self-motion. Front Integr Neurosci. 2011;5:90.
25. Nielsen FH, Hunt CD, Mullen LM, Hunt JR. Effect of dietary boron on mineral, estrogen, and testosterone metabolism in postmenopausal women. FASEB J. 1987;1(5):394, 7.
26. Nielsen FH. Boron in human and animal health. Plant Soil. 1994;193(2):199, 208.
27. Pizzorno L. Nothing boring about boron. Integr Med (Encinitas). 2015;14(4):35, 48.
28. Waldron KJ, Rutherford JC, Ford D, Robinson NJ. Metalloproteins and metal sensing. Nature. 2009;460(7257):823, 30.
29. Linder MC, Hazegh-Azam M. Copper biochemistry and molecular biology. Am J Clin Nutr. 1996;63(5):797S, 811S.
30. Pickart L, Vasquez-Soltero JM, Margolina A. GHK peptide as a modulator of gene expression. J Drugs Dermatol. 2015;14(3):273, 81.
31. Padayatty SJ, Katz A, Wang Y, et al. Vitamin C as an antioxidant: evaluation of its role in disease prevention. J Am Coll Nutr. 2003;22(1):18, 35.

32. Traber MG, Stevens JF. Vitamins C and E: beneficial effects from a mechanistic perspective. Free Radic Biol Med. 2011;51(5):1000, 13.

33. Frei B. Reactive oxygen species and antioxidant vitamins: mechanisms of action. Am J Med. 1994;97(3A):5S, 13S.

34. Kasai H. Analysis of 8-hydroxy-2′-deoxyguanosine as a marker of oxidative stress. Mutat Res. 1997;387(3):147, 63.

35. Morrow JD, Zackert WE, Yang JP, et al. Quantification of isoprostanes as indices of oxidant stress in vivo. Proc Natl Acad Sci U S A. 1999;96(26):15829, 34.

36. López-Lluch G, Hunt N, Jones B, et al. Calorie restriction induces mitochondrial biogenesis and bioenergetic efficiency. Proc Natl Acad Sci U S A. 2006;103(6):1768, 73.

37. Cantó C, Auwerx J. NAD+ as a signaling molecule modulating metabolism. Cell Metab. 2012;16(3):290, 5.

38. Balaban RS, Nemoto S, Finkel T. Mitochondria, oxidants, and aging. Cell. 2005;120(4):483, 95.

39. Harman D. Aging: a theory based on free radical and radiation chemistry. J Gerontol. 1956;11(3):298, 300.

40. Ordovas JM, Mooser V. Nutrigenomics and nutrigenetics. Curr Opin Lipidol. 2004;15(1):101, 8.

41. Fenech M, El-Sohemy A, Cahill L, et al. Nutrigenetics and nutrigenomics: leading the way toward personalized nutrition. J Sci Food Agric. 2011;91(2):199, 205.

42. Rajman L, Chwalek K, Sinclair DA. Therapeutic potential of NAD+ precursors in age-related diseases. Cell Metab. 2018;27(3):529, 47.

43. Wiehle RD, Fontenot GK, Wike J, et al. Testosterone restoration using enclomiphene citrate in men with secondary hypogonadism. BJU Int. 2013;112(8):1188, 1200.

44. Winters SJ, et al. Enclomiphene citrate for the treatment of secondary male hypogonadism. BJU Int. 2016;117(4):672, 6.

45. Wiehle RD, Whitten SJ, Meyer WR. Oral enclomiphene citrate raises testosterone and preserves sperm counts in obese hypogonadal men. BJU Int. 2016;117(4):677, 85.

46. Naghii MR, Mofid M, Asgari AR, et al. Comparative effects of daily and weekly boron supplementation on plasma steroid hormones and inflammatory biomarkers. J Trace Elem Med Biol. 2011;25(1):54, 8.

47. Mattson MP, Calabrese EJ. Hormesis: what it is and why it matters. Dose-Response. 2010;8(2):202, 15.

You can keep adding new references below 47 if you bring in more UCOS/peptide trial papers later.

2. Revised Appendix E with (Ref. X) Tags

Here's the top of Appendix E rewritten to match the new numbering. You can continue this pattern through the rest.

text

APPENDIX E: References & Bibliography

Organized by Chapter & Topic\\

Each entry includes its Master Reference number in parentheses, e.g., (Ref. 8).

• • •

Chapter 1, Mitochondrial Bioenergetics

\\\\Foundational mitochondrial science\\\\

- Mitchell P. Coupling of phosphorylation to electron and hydrogen transfer by a chemiosmotic type of mechanism. *Nature*\\. 1961;191(4784):144, 8. *(Ref. 1)*\\
- Mitchell P. Compartmentation and communication in living systems. *Eur J Biochem*\\. 1979;95(1):1, 20. *(Ref. 2)*\\
- Kroemer G, Zamzami N, Susin SA. Mitochondrial control of apoptosis. *Immunol Today*\\. 1997;18(1):44, 51. *(Ref. 6)*\\

\\\\ATP synthesis & electron transport\\\\

- Hatefi Y. The mitochondrial electron transport and oxidative phosphorylation system. *Annu Rev Biochem*\\. 1985;54:1015, 69. *(Ref. 3)*\\
- Yoshida M, Muneyuki E, Hisabori T. ATP synthase, a marvellous rotary engine of the cell. *Nat Rev Mol Cell Biol*\\. 2001;2(9):669, 77. *(Ref. 4)*\\
- Sazanov LA. A giant molecular extractor. *Science*\\. 2015;347(6217):34, 5. *(Ref. 5)*\\

\\|Magnesium & ATP\\|

- Romani AMP. Magnesium in health and disease. *Mol Aspects Med*\|. 2007;26(4, 5):193, 262. *(Ref. 7)*\|
- de Baaij JHF, Hoenderop JGJ, Bindels RJM. Magnesium in man: implications for health and disease. *Physiol Rev*\|. 2015;95(1):1, 46. *(Ref. 8)*\|
- Gröber U, Schmidt J, Kisters K. Magnesium in prevention and therapy. *Nutrients*\|. 2015;7(9):8199, 226. *(Ref. 9)*\|

• • •

Chapter 2, Magnesium Biochemistry

- Tardy AL, Pouteau E, Marquez D, et al. Vitamins and minerals for energy, fatigue and cognition. *Nutrients*\|. 2020;12(1):228. *(Ref. 12)*\|
- Lindberg JS, Zobitz MM, Poindexter JR, Pak CYC. Magnesium bioavailability from mineral water and synthetic magnesium oxide. *J Am Coll Nutr*\|. 1990;9(1):48, 55. *(Ref. 10)*\|
- Coudray C, Rambeau M, Feingold N, et al. Study of magnesium bioavailability from ten organic and inorganic Mg salts. *Magnesium Res*\|. 2005;18(4):215, 23. *(Ref. 11)*\|

• • •

Chapter 3, Epigenetics, B12, Folate, Homocysteine

- Stover PJ. Physiology of folate and vitamin B12 in health and disease. *Nutr Rev*\|. 2004;62 Suppl 1:S3, 12. *(Ref. 13)*\|
- Mattson MP, Shea TB. Folate and homocysteine metabolism in neural plasticity and neurodegenerative disorders. *Neuromolecular Med*\|. 2003;3(2):79, 94. *(Ref. 14)*\|
- Selhub J, Miller JW. The pathogenesis of homocysteinemia. *Am J Clin Nutr*\|. 1992;55(1):131, 8. *(Ref. 15)*\|
- Herrmann W, Obeid R. Homocysteine: a biomarker in neurodegenerative diseases. *Clin Chem Lab Med*\|. 2011;49(3):435, 41. *(Ref. 16)*\|
- Refsum H, Ueland PM, Nygård O, Vollset SE. Homocysteine and cardiovascular disease. *Annu Rev Med*\|. 1998;49:31, 62. *(Ref. 17)*\|

• • •

Chapter 4, Zinc & Immune Function

- Prasad AS. Zinc in human health: effect of zinc on immune cells. *Mol Med*\. 2008;14(5, 6):353, 7. *(Ref. 18)*\
- Shankar AH, Prasad AS. Zinc and immune function. *Am J Clin Nutr*\. 1998;68(2 Suppl):447S, 63S. *(Ref. 19)*\
- Eide DJ. Zinc transporters and the cellular trafficking of zinc. *Biochim Biophys Acta*\. 2006;1763(7):711, 22. *(Ref. 20)*\
- Vallee BL, Falchuk KH. The biochemical basis of zinc physiology. *Physiol Rev*\. 1993;73(1):79, 118. *(Ref. 21)*\

• • •

Chapter 5, Phosphorus, Creatine, Navigation

- Stryer L, Berg JM, Tymoczko JL. *Biochemistry*\. 7th ed. W.H. Freeman; 2011. *(Ref. 22)*\
- Wyss M, Kaddurah-Daouk R. Creatine and creatinine metabolism. *Physiol Rev*\. 2000;80(3):1107, 1213. *(Ref. 23)*\
- Cullen KE, Brooks JX. Proprioception and the predictive sensing of active self-motion. *Front Integr Neurosci*\. 2011;5:90. *(Ref. 24)*\

• • •

Chapter 6, Boron & Hormonal Regulation

- Nielsen FH, Hunt CD, Mullen LM, Hunt JR. Effect of dietary boron on mineral, estrogen, and testosterone metabolism in postmenopausal women. *FASEB J*\. 1987;1(5):394, 7. *(Ref. 25)*\
- Nielsen FH. Boron in human and animal health. *Plant Soil*\. 1994;193(2):199, 208. *(Ref. 26)*\
- Pizzorno L. Nothing boring about boron. *Integr Med (Encinitas)*\. 2015;14(4):35, 48. *(Ref. 27)*\
- Naghii MR, Mofid M, Asgari AR, et al. Comparative effects of daily and weekly boron supplementation on plasma steroid hormones and inflammatory biomarkers. *J Trace Elem Med Biol*\. 2011;25(1):54, 8. *(Ref. 46)*\

• • •

Chapter 7, Copper, GHK-Cu & Neural Function

- Waldron KJ, Rutherford JC, Ford D, Robinson NJ. Metalloproteins and metal sensing. *Nature*\. 2009;460(7257):823, 30. *(Ref. 28)*\
- Linder MC, Hazegh-Azam M. Copper biochemistry and molecular biology. *Am J Clin Nutr*\. 1996;63(5):797S, 811S. *(Ref. 29)*\
- Pickart L, Vasquez-Soltero JM, Margolina A. GHK peptide as a modulator of gene expression. *J Drugs Dermatol*\. 2015;14(3):273, 81. *(Ref. 30)*\

• • •

Chapter 8, Vitamin C & Oxidative Stress

- Padayatty SJ, Katz A, Wang Y, et al. Vitamin C as an antioxidant: evaluation of its role in disease prevention. *J Am Coll Nutr*\. 2003;22(1):18, 35. *(Ref. 31)*\
- Traber MG, Stevens JF. Vitamins C and E: beneficial effects from a mechanistic perspective. *Free Radic Biol Med*\. 2011;51(5):1000, 13. *(Ref. 32)*\
- Frei B. Reactive oxygen species and antioxidant vitamins: mechanisms of action. *Am J Med*\. 1994;97(3A):5S, 13S. *(Ref. 33)*\
- Kasai H. Analysis of 8-hydroxy-2′-deoxyguanosine as a marker of oxidative stress. *Mutat Res*\. 1997;387(3):147, 63. *(Ref. 34)*\
- Morrow JD, Zackert WE, Yang JP, et al. Quantification of isoprostanes as indices of oxidant stress in vivo. *Proc Natl Acad Sci U S A*\. 1999;96(26):15829, 35. *(Ref. 35)*\

• • •

\## Chapters 9, 10, Integration, NAD+, Aging

- López-Lluch G, Hunt N, Jones B, et al. Calorie restriction induces mitochondrial biogenesis and bioenergetic efficiency. *PNAS*\. 2006;103(6):1768, 73. *(Ref. 36)*\
- Cantó C, Auwerx J. NAD+ as a signaling molecule modulating metabolism. *Cell Metab*\. 2012;16(3):290, 5. *(Ref. 37)*\
- Balaban RS, Nemoto S, Finkel T. Mitochondria, oxidants, and aging. *Cell*\. 2005;120(4):483, 95. *(Ref. 38)*\

- Harman D. Aging: a theory based on free radical and radiation chemistry. *J Gerontol*\. 1956;11(3):298, 300. *(Ref. 39)*\
- Rajman L, Chwalek K, Sinclair DA. Therapeutic potential of NAD+ precursors in age-related diseases. *Cell Metab*\. 2018;27(3):529, 47. *(Ref. 42)*\

• • •

\## UCOS, Enclomiphene & Hormonal Voltage

- Wiehle RD, Fontenot GK, Wike J, et al. Testosterone restoration using enclomiphene citrate in men with secondary hypogonadism. *BJU Int*\. 2013;112(8):1188, 1200. *(Ref. 43)*\
- Winters SJ, et al. Enclomiphene citrate for the treatment of secondary male hypogonadism. *BJU Int*\. 2016;117(4):672, 6. *(Ref. 44)*\
- Wiehle RD, Whitten SJ, Meyer WR. Oral enclomiphene citrate raises testosterone and preserves sperm counts in obese hypogonadal men. *BJU Int*\. 2016;117(4):677, 85. *(Ref. 45)*\
- Mattson MP, Calabrese EJ. Hormesis: what it is and why it matters. *Dose-Response*\. 2010;8(2):202, 15. *(Ref. 47)*\

Appendix I

Index

Appendix K: Alphabetical Index

Appendix K: Alphabetical Index

Purpose and Use

This index provides an alphabetical listing of key terms, concepts, protocols, and topics discussed throughout "The Living Chip," along with the page numbers where they appear. Use this index to quickly locate specific information without searching through the entire book.

A

Adenine dinucleotide. See NAD+

ADP (adenosine diphosphate), XX, XX, XX

Aging, cellular

mitochondrial dysfunction and, XX

NAD+ decline in, XX, XX

telomere shortening, XX

ATP (adenosine triphosphate)

cellular energy currency, XX, XX

mitochondrial production, XX-XX

turnover rates, XX

Autophagy, XX, XX, XX

fasting and, XX

spermidine activation, XX

B

Boron, XX-XX

bone health and, XX

cognitive function, XX

dosing protocols, XX

BPC-157 peptide, XX, XX

[Continue through Z with all key terms]

M

Magnesium, XX-XX

ATP synthesis and, XX

cellular energy, XX, XX

deficiency symptoms, XX

dosing recommendations, XX

supplementation protocols, XX

Methylene blue, XX, XX

Mitochondria

ATP production, XX-XX

dysfunction, XX, XX

optimization strategies, XX-XX

MODS Max protocol, XX, XX

N

NAD+ (nicotinamide adenine dinucleotide), XX-XX

biosensors for, XX

decline with aging, XX

mitochondrial function and, XX

precursors (NMN, NR), XX, XX

UCOS protocol and, XX

Neuroplasticity, XX, XX

Nutritional optimization. See UCOS protocol

U

UCOS (Upstream Cellular Optimization Strategy), XX-XX

implementation guide, XX-XX
peptide protocols and, XX
principles, XX
results timeline, XX

Z

Zinc, XX-XX
cognitive function and, XX
immune system support, XX
neurological health, XX
supplementation guidelines, XX

How to Complete This Index:

1. Read through each chapter and identify important terms, concepts, protocols, and topics
2. Note the page number where each term appears
3. Organize alphabetically by main term
4. Use indentation for subtopics (as shown above)
5. Include cross-references (e.g., "See NAD+" or "See also Mitochondria")
6. Common index categories to include:

- Key nutrients and minerals (Magnesium, Zinc, Boron, etc.)
- Protocols (UCOS, MODS Max, etc.)
- Cellular processes (Autophagy, ATP synthesis, etc.)
- Peptides and compounds
- Conditions and symptoms
- Testing and biomarkers

Made in the USA
Las Vegas, NV
02 May 2026

46006159R20238